NURSING THEORIES

THEORIES

The Base for Professional Nursing Practice

FOURTH EDITION

Editor:

Julia B. George, RN, PhD
Professor and Chair
Department of Nursing
California State University, Fullerton
Fullerton, California

Appleton & Lange
Norwalk, Connecticut

Copyright © 1995 by Appleton & Lange
A Simon & Schuster Company
Copyright © 1990 by Appleton & Lange
Copyright © 1980, 1985 by Prentice-Hall, Inc., Englewood Cliffs, NJ

10 9 8 7 6 5

Prentice Hall International (UK) Limited, *London*
Prentice Hall of Australia Pty. Limited, *Sidney*
Prentice Hall Canada, Inc., *Toronto*
Prentice Hall Hispanoamericana, S.A., *Mexico*
Prentice Hall of India Private Limited, *New Delhi*
Prentice Hall of Japan, Inc., *Tokyo*
Simon & Schuster Asia Pte. Ltd., *Singapore*
Editora Prentice Hall do Brasil Ltda., *Rio de Janeiro*
Prentice Hall, *Englewood Cliffs, New Jersey*

Library of Congress Cataloging-in-Publication Data
Nursing theories : the base for professional nursing practice /
    editor, Julia B. George. — 4th ed.
        p.   cm.
    Includes bibliographical references and index.
    ISBN 0-8385-7056-9
    1. Nursing—Philosophy.   I. George, Julia B.
    [DNLM: 1. Nursing Theory.   WY 86 N9755 1995]
    RT84.5.N89   1995
    610.73'01—dc20
    DNLM/DLC
    for Library of Congress   94-41658
                                                                 CIP

Acquisitions Editor: David P. Carroll
Production Services: Rainbow Graphics, Inc.
Cover Designer: Janice Barsevich Beilawa

ISBN 0-8385-7056-9

90000

9 780838 570562

PRINTED IN THE UNITED STATES OF AMERICA

NURSING THEORIES

The Base for Professional Nursing Practice

FOURTH EDITION

CONTRIBUTORS

Janice Ryan Belcher, RN, PhD
Old Dominion University
Norfolk, Virginia

Agnes M. Bennett, RN, MS
Assistant Professor, Retired
Department of Nursing
Miami University
Oxford, Ohio

Susan Stanwyck Bowman, RN, MN
Professor
Department of Nursing
Humboldt State University
Arcata, California

Suzanne M. Falco, RN, PhD
Associate Professor
School of Nursing
The University of Wisconsin,
    Milwaukee
Milwaukee, Wisconsin

Lois J. Brittain Fish, RN, MSN
Supportive Home Services Specialist,
    Retired
Riverside School and R. T. Industries,
    Inc.
Troy, Ohio

Peggy Coldwell Foster, RN, MSN
Perinatal Clinical Nurse Specialist
Maternity Home Care Coordinator
Mercy Hospital Anderson
Cincinnati, Ohio

Noreen Cavan Frisch, RN, PhD
Professor and Chair
Department of Nursing
Humboldt State University
Arcata, California

Chiyoko Yamamoto Furukawa, RN,
    PhD
Professor, Retired
College of Nursing
University of New Mexico
Albuquerque, New Mexico

Julia Gallagher Galbreath, RN, CS, MS
Associate Professor
Edison State Community College
Piqua, Ohio

Julia B. George, RN, PhD
Professor and Chair
Department of Nursing
California State University, Fullerton
Fullerton, California

Janet S. Hickman, RN, EdD
Associate Professor, Director of
    Graduate Program
Department of Nursing
West Chester University
West Chester, Pennsylvania

Joan K. Howe, RN, MS
Lecturer in Nursing
Lima Technical College
Lima, Ohio

Mary Kathryn Leonard, RN, MS
Assistant Administrator
Southeast Volusia Hospital
New Smyrna Beach, Florida

Marie L. Lobo, RN, PhD, FAAN
Associate Professor
Graduate Program
College of Nursing
Medical University of South Carolina
Charleston, South Carolina

Charlotte Paul, RN, PhD
Professor and Chairperson
Director of Nursing Programs
Edinboro University of Pennsylvania
Edinboro, Pennsylvania

Susan G. Praeger, RN, EdD
Associate Professor
Wright State University-Miami Valley
  School of Nursing
Dayton, Ohio

Joan S. Reeves, RN, DrPH
Rush University
Chicago, Illinois

Barbara Talento, RN, EdD
Associate Professor Emeritus
Department of Nursing
California State University, Fullerton
Fullerton, California

CONTENTS

PREFACE

A unique knowledge base, and the means to communicate it, are requisite for a profession. Nursing continues to be deeply involved in developing its own unique knowledge base and in educating students about it. In identifying this base, various concepts, models, and theories specific to nursing have been recognized, defined, and developed. Although these concepts, models, and theories have been published in a variety of journals and in books by individual theorists, there is a need for them to gather this material in one volume and apply it to nursing practice.

This book is designed to consider the ideas of 21 nursing theorists and relate the work of each, where appropriate, to the nursing process of assessing, diagnosing, planning, implementing, and evaluating. It must be recognized that the book serves as a secondary source in relation to the statements and purposes of the individuals whose writings are discussed. It is intended as a tool for the thoughtful and considered application of nursing concepts and theories to nursing practice, and through three editions this book has served students in nursing programs in this country and around the world.

There are essentially three areas of focus. First, Chapters 1 and 2 present the place of concepts and theories in nursing and discuss the nursing process. These chapters provide a common base for the next twenty-two chapters and should be read first.

Next, Chapters 3 through 23 present the major components of the work of Florence Nightingale, Hildegard E. Peplau, Virginia Henderson, Lydia E. Hall, Dorothea E. Orem, Dorothy E. Johnson, Myra Estrin Levine, Imogene M. King, Martha E. Rogers, Callista Roy, Betty Neuman, Josephine E. Paterson and Loretta T. Zderad, Jean Watson, Rosemarie Rizzo Parse, Helen Erickson, Evelyn M. Tomlin, and Mary Ann P. Swain, Madeleine M. Leininger, Margaret Newman, and Anne Boykin and Savina Schoenhofer. Each chapter presents one theorist (or group of theorists). Selected theory chapters are followed by a brief summary of theory work done to build on or extend the original theory.

Although an effort has been made to present the information chronologically, these chapters may be read in any order. Each chapter gives the historical setting of the nurse theorist and the specific components identified as meaningful to nursing. This material is drawn from the work of each theorist or group of theorists. The components are then interpreted and discussed by the chapter authors in relation to the use of the theory in the nursing process and to the four basic concepts in nursing's metaparadigm: (1) the human or individual, (2) health, (3) society/environment, and (4) nursing. In addition, the work of each theorist is discussed in relation to the characteristics of a theory. This discussion is not to be considered a comprehensive critique of the work but rather an effort to give one view of the strengths and weaknesses of the work, and to stimulate the reader's thought processes about the characteristics of a theory and those of the particular work. The terms *theory, model, conceptual framework,* and *conceptual model* are not used consistently in the nursing literature. Thus the work being presented may meet the characteristics of a theory as described in this book and still not be generally accepted as a theory.

Chapter 24 is an aid to the reader for using several or all of these theories in nursing practice in a given situation. This chapter gives some examples of application of the components as a guide and stimulus to the reader's use of theory for professional nursing practice. Chapter 24 will be most meaningful if it is read after becoming familiar with the contents of Chapters 1 through 23. A glossary is also provided for quick reference to some common terms and to terms specific to the work of particular theories.

Some of the theorists, as appropriate to their times, used *she* to refer to the nurse, and *he* to refer to the recipient of care. In some chapters, it would have been awkward to change the theorist's use of such words. In these situations, we have indicated that the use is that of the original author. In like manner, we have tried to reflect the original author's use of the terms *patient* and *client.*

A special "thank you" is due the staff at Appleton & Lange for their help and encouragement during the process of developing the fourth edition of this book. They have been patient, understanding, and supportive.

Suggestions and comments from users of this text are requested and welcomed.

Julia B. George

AN INTRODUCTION TO NURSING THEORY

Janet S. Hickman

■ ■ ■

The purpose of this chapter is to provide the learner with the tools necessary for understanding and evaluating the nursing theories presented in this book. These tools include learning the language and definitions of theoretical thinking, acquiring a perspective of the historical development of nursing theories, and learning a method to analyze and evaluate nursing theories.

THE LANGUAGE OF THEORETICAL THINKING

Concepts

The basic unit in the language of theoretical thinking is the *concept.* Webster (1991) defines a concept as something conceived in the mind—a thought or a notion. Concepts are words that represent reality and enhance our ability to communicate about it. Concepts may be empirical or abstract, depending on their ability to be observed in the real world. Concepts are said to be *empirical* when they can be observed or experienced through the senses. A stethoscope is an example of an empirical concept; it can be seen and touched. *Abstract* concepts are those that are not observable, such as hope and infinity. All concepts become abstractions in the absence of the object. For example, once you have become familiar with a stethoscope, you are able to see the concept of a stethoscope in your mind without having one physically present. Abstractions such as hope or infinity are more difficult to picture, because one has never had the opportunity to observe or experience them through the senses.

To understand the presentations of nursing theories in this book, it will be of critical importance to look at the definitions of the concepts provided. Some of the theories will use concepts that you are familiar with, but they may be used in unfamiliar ways; others will introduce new concepts.

There is general agreement in the literature that nursing is concerned with four major concepts: person, health, environment, and nursing. Together these concepts make up the meta-paradigm of nursing. A meta-paradigm identifies the core content of a discipline.

In the meta-paradigm of nursing, each of the four concepts is presented as an abstraction. *Person* may represent one individual, a family, a community, or all of mankind. In this context, *person* is the recipient of nursing care. *Health* represents a state of well-being mutually decided on by the client and the nurse. *Environment* may represent the immediate surroundings, the community, or the universe and all it contains. *Nursing* is the science and art of the discipline.

All the nursing theories presented in this book address the concepts of the meta-paradigm of nursing. Some theories speak explicitly to these concepts, others only imply their presence.

Theories

Concepts are the elements used to generate theories. Kerlinger (1973) defines a theory as a set of interrelated concepts, definitions, and propositions that present a systematic way of viewing facts/events by specifying relations among the variables, with the purpose of explaining and predicting the fact/event. This definition can be broken down to the key ideas of *interrelated concepts, propositions specifying relations among the variables,* and *a stated purpose of explaining or predicting facts/events.* Simply stated, a theory suggests a direction in how to view facts and events.

Chinn and Kramer (1991) define theory as "a creative and rigorous structuring of ideas that project a tentative, purposeful, and systematic view of phenomena" (p. 79). An additional element of this definition is a focus on the tentative nature of theory. Theories cannot be equated with scientific laws, which predict the results of given experiments 100 percent of the time. Laws are the basis of most of the natural sciences. Because nursing is a human science, the rigor and objectivity of the laboratory are both inappropriate and impossible to duplicate. In the future, the predictability of nursing theories will become more reliable as the research base from which theories develop and in which theories are tested grows.

Meleis (1991) defines nursing theory as ". . . an articulated and communicated conceptualization of invented or discovered reality (central phenomena and relationships) in or pertaining to nursing for the purpose of describing, explaining, predicting, or prescribing nursing care" (p. 17). This definition adds the importance of communicating nursing theory and the purpose of prescription of nursing care.

Theories are composed of concepts (and their definitions) and propositions. Propositions explain the relationships between the concepts. For example, Nightingale *proposed* a beneficial relationship between fresh air and health. Theories are based on stated assumptions presented as givens. Theoretical assumptions, such as a value statement or ethic, may be taken as "truth" because they cannot be empirically tested. A theory may be presented as a model that provides a diagram or map of the theory's content.

Barnum (1994) states that a complete nursing theory is one that has context, content, and process. *Context* is the environment in which the nursing act takes place. *Content* is the subject of the theory. *Process* is the method by which the nurse acts in using the theory. The nurse acts on, with, or through the content elements of the theory.

Although some texts differentiate between "theories" and "conceptual models" of nursing, most authors believe that this is an artificial distinction. Meleis (1991) goes so far as to say, "These differences are tentative at best and hair-splitting, unclear, and confusing at worst" (p. 16). For the purposes of this text, the existing nursing conceptualizations presented *are* theories.

Levels of Theory

The level of a theory refers to the scope, or range, of phenomena to which the theory applies. The level of abstraction of the concepts in the theory is closely tied to its scope. Chinn and Kramer (1991) state that "theory may be characterized as *micro, macro, molecular, midrange, molar, atomistic,* and *holistic*" (p. 123). Micro, molecular, and atomistic suggest relatively narrow-range phenomena, whereas macro, holistic, and molar imply that the theory covers a broad scope. These labels are arbitrary and may differ in different disciplines. *Grand theory* is also a term used in the literature, meaning theory that covers broad areas of concern within a discipline. *Metatheory* is a term used to label theory about the theoretical process and theory development.

Another way of looking at levels of theory is to look at what it is that the theory does. For Dickoff, James, and Wiedenbach (1968), theory develops on four levels: factor-isolating, factor-relating, situation-relating, and situation-producing. Level 1, factor-isolating, is descriptive in nature. It involves naming or classifying facts/events. Level 2, factor-relating, requires correlating or associating factors in such a way that they meaningfully depict a larger situation. Level 3, situation-relating, explains and predicts how situations are related. Level 4, situation-producing, requires sufficient knowledge about how and why situations are related, so that when the theory is used as a guide, valued situations can be produced (Dickoff & James, 1968). When using this method, one speaks of the relative power of the theory, with Level 4 being the most powerful because it controls (or does more than describe, explain, or predict).

Worldviews

A worldview is one's philosophical frame of reference in looking at one's world. The worldview of the philosophy of science is that of logical empiricism. This worldview requires that all truths must be confirmed by sensory experiences. Logical empiricism requires objectivity and is relatively value free. Objectivity requires study of the smallest parts of phenomena by using the scientific method (Riegal et al., 1992). In this worldview, the whole is equal to the sum of its parts. In the literature, this worldview is also called the *received view* or the *positivist view*. It is from this view of nursing science that the nursing process was created.

One of the worldviews that opposes logical empiricism is that of the human science or the perceived view. A human science worldview focuses on human beings as wholes and on their lived experiences within a given context (Meleis, 1991).

Parse posits two worldviews of nursing related to the received and the perceived views. The description of the totality paradigm reflects the received view, whereas the description of the simultaneity paradigm reflects the perceived view (Parse, 1987). A basic difference in these paradigms is the perception of person. The totality paradigm looks at the bio-psycho-social-spiritual aspects of person, whereas the simultaneity paradigm views person as an irreducible whole in constant interrelationship with the universe. Theorists of the totality paradigm tend to define health as a state of well-being as measured against norms; simultaneity theorists view health as something the client determines individually.

CYCLICAL NATURE OF THEORY, RESEARCH, AND PRACTICE

It is important to understand that theory, research, and practice have an impact on one another in a cyclical way. Middle-range theory can be tested in clinical practice. The testing process for theory is clinical research. The research process may validate the theory, cause it to be modified, or invalidate it. The more research that is conducted about a specific theory, the more useful the theory is to practice. Practice is based on the theories of the discipline that are validated through research (see Fig. 1–1). Research findings are published in the periodical literature as well as in books.

Research may be based on the received or perceived worldview. Received view research is quantitative; statistical data represent empirical facts and events. The methodology of the research is based on the scientific method. Perceived view research is qualitative in nature and is based on the thoughts, feelings, and beliefs of the research subjects. A number of methodologies have been proposed to conduct qualitative research.

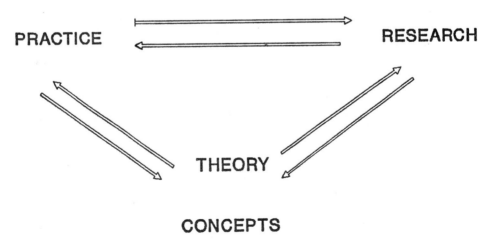

PRACTICE   RESEARCH

THEORY

CONCEPTS

Figure 1–1. Cyclical nature of theory, research, and practice.

According to Haase and Meyers (1988), quantitative and qualitative approaches differ in the following ways:

1. Quantitative methods assume a singular reality, whereas qualitative methods assume multiple interrelated realities.
2. Quantitative methods assume that objective reality is the appropriate domain. Qualitative methods assume that subjective experiences are also legitimate.
3. Quantitative methods are reductionistic, whereas the opposite methods take an ecological view—that is, they attempt to gain a full understanding of the reality.
4. Quantitative methods reveal the whole through its parts. Qualitative methods assume that the whole is greater than its parts.
5. Quantitative methods assume that discrepancies are to be accounted for or eliminated. Qualitative methods recognize that discrepancies may be existentially real.

HISTORICAL PERSPECTIVE

The history of theory development and theoretical thinking in nursing began with the writings of Florence Nightingale and continues in the 1990s. This section highlights significant events in this history.

Florence Nightingale

Nightingale's (1859/1992) *Notes on nursing* presents the first nursing theory that focuses on the manipulation of the environment for the benefit of the patient. Although Nightingale did not present her work as a "nursing theory," it has directed nursing practice for more than 100 years.

The Columbia School—The 1950s

In the 1950s the need to prepare nurses at the graduate level for administrative and faculty positions was recognized. Columbia University's Teachers College developed graduate education programs to meet these functional needs. The first theoretical conceptualizations of nursing science came from graduates of these programs. These include Peplau, Henderson, Hall, and Abdellah.

Theorists of the Columbia School operated from a biomedical model that focused primarily on what nurses do, on their functional roles. They considered patient problems and needs to be the practice focus. Independent of the Columbia theorists, Johnson (at the University of California, Los Angeles) suggested that nursing knowledge is based on a theory of nursing diagnosis that is different from medical diagnosis (Meleis, 1991).

The Yale School—The 1960s

In the 1960s theoretical thinking in nursing moved from focusing on a problem/need and the functional roles to focusing on the relationship between the nurse and the patient. The Yale School's theoretical position was influenced by the Columbia Teacher's College graduates who became faculty members there (Henderson, Orlando, and Wiedenbach).

Theorists of the Yale School view nursing as a process rather than an end in itself. They look at how nurses do what they do and how the patient perceives his or her situation. Theorists of this school include Orlando and Wiedenbach. Independent of the Yale School, Levine (1967) presented her four conservation principles of nursing.

In 1967 Yale faculty—Dickoff, James, and Wiedenbach (two philosophers and a nurse)—presented a definition of nursing theory and goals for theory development in nursing. Their paper was published in *Nursing Research* a year later and has become a classic document in the history of theoretical thinking in nursing (Dickoff et al., 1968).

It is important to note that it was during the 1960s that federal monies were made available for doctoral study for nurse educators. The resulting doctorally prepared individuals became the next wave of nurse theorists.

The 1970s

The 1970s were the decade in which many nursing theories were first presented. Most of these theories have been revised since their original presentations. Table 1–1 lists the theoretical publications of this decade.

The 1980s

In the 1980s, many nursing theories were revised on the basis of research findings that expanded them. In addition, the works of Dorothy Johnson, Rosemarie Rizzo Parse, Madeleine Leininger, and Erickson, Tomlin and Swain were added to the body of theoretical thought in nursing. The theoretical publications of the 1980s are presented in Table 1–2.

TABLE 1-1. NURSING THEORIES OF THE 1970s

Theorist	Year	Title
M. Rogers	1970	*An introduction to the theoretical basis of nursing*
I. King	1971	*Toward a theory for nursing: General concepts of human behavior*
D. Orem	1971	*Nursing: Concepts of practice*
M. Levine	1973	*Introduction to clinical nursing*
B. Neuman	1974	The Betty Neuman Health-Care Systems Model: A total person approach to patient problems
C. Roy	1976	*Introduction to nursing: An adaptation model*
J. Paterson & L. T. Zderad	1976	*Humanistic nursing*
M. Newman	1979	*Theory development in nursing*
J. Watson	1979	*Nursing: The philosophy and science of caring*

TABLE 1–2. NURSING THEORIES OF THE 1980S

Theorist	Year	Title(s)
		New
Johnson	1980	The behavioral model for nursing
R. Parse	1981	*Man–living–health: A theory for nursing*
	1985	Man–living–health: A man–environment simultaneity paradigm
	1987	*Nursing science: Major paradigms, theories, critiques*
	1989	Man–living–health: A theory of nursing
H. Erickson, E. Tomlin, & M. Swain	1983	*Modeling and role modeling*
		Revised/evolving
M. Leininger	1980	Caring: A central focus of nursing and health care services
	1981	The phenomenon of caring: Importance, research, questions and theoretical considerations
	1988	Leininger's theory of nursing: Cultural care diversity and universality
D. Orem	1980	*Nursing: Concepts of practice,* 2nd ed.
	1985	*Nursing: Concepts of practice,* 3rd ed.
	1991	*Nursing: Concepts of practice,* 4th ed.
M. Rogers	1980	Nursing: A science of unitary man
	1983	Science of unitary human beings: A paradigm for nursing
	1989	Nursing: A science of unitary human beings
C. Roy	1980	The Roy Adaptation Model
	1981	*Theory construction in nursing: An adaptation model*
	1984	*Introduction to nursing: An adaptation model,* 2nd ed.
	1989	The Roy Adaptation Model
I. King	1981	*A theory for nursing: Systems, concepts, process*
	1989	King's general systems framework and theory
B. Neuman	1982	*The Neuman Systems Model*
	1989	*The Neuman Systems Model,* 2nd ed.
M. Newman	1983	Newman's health theory
	1986	*Health as expanding consciousness*
J. Watson	1985	*Nursing: Human science and human care*
	1989	Watson's philosophy and theory of human caring in nursing
M. Levine	1989	The conservation principles: Twenty years later

The 1990s

In the 1990s, research studies that test and expand nursing theory are numerous. *Nursing Science Quarterly* (edited by Rosemarie Rizzo Parse and published by Chestnut House) is devoted exclusively to the presentation of theory-based research findings and theoretical topics.

Rogers published "Nursing: Science of Unitary, Irreducible, Human Beings: Update 1990," the latest refinement of her theory, in *Visions of Rogers' science-based nursing,* edited by Barrett. Barrett's (1990) text contains twenty-four additional chapters about Rogers' theory and its implications for practice, research. education, and the future.

In 1992 Parse changed the language of her theory from Man–Living–Health to the theory of Human Becoming (Parse, 1992). She explained that the reason for the change is that contemporary dictionary definitions of "man" tend to be gender-based, as opposed to meaning *mankind.* The assumptions and principles of the theory remain the same, only the language is new.

In 1993 Boykin and Schoenhofer published their theory of *Nursing as Caring.* They presented this theory as a grand theory with caring as a moral imperative for nursing

In 1994 Margaret Newman's second edition of her theory of health as expanding consciousness was published. This publication provided an update of her earlier work.

In 1995 Betty Neuman published her latest version of the Neuman systems model. This version is also an update rather than a major change in content.

Meleis (1992) presents six characteristics of the discipline of nursing that direct theory development in the twenty-first century:

1. The discipline of nursing is the human science underlying the discipline that is predicated on understanding the meanings of daily lived experiences as they are perceived by the members or the participants of the science.
2. There is increased emphasis on practice–orientation.
3. Nursing's mission is to develop theories to empower nurses, the discipline, and clients.
4. It is accepted that women may have different strategies and approaches to knowledge development than men do.
5. Nursing attempts to understand consumers' experiences for the purpose of empowering them to receive optimum care and to maintain optimum health.
6. The effort to broaden nursing's perspective includes efforts to understand the practice of nursing in third world countries (pp. 112–114).

Meleis (1992) forecasts that nursing theories will become theories for health, developed by nurses, physicians, occupational therapists and others. She also forecasts that the domain of nursing that focuses on environment–person interactions, energy levels, human responses, and caring will have long been accepted as a central and complementary perspective in providing health care to clients. She states that neglected aspects of care, such as advocacy, comfort, rest, access, sleep, trust, grief, symptom distress, harmony, and self-care will receive attention and will lead to collaborative programs of research and theory building.

Meleis (1992) also states that qualitative and quantitative research are *equally* essential for the development of the discipline of nursing. Theories may be single domain theories that describe, explain, or predict a phenomenon within a specific descriptive and explanatory context, or they may be prescriptive. Prescriptive theories reflect guidelines for caregivers and for providing appropriate actions. Meleis describes predictive theories of the future as having three components: levels and types of energy, mind–body wholeness, and environment–person connections.

CATEGORIES OF THEORIES

Nursing theories may be assigned to the categories of needs/problems, interaction, systems, and energy field. Assignment to a category is arbitrary, for many theories have elements of other categories within them. The nursing theories discussed in this text may be categorized as shown in Table 1–3.

Simply stated, needs/problem-oriented theorists focus on the needs and problems that clients have and seek to meet or correct them by using the nursing process. Interaction-oriented theorists focus on the communication process in the meeting of clients' needs. Systems theorists suggest that man is composed of many parts or subsystems that, when added together, are more than and different from their sum. Energy-field theorists believe that persons are energy fields in constant interaction with their environment or universe.

TABLE 1–3. CATEGORIES OF NURSING THEORIES

Needs/Problem-Oriented Theorists	Interaction-Oriented Theorists
Nightingale	Peplau
Abdellah	Orlando
Henderson	Wiedenbach
Orem	King
Hall	Paterson & Zderad
Watson	Erickson, Tomlin, & Swain
	Boykin & Schoenhofer

Systems-Oriented Theorists	Energy Field Theorists
Johnson	Rogers
Roy	Parse
Neuman	Newman
Levine	
Leininger	

CHARACTERISTICS OF A THEORY

Torres (1990) presented the following characteristics of a theory:

1. Theories can interrelate concepts in such a way as to create a different way of looking at a particular phenomenon. Theories are constructed from concepts, which are mental images representing reality. Torres (1990) states that a theory must identify more than one concept and that the relationship between these concepts must be clear. The concepts need to be explicitly defined so that one can picture the events and experiences that the theory is designed to describe, explain, or predict. For example, a needs-oriented theorist might identify the concepts of "self-care deficit" and "nursing." The concept of self-care deficit may be described as a client who experiences an inability to perform health promotion activities. Nursing may be defined in terms of actions that can be taken to assist the client to perform health promotion activities. Theories guide practice by directing the nurse to look for needs or deficits that the client may have.

2. Theories must be logical in nature. Torres (1990) defines logic as orderly reasoning. Interrelationships of concepts must be sequential and consistently used within the theory. There should not be any contradictions between the definitions of concepts, their relationships within the theory, and the goals of the theory. These relationships and goals should flow directly from the theoretical assumptions. For example, if "man–universe" is defined to be in continuous interaction, this concept must be consistent in *all* parts of the theory, from the assumptions to the practice methodology.

3. Theories should be relatively simple yet generalizable. A theory may be defined as "tight," or *parsimonious,* if it is stated in the most simple terms possible but at the same time describes, explains, or predicts a wide range of possible experiences in nursing practice. A theory of communication that can be explained simply and generalized to all person-to-person interactions would be considered parsimonious.

4. Theories can be the bases for hypotheses that can be tested or for theory to be expanded. Quantitative research tests hypotheses in clinical practice and uses statistical analyses to arrive at findings. These findings represent the testing of the precision of the theory in describing, explaining, or predicting reality. Qualitative research expands theory by using a different research methodology that focuses on the lived experiences of persons. These findings represent determining, identifying, and exploring themes in the reality lived by the persons who participate in the studies.

5. Theories contribute to and assist in increasing the general body of knowledge within the discipline through the research implemented to validate them. Theories that can be tested, whether by quantitative or qualitative research methods, contribute to the general body of knowledge of the discipline of nursing. Validation of the theories enhances the ability of the nurse to describe, explain, predict, or control nursing practice.

6. Theories can be used by practitioners to guide and improve their practice. Torres (1990) states that one of the most significant characteristics of a theory is its usefulness to the practitioner. Theories guide practice by describing, explaining, or predicting events in clinical practice.

7. Theories must be consistent with other validated theories, laws, and principles but will leave open unanswered questions that need to be investigated. Torres (1990) states that the logic of theories and their assumptions must be based on underlying laws, previously validated knowledge, and humanitarian values that are generally accepted as good and right. However, the tentative nature of theory continues to raise questions that challenge aspects of knowledge that have not yet been challenged.

The authors of this text will compare the work of each nurse theorist with these characteristics of a theory.

ANALYSIS AND EVALUATION OF THEORY

There is a variety of methods for analyzing and evaluating nursing theories. Generally speaking, analysis of a theory refers to examining the content of the theory, whereas evaluation refers to a critique or judgment about the theory.

Chinn and Kramer (1991) offer a fairly simple approach to theory analysis and evaluation. They suggest that one should consider the following five criteria: clarity (semantic and structural), simplicity, generality, empirical applicability, and consequences.

Fawcett (1989) differentiates between analysis and evaluation. She developed this framework for analysis and evaluation of conceptual models, but it can readily be applied to theories. For analysis, Fawcett proposes a consideration of the historical evolution of the theory, the approach to model development, content, and source of concern. For evaluation, she proposes evaluation of the explicitness of the assumptions, degree of comprehensiveness of content, logical congruence, ability of the model to test and generate hypotheses, how much the model contributes to nursing's knowledge development and social conditions.

Barnum (1990) proposes evaluative criteria for internal criticism (internal construction) and external criticism (the theory and its relationships to people, nursing, and health). The criteria for internal criticism are clarity, consistency, adequacy, logical development, and levels of theory development. The criteria for external criticism are reality convergence, utility, significance, discrimination, scope of the theory, and complexity.

Meleis (1991) suggests a model that defines evaluation as encompassing description, analysis, critique, and testing. This model is too detailed for presentation here. The reader is referred to the reference citation for further study about this model.

SUMMARY

When concepts are interrelated, they provide the building blocks of theory. Theories guide nursing practice by describing, explaining, or predicting phenomena. Nursing theories interrelate the four concepts of the meta-paradigm of nursing; person, environment/society, health, and nursing. Nursing research using quantitative and qualitative methods expands or tests theory.

Theory development in nursing began with Nightingale and was revived in the 1950s. Nursing theories can be arbitrarily categorized into theories which are oriented to needs, interactions, systems, and energy fields.

The characteristics of a theory were discussed and methods for analysis and evaluation were presented in this chapter.

REFERENCES

Barnum, B. J. S. (1994). *Nursing theory: Analysis, application, and evaluation* (4th ed.). Philadelphia: Lippincott.

Barrett, E. A. M. (1990). *Visions of Rogers' science based nursing.* New York: National League for Nursing.

Boykin, A., & Schoenhofer, S. (1993). *Nursing as Caring: A model for transforming practice.* New York: National League for Nursing.

Chinn, P. L., & Kramer, M. K. (1991). *Theory and nursing: A systematic approach* (3rd ed.). St. Louis: Mosby.

Dickoff, J., & James, P. (1968). A theory of theories: A position paper. *Nursing Research, 17,* 197–203.

Dickoff, J., James, P., & Wiedenbach, E. (1968). Theory in a practice discipline, Part 1—Practice-oriented theory. *Nursing Research, 17,* 415–435.

Erickson, H. C., Tomlin, E. M., & Swain, M. A. P. (1983). *Modeling and role-modeling.* Lexington, SC: Pine Press.

Fawcett, J. (1989). *Analysis and evaluation of conceptual models of nursing* (2nd ed.). Philadelphia: Davis.

Haase, J. E., & Meyers, S. T. (1988). Reconciling paradigm assumptions of qualitative and quantitative research. *Western Journal of Nursing Research, 10,* 132.

Johnson, D. E. (1980). The Behavioral System Model for Nursing. In J. P. Riehl, & C. Roy (Eds.), *Conceptual models for nursing practice* (2nd ed.) (pp. 207–216). New York: Appleton-Century-Crofts. [out of print]

Kerlinger, F. N. (1973). *Foundations of behavioral research* (2nd ed.). New York: Holt, Rinehart & Winston.

King, I. (1971). *Toward a theory for nursing: General concepts of human behavior.* New York: Wiley. [out of print]

King, I. M. (1981). A theory for nursing: System, concepts, process. New York: Wiley. (Reissued 1991, Albany, NY: Delmar.)

King, I. M. (1989). King's general systems framework and theory. In J. Riehl-Sisca (Ed.), *Conceptual models for nursing practice* (3rd ed.) (pp. 149–158). Norwalk, CT: Appleton & Lange.

Leininger, M. M. (1980). Caring: A central focus of nursing and health care services. *Nursing and Health Care, 1,* 135–143.

Leininger, M. M. (1981). The phenomenon of caring: Importance, research questions, and theoretical considerations. In M. M. Leininger (Ed.), *Caring: An essential human need* (pp. 3–15). Thorofare, NJ: Slack. [out of print]

Leininger, M. M. (1988). Leininger's theory of nursing: Culture care diversity and universality. *Nursing Science Quarterly, 1,* 152–160.

Levine, M. E. (1967). The four conservation principles. *Nursing Forum, 6,* 45–59.

Levine, M. E. (1973). *Introduction to clinical nursing.* Philadelphia: Davis. [out of print]

Levine, M. E. (1989). *The conservation principles: Twenty years later.* In J. Riehl-Sisca (Ed.), *Conceptual models for nursing practice* (3rd ed.) (pp. 325–337). Norwalk, CT: Appleton & Lange.

Meleis, A. I. (1991). *Theoretical nursing: Development and progress* (2nd ed.). Philadelphia: Lippincott.

Meleis, A. I. (1992). Directions for nursing theory development in the 21st century. *Nursing Science Quarterly, 5,* 112–117.

Neuman, B. (1974). The Betty Neuman Health Care Systems Model: A total person approach to patient problems. In J. P. Riehl, & C. Roy (Eds.), *Conceptual models for nursing practice.* (pp. 99–114). New York: Appleton-Century-Crofts. [out of print]

Neuman, B. (1982). *The Neuman systems model.* Norwalk, CT: Appleton-Century-Crofts. [out of print]

Neuman, B. (1989). *The Neuman systems model* (2nd ed.). Norwalk, CT: Appleton & Lange. [out of print]

Neuman, B. (1995). *The Neuman systems model* (3rd ed.) Norwalk, CT: Appleton & Lange.

Newman, M. A. (1979). *Theory development in nursing.* Philadelphia: Davis.

Newman, M. A. (1983). Newman's health theory. In I. W. Clements, & F. B. Roberts (Eds.), *Family health: A theoretical approach to nursing care* (pp. 161–175). New York: Wiley. [out of print]

Newman, M. A. (1986). *Health as expanding consciousness.* St. Louis: Mosby.

Newman, M. A. (1994). *Health as expanding consciousness.* (2nd ed.) New York: National League for Nursing.

Nightingale, F. (1992). *Notes on nursing.* (Com. ed.). Philadelphia: Lippincott. (Original work published in 1859.)

Orem, D. (1971). *Nursing: Concepts of practice.* New York: McGraw-Hill. [out of print]

Orem, D. (1980). *Nursing: Concepts of practice* (2nd ed.). New York: McGraw-Hill. [out of print]

Orem, D. (1985). *Nursing: Concepts of practice* (3rd ed.). New York: McGraw-Hill. [out of print]

Orem, D. (1991). *Nursing: Concepts of practice* (4th ed.). St. Louis: Mosby.

Parse, R. R. (1987). *Nursing science: Major paradigms, theories, and critiques.* Philadelphia: Saunders.

Parse, R. R. (1989). Man–Living–Health: A theory of nursing. In J. Riehl-Sisca (Ed.), *Conceptual models for nursing practice* (3rd ed.) (pp. 253–257). Norwalk, CT: Appleton & Lange.

Parse, R. R. (1992). Human Becoming: Parse's theory of nursing. *Nursing Science Quarterly, 5,* 35–42.

Paterson, J. G., & Zderad, L. T. (1976). *Humanistic nursing.* New York: Wiley. (Reissued 1988, New York: National League for Nursing.)

Riegal, B., Omery, A., Calvillo, E., Elsayed, N. G., Lee, P., Shuler, P., & Siegal, B. E. (1992). Moving beyond: A generative philosophy of science. *Image, 24,* 115–120.

Rogers, M. E. (1970). *An introduction to the theoretical basis of nursing.* Philadelphia: Davis. [out of print]

Rogers, M. E. (1980). Nursing: A science of unitary man. In J. P. Riehl, & C. Roy (Eds.), *Conceptual models for nursing practice* (2nd ed.) (pp. 329–337). New York: Appleton-Century-Crofts. [out of print]

Rogers, M. E. (1983). Science of unitary human beings: A paradigm for nursing. In I. W. Clements, & F. B. Roberts (Eds.), *Family health: A theoretical approach to nursing care* (pp. 219–228). New York: Wiley. [out of print]

Rogers, M. E. (1989). Nursing: A science of unitary human beings. In J. Riehl-Sisca (Ed.), *Conceptual models for nursing practice* (3rd ed.) (pp. 181–188). Norwalk, CT: Appleton & Lange.

Rogers, M. E. (1990). Nursing: Science of unitary, irreducible human beings. In E. A. M. Barrett (Ed.), *Visions of Rogers' science based nursing* (pp. 5–11). New York: National League for Nursing.

Roy, C. (1976). *Introduction to nursing: An adaptation model.* Englewood Cliffs: Prentice-Hall. [out of print]

Roy, C. (1980). The Roy Adaptation Model. In J. P. Riehl, & C. Roy (Eds.), *Conceptual models for nursing practice* (2nd ed.) (pp. 179–188). New York: Appleton-Century-Crofts. [out of print]

Roy, C. (1984). *Introduction to nursing: An adaptation model* (2nd ed.). Norwalk, CT: Appleton-Century-Crofts.

Roy, C. (1989). The Roy Adaptation Model. In J. Riehl-Sisca (Ed.), *Conceptual models for nursing practice* (3rd ed.) (pp. 105–114). Norwalk, CT: Appleton & Lange.

Roy, C., & Roberts, S. (1981). *Theory construction in nursing: An adaptation model.* Englewood Cliffs: Prentice-Hall. [out of print]

Torres, G. (1990). The place of concepts and theories within nursing. In J. B. George (Ed.), *Nursing theories: The base for professional nursing practice* (3rd ed.) (pp. 1–12). Norwalk, CT: Appleton & Lange.

Watson, J. (1979). *Nursing: The philosophy and science of caring.* Boston: Little, Brown. [out of print]

Watson, J. (1985). *Nursing: Human science and human care.* Norwalk, CT: Appleton-Century-Crofts. (Reissued 1988, New York: National League for Nursing.)

Watson, J. (1989). Watson's philosophy and theory of human caring. In J. Riehl-Sisca (Ed.), *Conceptual models for nursing practice* (3rd ed.) (pp. 219–236). Norwalk, CT: Appleton & Lange.

Webster's ninth new collegiate dictionary. (1991). Springfield, MA: Merriam.

AN OVERVIEW OF THE NURSING PROCESS

Charlotte Paul
*Joan S. Reeves**

■ ■ ■

This chapter is based on the assumption that professional nursing practice is interpersonal in nature. Recognizing the importance and effect of the nurse's relationship with the client/patient, professional nurses use this knowledge throughout the nursing process.

It is also assumed that professional nurses view human beings as holistic, thereby acknowledging that mind and body are not separate but function as a whole. People respond as unique whole beings. What happens in one part of the mind or body affects the person as a whole entity.

Given these two assumptions, it would be impossible for a nurse to view a client/patient as "the hysterectomy in room 201" or "the paranoid in bed 2." The woman who experiences a hysterectomy may have physiological, spiritual, and psychological health problems (ie, physiological and psychological adjustments to induced menopause). She may need to make spiritual adjustments if her life style includes a religious orientation related to a life of childbearing. The person with symptoms of paranoia may refuse to eat, causing physiological changes related to malnutrition. These two assumptions—that nursing is interpersonal in nature and that professional nurses view human beings as holistic—give guidance and direction to the use of the nursing process.

The nursing process is the underlying scheme that provides order and direction to nursing care. It is the essence of professional nursing practice. It is the "tool" and methodology of the nursing profession, and as such it helps nurses in arriving at decisions and in predicting and evaluating consequences. The nursing process is a deliberate intellectual activity by which the practice of nursing is approached in an orderly, systematic manner. Each of these terms for defining the process can be further delineated as follows:

---

*Gratitude is expressed to Marjorie Stanton for her contributions to this chapter in earlier editions.

Adjective	Definition
• *Deliberate*	Careful, thoughtful, intentional
• *Intellectual*	Rational, knowledgeable, reasonable, conceptual
• *Activity*	The state or condition of functioning, initiating, changing, behaving
• *Orderly*	A methodical, efficient, logical arrangement
• *Systematic*	Purposeful, pertaining to classification

The nursing process was developed as a specific method for applying a scientific approach or a problem-solving approach to nursing practice (Christensen & Kenney, 1990; Oermann, 1991; Wilkinson, 1992). Problem-solving approaches are not unique to nursing. For example, health planners have long used a health-planning process that is a problem-solving approach aimed at planned social change (Blum, 1981). Physicians use a specific process of gathering assessment data to make a medical diagnosis. The nursing process deals with problems specific to nurses and their clients/patients. In nursing, the client/patient may be an individual, family, or community, and the nursing process has been adapted for use with each type of client/patient (Christensen & Kenney, 1990).

Students of nursing using the nursing process are learning to behave as professional nurses in practice behave. Since the nursing process is the essence and tool (methodology) of professional nursing practice, students must become familiar with and adept at using it as their basis for practice. The nursing process also provides a means for evaluating the quality of nursing care given by nurses and assures their accountability and responsibility to the client/patient. To use the nursing process effectively, nurses need to understand and apply appropriate concepts and theories from nursing, the biological, physical, and behavioral sciences, and the humanities. These concepts and theories provide a rationale for decision making, judgments, interpersonal relationships, and actions. These concepts and theories provide the framework for nursing care.

FIVE PHASES

In earlier writings about the nursing process, many authors agreed that four phases, components, steps, or stages were necessary: assessment, including nursing diagnosis or problem identification; planning; intervention or implementation; and evaluation (Bower, 1977; Marriner, 1975; Mitchell, 1973; Yura & Walsh, 1973). However, in recent years, most authors include nursing diagnosis as a separate phase (Christensen & Kenney, 1990; Lindberg, Hunter, & Kruszewski, 1994; Oermann, 1991; Wilkinson, 1992). Because nursing diagnosis is considered an essential component of the nursing process, this book considers the following phases or components:

1. Assessment
2. Nursing diagnosis
3. Planning
4. Implementation
5. Evaluation

Although this listing suggests a forward movement of the process through each discrete phase, such movement does not always occur in the actual process. In fact, most nurses blend the phases in their practice. Assessment must always begin the process, and assessment leads to one or more nursing diagnoses. The assessment phase includes collection and analysis of data. Nursing diagnoses are derived from the assessment. However, during the diagnosis, planning, implementation, and evaluation phases, *reassessment* can lead to immediate changes in each of these four stages. Reassessment, the further collection and analysis of data, is a continuous, ongoing process; it is not to be confused with evaluation, which measures outcomes. Reassessment may also lead to a change in diagnosis, which could lead to a change in planning, implementation, and evaluation as the process continues (see Fig. 2–1).

Assessment

Assessment is the first phase in the nursing process and has two subphases: data collection and data analysis or synthesis. Assessment consists of the systematic and orderly collection and analysis of data about the health status of the client/patient for the purpose of making the nursing diagnosis. It always leads to one or more nursing diagnoses. Thus, insufficient or incorrect assessment could lead to incorrect nursing diagnoses, which could mean inappropriate planning, implementation, and evaluation. Therefore, the importance of accurate assessment cannot be overemphasized. It is vital to the process and is the basis for all other phases. Although assessment is the first phase, it may also occur as reassessment during any other phase of the process when new data are obtained.

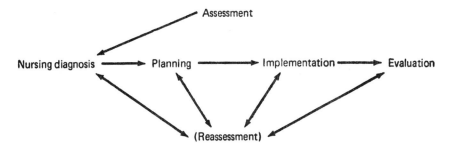

Figure 2–1. The nursing process.

The systematic and orderly collection of data is essential for the nurse to know if sufficient data have been collected. It also provides a method of quick retrieval of information about the client/patient for auditing professional practice and for doing nursing research. In addition, it serves as a means for communicating information to other health care providers. Several authors have included guidelines for the systematic collection of data (Christensen & Kenney, 1990; McFarland & McFarlane, 1993; Oermann, 1991; Wilkinson, 1992). The American Nurses' Association's (ANA) (1973) *Standards of nursing practice* also provides information to aid in the collection and organization of data. A holistic view during the assessment phase ensures that the biological, psychological, social, cultural, and spiritual spheres of the client are considered. Any assessment guidelines should include the following:

- Biographical data
- A health history, including family members
- Subjective and objective data about the current health status, including physical examination and reasons for contact with health care professional, medical diagnosis if the client/patient has a medical problem, and results of diagnostic studies
- Social, cultural, and environmental data
- Behaviors that may place a person at risk for potential disease/ problems

By using these guidelines, the data collected are classified into discrete areas that can be compared, contrasted for relationships, and clustered during the analysis of the data.

The biographical data are generally provided during an interview with the client or the person responsible for the client (Christensen & Kenney, 1990; Wilkinson, 1992). Such data are necessary to appropriately assess the client as an individual and may provide clues to the client's health status. For example, the age of clients suggests the appropriate growth and development status.

A health history is information from the client about past and present occurrences that have, or may have, an effect on his or her present or future state of health. The history is obtained through interviewing the client, the individual responsible for the client (ie, a parent), or both, and by reviewing previous health records of the client if such records are available. If able, clients may fill out part of the biographical data and health history forms. Interviewing the client is essential for discerning clues and cues and for beginning the establishment of a therapeutic relationship. Depending on the situation, the health history of other family members may be obtained from the client and/or these members. If the nurse is visiting the client in the home setting, data on the environment can be obtained from the client and through the nurse's observation.

The current health status of the client is also ascertained through interviewing the client or the person responsible for the client (subjective data) and through examination and observation of the client to obtain data that can be seen or measured objectively (objective data). For example, a client's description of pain is considered subjective data, whereas vital signs are an example of an objective measurement of physiological data (Marelli, 1992; Oermann, 1991; Wilkinson, 1992). When possible, objective data should be obtained to verify subjective data. For example, the client complains of abdominal pain (subjective data), which the nurse verifies by observation of the position of the client and palpation of the abdomen for tenderness or rigidity (objective data).

Situation. Mrs. James has come to the ambulatory medical clinic because "I just don't feel well." Her medical diagnosis is general malaise. An excerpt of the assessment data collected by the nurse for Mrs. James might look like Table 2–1.

After the data are collected, analysis of the data takes place. This is the professional nurse's responsibility and *must* occur to make a nursing diagnosis. The nurse examines the data to identify, compare, and contrast the relationship of one piece of data to another. The collected data are also compared to societal norms, while maintaining sensitivity to cultural differences, to identify actual or potential health problems. For example, a four-year-old who is unable to walk does not meet the developmental standards for four-year-olds; this is an illustration of an actual health problem.

It is during the analysis subphase of assessment that the nurse uses her or his knowledge of various theories and concepts to cluster the collected data. Clustering the data is the grouping of data pieces that fit together and show relationships. Nursing diagnoses are derived from clusters of data that show

TABLE 2–1. ASSESSMENT OF MRS. JAMES

Biographical Data	Health History	Subjective Data	Objective Data
Client—Mrs. James Age 45 Housewife Husband Philip, age 46 electrical helper Daughters Ann, age 18 Jean, age 15	Italian/Spanish heritage. Mother of Mrs. James had diabetes in older years. "All family are overweight." Shops at local fast-food market. Usually shops daily. Mrs. James responsible for cooking. Family does not have regular mealtimes.	"Fingernails break easily." Favorite foods are pizza, pasta with butter, french fries, biscuits with gravy. Drinks are coffee and diet cola. Dislikes milk, meats, and vegetables.	Height—5'2" Weight—180 lb Skin pale, dry to touch. Hair lifeless and dry to touch. Nails are ragged and broken.

TABLE 2–2. COMPARISON AND RELATIONSHIP
OF DATA FOR MRS. JAMES

Biographical Data	Health History	Current Health Status
45 years old	Mother had adult onset diabetes	Height—5'2" Weight—180 lb

relationships, make sense, and lead to a logical conclusion. The clustering of data in Table 2–2 indicates that the client may have a potential health problem in relation to diabetes. The identification of this potential problem is based on age, family history of diabetes, and obesity.

When analyzing the data related to age, the nurse needs to know what is expected of people during each stage of development. Abraham Maslow's (1954) hierarchy of needs, E. H. Erikson's (1963) eight stages of man, and other sources in the literature are useful references to consider in looking at the data.

Identification of gaps in the data should occur during the analysis subphase to ensure that all important information has been supplied and that the nursing diagnoses are based on actual data and not on inaccurate assumptions. To accomplish this one can ask, "What additional data do I need to collect? How should the data be organized in order to develop the care plan for the client?" For example, if a young child is assessed without the assessor's talking to the parent or the person responsible for the child, the nurse immediately knows that there are gaps in the data.

An analysis of the data should also give clues to the kinds of patterns that are developing. In the case of Mrs. James, there is a pattern of poor eating habits, poor selection of foods, and little understanding of diet for good health. These patterns may be handed down from generation to generation.

Nursing Diagnosis

Nursing diagnosis, the second phase of the nursing process, is recognized in the ANA (1980) definition of nursing as "the diagnosis and treatment of human responses to actual or potential health problems" (p. 3). The North American Nursing Diagnosis Association (NANDA) defines nursing diagnosis as "a clinical judgment about individual, family or community responses to actual or potential health problems/life processes. Nursing diagnoses provide the basis for selection of nursing interventions to achieve outcomes for which the nurse is accountable" (Kim, McFarland, & McLane, 1993, p. 395). The diagnostic statement identifies the client's actual or potential health problem, deficit, or concern, which can be affected by nursing actions. It describes a group of data with interpretation based upon the client's ability to meet basic needs. Models for these diagnostic statements have been provided by many authors, based on the taxonomy developed by NANDA (Cox et al., 1993; Doenges & Moorhouse, 1993; Gordon, 1991; Kim, McFarland, & McLane,

1993; McFarland & McFarlane, 1993; Sparks & Taylor, 1993; Wilkinson, 1992). For most clients, there will be more than one nursing diagnosis.

These diagnostic statements are derived from the nurse's inferences, which are based on the assessed and validated data coupled with nursing, scientific, and humanistic concepts and theories. As one proceeds through the analysis of data, certain patterns develop, and the use of relevant concepts and theories becomes appropriate. Nursing diagnoses are formulated after conclusions or decisions have been reached based on analysis of the data. Each nursing diagnosis can be considered a client-related behavioral statement that identifies the area for focus of nursing action. A diagnosis may deal with an actual (present-oriented) or a potential (future-oriented) health problem. It is based on conclusions reached in the assessment phase.

After the nursing diagnoses are identified, they should be ranked in order of priority. This ranking should consider both the client's and the nurse's opinions. Those areas that have the greatest impact on the client, the family, or both should receive particular attention. The nurse also determines priorities based on past nursing experience and on scientific knowledge of the needs and functions of human beings. Therefore, a continuum of priorities of nursing diagnoses is developed that is based on the degree of threat to the level of wellness of the client.

The nursing diagnosis can be considered a decisive statement concerning the client's nursing needs. It is important to remember that diagnoses are based on the client's concerns as well as on actual or potential problems that may be symptoms of physiological disorders or of behavioral, psychosocial, or spiritual problems.

Situation. Mrs. James's medical diagnosis has been altered to "adult onset diabetes mellitus." She asks the nurse if this means she will need to make any changes in how she lives. She says she remembers her mother "took some kind of shots."

For Mrs. James, an actual health problem can be identified as a lack of information regarding diabetes management. This identification is based on data about her height, weight, family nutrition patterns, and the status of her integumentary system. In this case, the nursing diagnosis could be *Knowledge deficit (diabetes management) related to lack of information regarding cause, effect, and therapeutic action* (Kim, McFarland, & McLane, 1993). This statement indicates that the client has inadequate information, as determined from assessed and validated data.

The nursing diagnosis also states the categories in which lack of information is pertinent, which assists the nurse in developing a plan of action. Another, more specific diagnosis would be *Nutrition, altered: high risk for more than body requirements* (Kim, McFarland, & McLane, 1993). This statement identifies the need to investigate the client's eating habits, her motivation to change, and her knowledge of nutritional needs.

Other nursing diagnoses for Mrs. James may deal with potential problems that can be identified through assessment or reassessment. These problems are related to significant risk factors that can be modified to reduce the impact of the illness. In this case, a nursing diagnosis could be *Knowledge deficit (diabetic skin care) related to lack of information regarding special skin care, peripheral circulation, and the healing process* (Kim, McFarland, & McLane, 1993). This nursing diagnosis establishes the potential problem and identifies the categories where lack of knowledge can create problems, thus assisting the nurse in developing the plan for care. Another way to state this diagnosis could be *Skin integrity, impaired, high risk for* (Kim, McFarland, & McLane, 1993). This diagnosis implies the need to evaluate the knowledge base of the client about special skin care and the healing process in persons with diabetes. These diagnoses, the needs, and the problem categories they represent are shown in Table 2–3. It is important to keep in mind that a nursing diagnosis is a statement of a health problem, or potential health problem, that a licensed nurse can treat. It is a problem for which the nurse will assume responsibility and accountability regarding the outcome.

Planning

Planning is the third phase of the nursing process. The plan for providing nursing care can be described as the determination of what can be done to assist the client. Planning involves the mutual setting of goals and objectives, judging of priorities, and designing methods to resolve actual or potential problems (Christensen & Kenney, 1990; Wilkinson, 1992).

The first subphase of planning is setting goals and objectives, which are derived from the nursing diagnoses and are established for each nursing diagnosis listed. The plan is a written document for nursing action designed to help the caregiver give quality client care. The plan contains relevant nursing diagnoses, expected outcomes, nursing interventions, and evaluation information. In addition, it becomes a permanent part of the client's record.

In preparing to write the plan, the client and his or her family should be consulted before formulating the goals and objectives, which should be realistic and attainable, supportive of the client's needs, and mutually acceptable. It is important to consider the need for objectives that can be defined and stated concisely in an "act-of-being" phrase. This phrase should contain a performer (the client), a performance (action), and a change in behavior to be accomplished (objective). This expected end behavior needs to be identified and placed in the proper time frame, and can be used for evaluation.

Goals are stated in broad terms to identify effective criteria for evaluating nursing action. These goals can pertain to rehabilitation, prevention of complications associated with stressors, the ability of the client to adapt to these stressors, or all three. Other goals may deal with the achievement of the highest health potential for a client. A sample goal statement would be, "Mrs. James will have an adequate understanding of the basic food groups and their relationship to recommended daily allowance (RDA) requirements within one month."

Objectives are determined from the goals and need to be stated in terms of observable behaviors. Objectives should define the conditions under which

TABLE 2–3. CLASSIFICATION OF NURSING DIAGNOSES

Nursing Diagnosis Statement	Type of Need	Problem Category	
		Actual (present)	*Potential (future)*
I.			
Inadequate information relating to diabetes management; lack of information regarding cause, effect, and therapeutic action associated with diabetes management (more specific nutritional needs)	Biopsychosocial	Lack of information regarding diabetes management	
or			
Alterations in nutrition (eating and drinking)	Biological	Lack of knowledge pertaining to nutrition, eating habits; lack of motivation to change	
II.			
Inadequate knowledge relating to diabetic skin care: lack of information regarding special skin care, peripheral circulation, and the healing process	Biopsychosocial		Lack of knowledge regarding the need for special skin care
or			
Potential for alterations in skin integrity	Biological		Implies the need to evaluate knowledge base of client regarding special skin care and healing process in diabetes

the expected end behaviors are to occur and should specify the performance level and specific behaviors that will be accepted as evidence that desired outcomes have been met. The behaviors in question refer to psychological, physiological, social, cultural, and intellectual activities and other observable responses. Objectives related to the goal for Mrs. James could be:

1. Identify the basic food groups from a chart by the end of Week 1.
2. Prepare a shopping list to include at least two necessary foods from each group by the end of Week 1.

3. Prepare family menus for three days using the basic food groups as a guide by Week 2.
4. Make substitutions in family menus for three days using the basic food groups pyramid as a guide by Week 3.
5. Evaluate eating patterns of family for one week using the basic food groups pyramid as a guide and identify at least two problem areas to discuss with nurse by Week 4.

Desired behavioral outcomes (objectives) should be stated in a manner that everyone can understand without having to seek clarification. Robert Mager, in his classic book on preparing objectives, indicates that a meaningfully stated outcome would be one that communicates to the staff the intent of the individual who stated it. "The statement which communicates best will be one which describes the terminal behavior of the learner well enough to prevent misinterpretation" (Mager, 1962, p. 11).

Time is another consideration when specifying desired outcomes. The time limits should be precise for evaluation purposes but should not be so rigid that changes cannot readily be made. Changes in time limits are based on reassessment of the priorities and necessary outcomes. It is important to remember to state the desired outcomes in terms of client behaviors rather than nurse behaviors, in keeping with the standards of nursing practice developed by the ANA (American Nurses' Association, 1973).

The second subphase in nursing care planning is the identification of nursing actions for each nursing diagnosis. Each nursing action is based on carefully thought out scientific rationale and specifies what kind of nursing care is to be done to meet the client's problem effectively. Nursing actions should be spelled out precisely. These actions are part of the scheme for providing good nursing care.

Nursing actions can be said to be hypotheses established for testing if they contribute to the solution of the problem. It is up to the nurse with the client, the family, or both to select appropriate actions to produce desired results. In selecting these nursing actions, it is important to analyze the available options and to determine the probability of success in reaching the objective. Sometimes compromises must be made to provide the best care for the client, and the nurse needs to be aware of this when specifying nursing actions.

The nursing care plan deals with actual and potential problems. Nursing actions are based on scientific principles and theories of nursing, and they need to be specific. The plan serves as a means for resolving the problems and for meeting established goals in an orderly fashion. Also, it provides a means for organization, giving direction and meaning to the nursing action used in helping the client, the family, or both to resolve the health problems. A plan of action is necessary because it aids in the efficient use of time. It saves both time and energy by providing essential data for those individuals who are responsible for giving care.

Since the client's condition is continuously changing, the written nursing care plan needs to reflect these changes. Therefore, planning becomes a continuous process based on evaluation and reassessment. The written plan is the most efficient way of keeping all individuals involved in the client's care informed of modifications in the plan of nursing care.

Implementation

After planning, implementation is the next, or fourth, phase of the nursing process. Implementation refers to the actions initiated to accomplish the defined goals and objectives. Implementation is often considered as the actual giving of nursing care. It is putting the plan into action. Other terms used to describe this part of the process are *action* or *intervention.* The words *implementation* and *intervention* are not synonymous. Implementation refers to putting a plan into action; intervention speaks to involvement in the affairs of another, a coming between the other and a problematic situation. Therefore, the term *implementation* seems more appropriate to describe this phase of the process if nursing actions are to follow from mutually established goals and objectives. The implementation phase encompasses all nursing actions directed toward resolving the problem and meeting the health care needs of the client. It is an ongoing process through which the nurse is reassessing, reviewing, and modifying the plan of care, and if necessary seeking assistance in meeting the client's health care needs.

Since the nursing process is interpersonal in nature, it must take place between the nurse and the client. The client may be a person, a group, a family, or even a community. The beliefs that the nurse and the client have about human beings, nurses, and clients, and about interactions between nurses and clients will affect the types of actions that both consider appropriate. If human beings are considered unique, then nursing actions should reflect this uniqueness. Therefore, the philosophy of nursing that a nurse develops will affect the nursing actions that he or she uses in meeting the needs of clients. Yura and Walsh (1973) indicated that the implementation phase of the nursing process draws heavily on the intellectual, interpersonal, and technical skills of the nurse. Wilkinson (1992) supports the importance of critical thinking throughout the nursing process. Although the focus is on action, the action is intellectual, interpersonal, and technical in nature.

The implementation phase begins when the nurse considers various alternative actions and selects those most suitable to achieve the planned goals and objectives. Just as goals and objectives have priorities in the plan, actions may also have priorities. Nursing actions may be carried out by the nurse who developed the nursing care plan or by other nurses or nursing assistants. Nursing actions may also be carried out by the client or family. To carry out a nursing action, the nurse refers to the written plan for specific information. Many nursing actions fall into the broad categories of counseling, teaching, providing physical care, carrying out delegated medical therapy, coordination of resources, referral to other sources of help, and therapeutic communication (verbal and nonverbal).

According to the goals and objectives for Mrs. James, as discussed on pages 22–24, several nursing actions could be implemented. For example, under Objective 1 (identify the basic food groups from a chart), the following actions could be considered:

1. Establish an agreed upon time when Mrs. James and her family could meet with the nurse in their home during the next week.
2. Establish a baseline knowledge about Mrs. James's and the family members' understanding of basic food groups.
3. Take chart and booklets containing information about the basic food groups to Mrs. James's home.
4. Teach family about using the basic food groups for good nutrition (base teaching on information gained from baseline knowledge).
5. Focus on the value of the food groups for each family member based on age, height, weight, and activity.
6. Request a return demonstration in which Mrs. James and other family members will identify foods by placing the food in a food group and will state why each food group is important.

In Campbell's (1980) study of nursing diagnoses and nursing actions, seven categories of nursing actions were developed. These are: assertive, hygienic, rehabilitative, supportive, preventive, observational, and educative. Wilkinson (1992) speaks to doing, delegating, and recording. Both point out that almost all nursing actions are initiated by nurses without medical direction. Nurses initiate and carry out all activities that fall within the nursing domain. In the hospital setting, nurses are also asked to assist physicians in carrying out medical prescriptions and to follow institutional policies. Therefore, nurses need to be clear about their dependent and independent functions.

For every nursing action, the client responds as a total person; that is, as a whole. The concept of *holism*, which states that a person is more than the sum of that person's parts, means that the nurse may be treating a person's leg but the person will respond as a whole person (Leddy & Pepper, 1993). The concept is useful in thinking about the consequences of any nursing actions. For example, the simple action of turning the patient every two hours will have a variety of consequences. Some of these consequences could or should be: (1) increased circulation, (2) improved muscle tone, (3) improved breathing, (4) less flatus (gas) in the intestinal track, (5) prevention of pressure sores, (6) increased or decreased pain, (7) opportunity for communication with caregiver, (8) increased ability to socialize with patient in next bed, and (9) increased or decreased ability to reach articles at bedside. There may be other consequences that could not have been predicted, such as an opportunity to express values or beliefs. Therefore, in planning nursing actions, it is important to consider the cluster of consequences of both positive and negative value that can be expected to occur with and following each action (Oermann, 1991). Using this knowledge will help the nurse select the most appropriate actions. Although not all consequences are predictable for a specific client, it is possible to develop a general knowledge of expected consequences. Knowledge of consequences is an important aspect of the implementation phase of the nursing process. The implementation phase is completed when the nursing actions are finished and the results are recorded against each diagnosis.

Evaluation

Evaluation is the fifth and final phase of the nursing process. It may be defined as the appraisal of the client's behavioral changes that are a result of the action of the nurse (Christensen & Kenney, 1990; Leddy & Pepper, 1993; Wilkinson, 1992). Although evaluation is considered to be the final phase, it frequently does not end the process. As mentioned earlier in this chapter, evaluation may lead to reassessment, which in turn may result in the nursing process beginning all over again. The main questions to ask in evaluation are: Were the goals and objectives met? Were there identifiable changes in the client's behavior? If so, why? If not, why not? Were the consequences of nursing actions predicted? These questions help the nurse to determine which problems have been solved and which problems need to be reassessed and replanned. Unsolved problems cannot be assumed to reflect faulty or inadequate data collection; rather, each part of the nursing process may need to be evaluated to determine the cause of ineffective actions.

The key to appropriate evaluation of nurse–client actions lies in the planning phase of the nursing process. When objectives are described in behavioral terms with clearly stated expected outcomes, it is easy to determine whether or not the nurse–client actions were successful. These objectives become the criteria for evaluating nurse–client actions. Just as goals should be mutually set with a client whenever possible, it is also important for the nurse and client to mutually establish the objectives (criteria for evaluation).

According to Wilkinson (1992), evaluation consists of the following five steps:

1. Review the goals or predicted outcomes.
2. Collect data about the client's responses to nursing actions.
3. Compare actual outcomes to predicted outcomes and decide if goals have been met.
4. Record the conclusion.
5. Relate nursing plans to client outcomes.

The first three steps are specific to client outcomes. Step 1 has been briefly discussed in relation to the planning phase of the process. In addition to stating the desired behavior change, it is also important for the nurse to decide how the change will be measured (predicted outcome) and when it will be measured.

Step 2 involves the collection of evidence (data). Although data are collected in both assessment and evaluation, the data collected during evaluation are used differently from data collected during assessment. In assessment, data are collected for the purpose of making a nursing diagnosis. In evaluation, data are collected as evidence to determine whether the goals and objectives were met. This is an important difference to note in using the nursing process.

Step 3 in evaluation is the one that is often the most difficult because it is easy to use different measurements in making judgments. For example, if a nurse observed that a client "ate well," would this mean the same thing to the client or to another nurse? "Ate well" could be interpreted to mean that the client was able to chew, swallow, and digest the food with no difficulty, or it could refer to the amount and kind of food consumed. Therefore, in evaluation it is not only important to determine the criteria (objectives) and be specific in predicting outcomes, it is also important to determine the exact way(s) in which evidence is gathered and interpreted to ascertain whether the criteria were met.

In the situation regarding Mrs. James, objectives can be mutually set in measurable terms. Using Wilkinson's (1992) Step 1, it is possible to predict outcomes for measuring the first objective (identify the basic food groups from a chart). The predicted outcomes could include eighteen out of twenty foods correctly identified. If at the end of Week 1, Mrs. James can identify nineteen foods correctly by food groups, then Objective 1 can be evaluated as "accomplished." Specific evidence has been collected (Step 2) and compared to the predicted outcome (Step 3). The actual outcome exceeded the predicted outcome.

Under Objective 2 (prepare a shopping list to include at least two foods from each group by the end of Week 1), the predicted outcomes could be the following:

1. The shopping list will include all foods essential for preparing three meals per day for seven days.
2. Two foods from each food group will be included on the shopping list.

In looking at the shopping list, the nurse may discover that no dairy foods are included, therefore creating a limited use of one food group. (Mrs. James revealed that her husband did not like dairy foods.) This information is then included as reassessment data, and the nurse collects information about foods containing calcium that the family can eat. By evaluating the family eating patterns (Objective 5), the nurse obtains information to enable him or her to help Mrs. James in choosing foods rich in vitamins and minerals, thereby meeting Objective 2.

When predicted outcomes are not reached, reassessment should occur, and the process begins again. If the evaluation shows that the nurse–client objectives have been met, the nursing process is complete.

Evaluation based on behavioral changes is *outcome evaluation*. There are two other types of evaluation, both of which are reflected in Wilkinson's (1992) evaluation steps. *Structure evaluation* relates to such things as appropriate equipment to assess the client or to carry out the plan and to record evaluation conclusions (Step 4). For example, if the scales were inaccurate, then correct data could not be obtained. Structure evaluation may also relate to the organization within which the nurse works. The nurse may be unable to carry out the nursing process appropriately because of agency limitations on time; this must be considered part of the evaluation.

Process evaluation, which focuses on the activities of the nurse, can be done during each phase of the nursing process, or it may be carried out at the end of the process (Step 5). The following are examples of process evaluation questions that can be used in evaluating each phase of the process.

Assessment

1. Were historical data that might be related to health problems collected?
2. Was a physical examination carried out and the results recorded?
3. Was the analysis logical? Did it make use of the collected data? Were significant findings mentioned in the analysis?

Diagnosis

1. Was the diagnosis based on the analysis?
2. Is the diagnosis a logical conclusion from the data collected?

Planning

1. Are goals and objectives stated?
2. Does the plan rationally follow from the diagnosis?
3. Were goals and objectives mutually established with the client?

Implementation

1. What activities did the nurse carry out?
2. What activities did the client carry out?
3. Were the activities consistent with the objectives?

Evaluation

1. Were the predicted outcomes achieved?
2. What evaluation methods were used?
3. Were the conclusions recorded?

The nurse and the client are responsible for carrying out outcome evaluation. Structure and process evaluations are typically carried out by the nurse, others in nursing administration, or both within an agency.

SUMMARY

In summary, the nursing process is the tool or methodology of professional nursing that helps nurses arrive at decisions and helps them predict and evaluate consequences. To use the nursing process successfully, a nurse needs to apply concepts and theories from nursing; from biological, physical, and behavioral sciences; and from the humanities, to provide a rationale for decision making, judgments, interpersonal relationships, and actions. The five components considered necessary to the nursing process are: assessment, nursing diagnosis, planning, implementation, and evaluation.

Students who are learning about the use of the nursing process need to use many references to augment their knowledge and skills as they proceed. The citations in this chapter reflect both historical and current materials.

REFERENCES

American Nurses' Association. (1973). *Standards for nursing practice*. Kansas City: Author.

American Nurses' Association. (1980). *Nursing: A social policy statement*. Kansas City: Author.

Blum, H. L. (1981). *Planning of health* (2nd ed.). New York: Human Sciences.

Bower, E. L. (1977). *The process of planning nursing care—A model for practice*. St. Louis: Mosby.

Campbell, C. (1980). *Nursing diagnosis and intervention in nursing practice*. New York: Wiley.

Christensen, P. J., & Kenney, J. W. (1990). *Nursing process—Application of conceptual models* (3rd ed.). St. Louis: Mosby.

Cox, H. C., Hinz, M. D., Lubno, M. A., Newfield, S. A., Ridenour, N. A., Slater, M. M., & Sridaromont, K. (1993). *Clinical applications of nursing diagnosis* (2nd ed.). Philadelphia: Davis.

Doenges, M. E., & Moorhouse, M. F. (1993). *Nurse's pocket guide: Nursing diagnoses with interventions* (4th ed.). Philadelphia: Davis.

Erikson, E. H. (1963). *Childhood and society*. New York: Norton & Coe.

Gordon, M. (1991). *Manual of nursing diagnoses*. St. Louis: Mosby.

Kim, M. J., McFarland, G. K., & McLane, A. M. (1993). *Pocket guide to nursing diagnoses* (5th ed.). St. Louis: Mosby.

Leddy, S., & Pepper, J. M. (1993). *Conceptual bases of professional nursing* (3rd ed.). Philadelphia: Lippincott.

Lindberg, J. B., Hunter, M. L., & Kruszewski, A. Z. (1994). *Introduction to nursing: Concepts, issues, and opportunities* (2nd ed.). Philadelphia: Lippincott.

McFarland, G. K., & McFarlane, E. A. (1993). *Nursing diagnosis & intervention*. St. Louis: Mosby.

Mager, R. (1962). *Preparing instructional objectives*. Palo Alto, CA: Fearon.

Marrelli, T. M. (1992). *Nursing documentation handbook*. St. Louis: Mosby.

Marriner, A. (1975). *The nursing process: A scientific approach to nursing care.* St. Louis: Mosby.

Maslow, A. (1954). *Motivation and personality.* New York: Harper & Row.

Mitchell, P. H. (1973). *Concepts basic to nursing.* New York: McGraw-Hill.

Oermann, M. H. (1991). *Professional nursing practice: A conceptual approach.* Philadelphia: Lippincott.

Sparks, S. M., & Taylor, C. M. (1993). *Nursing diagnosis reference manual* (2nd ed.). Springhouse, PA: Springhouse.

Wilkinson, J. M. (1992). *Nursing process in action: A critical thinking approach.* Redwood City, CA: Addison-Wesley.

Yura, H., & Walsh, M. B. (1973). *The nursing process: Assessing, planning, implementing, evaluating* (2nd ed.). New York: Appleton-Century-Crofts.

FLORENCE NIGHTINGALE

Marie L. Lobo

■ ■ ■

Florence Nightingale was born in Florence, Italy, on May 12, 1820, during one of her parents' extensive trips abroad. As she grew up, her father provided her with a very broad education, which was unusual for Victorian women. According to her biographer, Sir Thomas Cook, Nightingale was a linguist; had a broad knowledge of science, mathematics, literature, and the arts; was well read in philosophy, history, politics and economics; and as well was knowledgeable about the workings of government. She wanted to do more with her life than become an idle wife of an aristocrat. She had a strong belief in God, and for a time believed she had a religious calling.

Nightingale became a heroine in Great Britain as a result of her work in the Crimean War. Her description of the very poor sanitary conditions in the hospital wards at Scutari is overwhelming. She fought the bureaucracy for bandages, food, fresh bedding, and cleaning supplies for the invalid soldiers. At times she bought supplies with her own money. She demonstrated great concern for the well-being of the English soldier—well, injured, or sick—including assisting with the establishment of a laundry, a library, assistance with letter writing, a banking system so the soldiers could save their pay, and a hospital for the families who accompanied the soldiers to war. As well, she provided comfort to the critically ill and dying. Her managerial skills were often greater than those of many officers in the army. She spent the years after the Crimea establishing schools of nursing and influencing public policy by lobbying her acquaintances about various of her concerns.

Nightingale was romanticized by Henry Wadsworth Longfellow in his poem *The Lady with the Lamp*. Although this poem was meant to honor Nightingale, it may have done a great disservice to her because it ignored her superb management skills and ability to provide nursing care to both healthy and ill soldiers. Nightingale died on August 13, 1910, and she is honored each year in a commemorative service at St. Margaret's Church, East Wellow, Great Britain, where she is buried.

Nightingale is viewed as the mother of modern nursing. She synthesized information gathered in many of her life experiences to assist her in the development of modern nursing. Her place in history has been established. To understand how Nightingale developed her conceptualization of nursing it is helpful to review her roots. As noted, she was highly educated for a woman of the Victorian era. In seeking to use her knowledge, she was frustrated by prevailing social norms. Her desire to have a position that was useful to society was incompatible with nineteenth-century upper-class British society's expectations of women. While Nightingale was struggling with decisions about her life, the seeds of modern nursing were being planted in Germany.

Germany was the site of the first organized nursing school. In 1836 Pastor Theodor Fliedner, a protestant pastor in Kaiserswerth, Germany, opened a hospital in a "vacant textile factory with one patient, one nurse, and a cook" (Hegge, 1990, p. 74). When Fliedner realized there was no work force for the hospital, he designed a school of nursing. The physician for Fliedner's hospital spent one hour a week teaching the nursing students. Gertrude Reichardt, the physician's daughter, taught anatomy and physiology, although her only experience had been gained at her father's side. Reichardt became the first matron of the Deaconess School of Nursing. Local peasant girls were taught hygiene, manners, and ladylike behavior as well as how to read, write, and calculate. There were no textbooks for nursing until 1837, when a German physician prepared a handbook.

Nightingale visited Kaiserswerth for 14 days in 1850 after a trip to Egypt. She applied for admission to the school with a 12-page, handwritten "curriculum" stating her reasons for wanting to be a nurse and entered the nursing program July 6, 1851, as the 134th nursing student to attend the Fliedner School of Nursing. She left Kaiserswerth on October 7, 1851, and was deemed to be educated as a nurse (Hegge, 1990). During the three months she spent studying with the sisters of Kaiserswerth, she developed skills in both nursing care and management which she took back to England.

When Nightingale returned to England, she used the information from Kaiserswerth to champion her cause as a reformer for the health and well-being of the citizens. Her reform efforts occurred in part because she was frustrated with the conditions in England that limited women's life choices to "indolence, marriage, or servitude," as well as with the two existing social conditions of most of England's citizens: abject poverty or affluence (Nightingale, 1860).

In 1854 Nightingale went to the front of the Crimean War at the request of her friend, Sir Sidney Herbert, Secretary at War. She arrived in Scutari on November 5, 1854, accompanied by 38 nurses. Nightingale's 19-month stay at Scutari was difficult. The idea of women being involved in the affairs of the military was difficult for many to accept. The hospital barracks were infested with fleas and rats, and sewage flowed under the wards. The mortality rate at the hospital was 42.7 percent of those treated, a mortality rate which was higher from disease than from war injuries (Cohen, 1984). Six months after Nightingale came to Scutari the mortality rate at the hospital dropped to 2.2 percent. Nightingale achieved this drop in mortality by attending to the environment of the soldiers. One year and nine months after she landed at Scutari, on August 5, 1856, Nightingale returned from the Crimea. She sneaked into England to avoid a hero's welcome.

After her return to England, Nightingale used her knowledge of data concerning the health and well-being of soldiers to influence the decisions of the War Department by providing information to Sir Sidney Herbert. Many of the position papers and reports, although officially submitted by Sir Sidney Herbert, Secretary at War, were virtually intact manuscripts written by Nightingale. Because of the position of women in Victorian England, she was not permitted to submit her findings under her own name.

Nightingale was also a skilled statistician who used statistics to present her case for hospital reform. According to Cohen "the idea of using statistics for such a purpose—to analyze social conditions and the effectiveness of public policy—is commonplace today, but at that time it was not" (Cohen, 1984, p. 132). Nightingale was regarded as a pioneer in the graphic display of statistics and was elected a fellow of the Royal Statistical Society in 1858. In 1874 an honorary membership in the American Statistical Association was bestowed on her (Agnew, 1958; Nightingale, 1859/1992). Given her reliance on observable data to support her position, it can be said that Nightingale was the first nurse researcher.

NIGHTINGALE'S APPROACH TO NURSING

Nightingale used her broad base of knowledge, her understanding of the incidence and prevalence of disease, and her acute powers of observation to develop an approach to nursing as well as to the management and construction of hospitals. Nightingale's main focus was the control of the environment of individuals and families, both healthy and ill. She discussed the need for ventilation and light in sickrooms, proper disposal of sewage, and appropriate nutrition. Her most frequently cited work, *Notes on nursing,* was written not as a nursing text but to "give hints for thought to women who have personal charge of the health of others" (Nightingale, 1859/1992, preface). She did not intend for *Notes on nursing* to become a manual for teaching nurses to nurse. Rather, *Notes on nursing* is a thought-provoking essay on the organization and manipulation of the environment of those persons requiring nursing care. Nightingale stated that her purpose was "everyday sanitary knowledge, or the knowledge of nursing, or in other words, of how to put the constitution in such a state as that it will have no disease, or that it can recover from disease" (Nightingale, 1859/1992, preface). She wanted women to teach themselves to nurse and viewed *Notes on nursing* as hints to enable them to do this. Nightingale viewed disease as a reparative process, a thought that is reflected in the American Nurses' Association *Social policy statement* that nursing is the diagnosis and treatment of human responses to actual or potential health problems (American Nurses' Association, 1980).

Although *Notes on nursing* is Nightingale's most accessible work, she also wrote *Notes on hospitals* and *Introductory notes on lying-in institutions* (the first maternity centers) as well as numerous letters (Vicinus & Nergaard, 1990). In her volumes of writing she provided much information on the influence of the environment on the human being and the critical nature of balance between the human and his or her environment. For example,

Nightingale did not view pregnancy as a disease and recommended facilities away from those treating diseases in which women could bear their babies. She analyzed data from the Midwifery Department of King's College Hospital concerning the mortality rate in childbearing and recommended environmental changes and handwashing to decrease puerperal fever, then the leading cause of maternal death (Nightingale, 1871).

NIGHTINGALE'S ENVIRONMENTAL MODEL

Webster (1991) defines environment as the surrounding matters that influence or modify a course of development. According to Miller (1978) the system must interact and adjust to its environment. Nightingale viewed the manipulation of the physical environment as a major component of nursing care. She identified ventilation and warmth, light, noise, variety, bed and bedding, cleanliness of rooms and walls, and nutrition as major areas of the environment the nurse could control. When one or more aspects of the environment are out of balance, the client must use increased energy to counter the environmental stress. These stresses drain the client of energy needed for healing. These aspects of the physical environment are also influenced by the social and psychological environment of the individual. Nightingale addressed these aspects of the environment in chapters titled "Chattering hopes and advices" and "Variety." Although Nightingale did not address political activism in *Notes on nursing*, her life was a model of political involvement. She was very knowledgeable about current affairs and wrote many letters attempting to influence the health of individuals, families, and communities.

Health of Houses

In *Notes on nursing* Nightingale discussed the importance of the health of houses as being closely related to the presence of pure air, pure water, efficient drainage, cleanliness, and light. To support the importance of hospital-based nursing attending to these, Nightingale (1859/1992) said, "Badly constructed houses do for the healthy what badly constructed hospitals do for the sick. Once insure that the air is stagnant and sickness is certain to follow" (p. 15). Nightingale also noted that the cleanliness outside the house affected the inside. Just as Nightingale noted that dung heaps affected the health of houses in her time, so too can modern families be affected by toxic waste, contaminated water, and polluted air.

Ventilation and Warming

In her chapter on ventilation and warming, Nightingale (1859/1992) stated it was essential to "keep the air he breathes as pure as the external air, without chilling him" (p. 8). She urged the caregiver to consider the source of the air in the patient's room. The air might be full of fumes from gas, mustiness, or open sewage if the source was not the freshest. Nightingale believed that the person who repeatedly breathed his or her own air would become sick or remain sick. In the twentieth century we have buildings that are sealed in such a manner that fresh air is difficult to receive, and a new problem, labeled *building sickness,* has evolved.

Nightingale (1859/1992) was very concerned about "noxious air" or "effluvia" or foul odors that came from excrement. In many public places, as well as hospitals, raw sewage could be found near patients, in ditches under or near the house, or contaminating drinking water. Her concerns about "effluvia" also included bedpans, urinals, and other utensils used to discard excrement. She also criticized "fumigations," for she believed that the offensive source, not the smell, must be removed.

The importance of room temperature was stressed by Nightingale. The patient should not be too warm or too cold. The temperature could be controlled by appropriate balance between burning fires and ventilation from windows. Today buildings often are constructed to be climate-controlled in such a manner that the client or the nurse cannot control the temperature of the individual room. In shared rooms the climate control may not satisfy either patient, with one wanting the room colder and another wanting it warmer, as each individual interacts with the environment.

Light

Nightingale (1859/1992) believed that second to fresh air the sick needed light. She noted that direct sunlight was what patients wanted. Although acknowledging a lack of scientific information, she noted that light has "quite real and tangible effects upon the human body" (pp. 47–48). She noted that people do not consider the difference between light needed in a bedroom (where individuals sleep at night) and light needed in a sickroom. To a healthy sleeper it does not matter where the light is because he is usually in his room only during hours of darkness. She noted that the sick rarely lie with their face toward the wall but are much more likely to face the window, the source of the sun. Again, modern hospitals may be constructed in such a manner that daylight is rarely available. This is particularly the case in neonatal intensive care units, and for many years was also true in the construction of adult intensive care units. The lack of appropriate environmental stimuli can lead to intensive care psychosis or a confusion related to the lack of the accustomed cycling of day and night.

Noise

Noise was also of concern to Nightingale, particularly those noises that could jar the patient. She stated that patients should never be waked intentionally or accidentally during the first part of sleep. She asserted that whispered or long conversations about patients are thoughtless and cruel. She viewed unnecessary noise, including noise from female dress, as cruel and irritating to the patient. Nurses today do not wear crinoline petticoats, but they do wear jewelry and carry keys that jingle and make other noises. Other more modern noises include the snapping of rubber gloves, the clank of a stethoscope against metal bed rails, and radios and TVs. Modern health care facilities contain much equipment that issue alarms, beeps, and other noises that startle or jar a patient from sleep to wakefulness. Nightingale was very critical of noises that annoyed the patient, such as a window shade blowing against the window frame. She viewed it as the nurse's responsibility to assess and stop this kind of noise.

Variety

Nightingale believed that variety in the environment was a critical aspect affecting the patient's recovery. She discussed the need for changes in color and form, including bringing the patient brightly colored flowers or plants. She also advocated rotating 10 or 12 paintings and engravings each day, week, or month to provide variety for the patient. She wrote that "volumes are now written and spoken upon the effect of the mind upon the body. Much of it is true" (Nightingale, 1859/1992, p. 34). The increasing research being done on the interaction between mind and body has supported this observation. Nightingale also advocated reading, needlework, writing, and cleaning as activities to relieve the sick of boredom.

Bed and Bedding

Nightingale (1859/1992) viewed bedding as an important part of the environment. Although her view has not been substantiated by data, she noted that an adult in health exhales about three pints of moisture through the lungs and skin in a 24-hour period. This organic matter enters the sheets and stays there unless the bedding is changed and aired frequently. She believed that the bed should be placed in the lightest part of the room and placed so the patient could see out of a window. She reminded the caregiver never to lean against, sit upon, or unnecessarily shake the bed of a patient. In modern hospitals mattresses are usually covered with plastic or other materials that can be washed to remove drainage, excreta, or other matter. These mattresses often cause the patient to perspire, leading to damp bed clothing. Sheets also do not fit tightly on these mattresses, leading to wrinkles that can result in pressure points on the skin of the patient lying in bed. Modern technology may also interfere with providing a comfortable bed environment for the patient. Multiple intravenous pumps, ventilators, and monitors attached to a patient may impede comfort. It remains important for the nurse to keep bedding clean, neat, and dry and to position the patient for maximum comfort.

Personal Cleanliness

Nightingale viewed the function of the skin as important, believing that many diseases "disordered," or caused breaks in the skin. She thought this was particularly true of children and that the excretion that comes from the skin must be washed away. She believed that unwashed skin poisoned the patient and noted that bathing and drying the skin provided great relief to the patient, saying, "Just as it is necessary to renew the air round a sick person frequently, to carry off morbid effluvia from the lungs and skin, by maintaining free ventilation, so is it necessary to keep pores of the skin free from all obstructing excretions" (Nightingale, 1859/1992, p. 53). She also believed that personal cleanliness extended to the nurse and that "every nurse ought to wash her hands very frequently during the day" (p. 53).

Nutrition and Taking Food

Nightingale addressed the variety of food presented to the patient and discussed the importance of variety in the food presented. She found that the attention provided to the patient affected how the patient ate. She noted that individuals desire different foods at different times of the day and that frequent small servings may be more beneficial to the patient than a large breakfast or dinner. She observed that patients may desire a different pattern of taking foods, such as eating breakfast foods at lunch, and that chronically ill patients may be starved to death because their incapacitation can make them unable to feed themselves. She urged that no business be done with patients while they are eating because this was distraction.

Chattering Hopes and Advices

Nightingale did not speak to the social and psychological environment of the patient to the same degree that she addressed the physical environment. However, she included a chapter on "Chattering hopes and advices," which discussed what is said to the patient. She wrote that the chapter heading might seem "odd" but that to falsely cheer the sick by making light of their illness and its danger is not helpful. She considered it stressful for a patient to hear opinions after only brief observations had been made. False hope was depressing to patients, she felt, and caused them to worry and become fatigued. Nightingale encouraged the nurse to heed what is being said by visitors, believing that sick persons should hear good news that would assist them in becoming healthier.

Social Considerations

Nightingale (1859/1992) supported the importance of looking beyond the individual to the social environment in which he or she lived. She was an epidemiologist who looked at not only the numbers of people who died but also what was unique about a given house or street. She observed that generations of families lived and died in poverty. Using her statistical data, she wrote letters and position papers and sent them to her acquaintances in the government in an effort to improve undesirable living conditions. Nightingale was a role model for political activism by nurses.

Nightingale was also an excellent manager. She demonstrated her management skills at Scutari and wrote about them in many of her nursing-related books. In *Notes on nursing* (1859/1992), she discussed "petty management" or ways to assure that "what you do when you are there, shall be done when you are not there" (p. 20). She believed that the house and the hospital needed to be well managed—that is, organized, clean, and with appropriate supplies.

NIGHTINGALE'S ENVIRONMENTAL MODEL AND NURSING'S METAPARADIGM

Nightingale did not invent or define the four major concepts used to organize nursing theory. They evolved from an analysis of nursing curricula (Falco, 1989). Although we have applied our modern conventions to her framework, not all the concepts were addressed specifically by Nightingale. This is not a criticism of Nightingale's thinking but a reality of the development of nursing thought. Therefore, Nightingale's writings were analyzed to identify her definitions of these concepts.

Nursing. "What nursing has to do . . . is to put the patient in the best condition for nature to act upon him" (Nightingale, 1859/1992, p. 74). Nightingale viewed medicine and surgery as removing obstructions to health to allow nature to return the person to health. Nightingale stated that nursing "ought to signify the proper use of fresh air, light, warmth, cleanliness, quiet, and the proper selection and administration of diet—all at the least expense of vital power to the patient" (p. 6). She reflected the art of nursing in her statement that, "the art of nursing, as now practised, seems to be expressly constituted to unmake what God had made disease to be, viz., a reparative process" (p. 6).

Based on her definition of nursing, the following definitions of human beings, environment, and health can be deduced.

Human Beings. Humans beings are not defined by Nightingale specifically. They are defined in relationship to their environment and the impact of the environment upon them.

Environment. The physical environment is stressed by Nightingale in her writing. As noted, she focused on ventilation, warmth, noise, light, and cleanliness. Nightingale's writings reflect a community health model in which all that surrounds human beings is considered in relation to their state of health. She synthesized immediate knowledge of disease with the existing sanitary conditions in the environment.

Health. Nightingale (1859/1992) did not define health specifically. She believed, however, that pathology teaches the harm disease has done, and nothing more. She stated, "We know nothing of health, the positive of which pathology is the negative, except from observation and experience" (p. 74). She believed "nature alone cures" (p. 74). Given her definition that of the art of nursing is to "unmake what God had made disease" (p. 6), then the goal of all nursing activities should be client health. She believed that nursing should provide care to the healthy as well as the ill and discussed health promotion as an activity in which nurses should engage.

One way of organizing Nightingale's environmental model can be seen in Figure 3–1. Note that the client, the nurse, and the major environmental concepts are in balance; that is, the nurse can manipulate the environment to compensate for the client's response to it. The goal of the nurse is to assist the patient in staying in balance. If the environment of a client is out of balance, the client expends unnecessary energy. In Figure 3–2 the client is experiencing stress because of noise in the environment. Nursing observations focus on the client's response to noise; nursing interventions focus on reducing the noise and decreasing the client's unnecessary energy expenditure. The nurse's role is to place the client in the best position for nature to act upon him, thus encouraging healing.

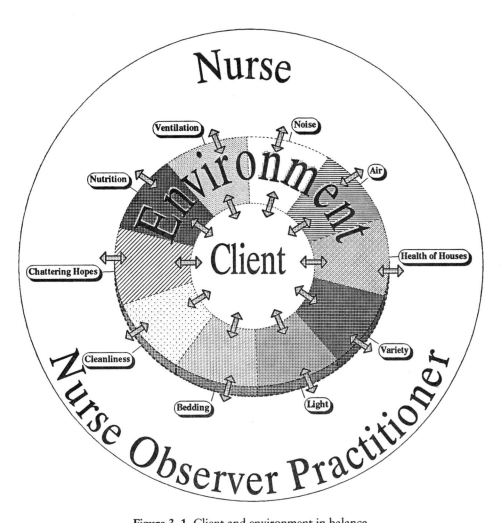

Figure 3–1. Client and environment in balance.

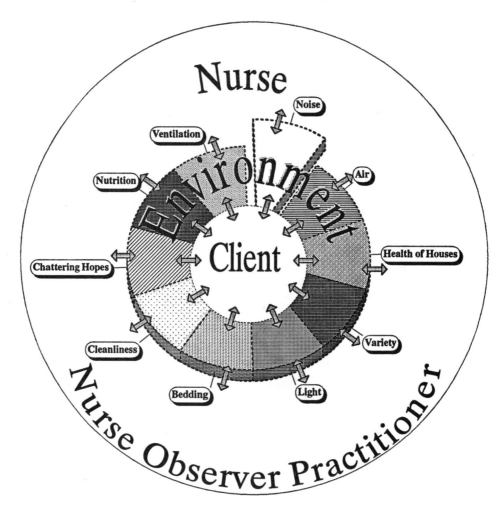

Figure 3–2. Client expending unnecessary energy by being stressed by environment (noise).

NIGHTINGALE AND THE NURSING PROCESS

In the *assessment* of clients Nightingale (1859/1992) advocated two essential behaviors by the nurse. The first is to ask the client what is needed or wanted. If the patient is in pain, ask where the pain is located. If the patient is not eating, ask *when* he or she would like to eat and *what* food is desired. Find out what the patient believes is wrong. Nightingale warned against asking leading questions and advocated asking precise questions. She recommended asking questions such as "How many hours' sleep has _____ had? and at what hours of the night?" (p. 61) instead of "Has he had a good night?" Nightingale also warned that the individual asking the questions needed to be concerned about the shyness of the patient in answering questions.

The second area of assessment that Nightingale (1859/1992) advocated was the use of observation. She used precise observations concerning all aspects of the client's physical health and environment. She stated "the most important practical lesson that can be given to nurses is to teach them what to observe—how to observe—what symptoms indicate improvement—what is the reverse—which are of importance—which are of none—which are evidence of neglect—and of what kind of neglect" (p. 59). Nurses must make the observations because clients may be too weak or shy to make them. Observations revolve around Nightingale's environmental model, that is, the impact of the environment on the individual. For example, how do light, noise, smells, and bedding affect the client?

An assessment guide can be structured from Nightingale's environmental model. The major environmental concepts guide the structure of the assessment tool, leading to examining the impact of the environment on clients and integrating the expanding body of scientific knowledge concerning the effects of a balanced or unbalanced environment.

Nursing diagnoses are based on an analysis of the conclusions gained from the information in the assessment. Nightingale believed data should be used as the basis for forming any conclusion. It is important that the diagnosis be the clients' response to their environment and not the environmental problem. Nursing diagnoses reflect the importance of the environment to the health and well-being of the client.

Planning includes identifying the nursing actions needed to keep clients comfortable, dry, and in the best state for nature to work on. "The value of informed action, based on extensive knowledge is well illustrated by the Nightingale personality" (Palmer, 1980). Planning is focused on modifying the environment to enhance the client's ability to respond to the disease process.

Implementation takes place in the environment that affects the client and involves taking action to modify that environment. All factors of the environment should be considered, including noise, air, odors, bedding, cleanliness, light—all the factors that place clients in the best position for nature to work upon them.

Evaluation is based on the effect of the changes in the environment on the clients' ability to regain their health at the least expense of energy. Observation is the primary method of data collection used to evaluate the client's response to the intervention.

Application of Nightingale's Work in the Nursing Process

Assessment. Nancy Smith, a 10-year-old African American female from a rural area, was injured in an accident related to farm machinery. She had a head injury and although she was "conscious," she was not oriented to place and time. She had multiple abrasions, multiple bruises, and a deep leg wound containing dirt and debris from the farm equipment that injured her. She was transported to the regional children's hospital by helicopter. After triage in the emergency department and surgery, she was admitted to a crowded pediatric intensive care unit (PICU). In the PICU the lights were on 24 hours a day, noises from equipment permeated the unit, and visits by her parents were restricted. Today, after two days and nights of interrupted sleep, Nancy has become increasingly confused but does not have physiological evidence of increased intracranial pressure. Her leg has become infected, requiring increased intravenous antibiotics and dressing changes twice a day.

Analysis of Data. Data gaps include information about family structure; who lives in the household; who was present when injury occurred; Nancy's school performance; economic resources available to the family, including insurance; Nancy's nutritional status; and evaluation of her growth and development in relation to developmental standards. Of primary concern are Nancy's lack of sleep and the infected wound.

Nursing Diagnosis. Sleep disruption related to environmental light and noise and separation from family.

Planning and Implementation. Nursing actions focus on changing the environment to support more normal sleep patterns, that is, being awake during the day and sleeping at night. During the day, both natural and artificial light is plentiful around Nancy's bed. She also is encouraged to listen to her favorite music or watch her favorite television show to expose her to normal sounds. Her parents are encouraged to visit more often and to talk with her about the future when she will return to home and school. The nurse teaches Nancy about her dressing change and enourages her to participate as much as possible to help her become more comfortable in this new environment. At night sleep is supported by dimming the lights, reducing noise including turning down the volume of alarms, and keeping to a minimum activities and procedures that would awaken Nancy.

Evaluation. Criteria for evaluation: after two nights of uninterrupted sleep, normal sounds, and parental encouragement, Nancy will demonstrate increased orientation to place by being able to identify that she is in the hospital. Nancy will begin participating in her dressing changes by the third day of the care plan.

NIGHTINGALE AND THE CHARACTERISTICS OF A THEORY

1. Theories can interrelate concepts in such a way as to create a different way of looking at a particular phenomenon. When nursing situations are viewed from a Nightingale perspective, using her environmental model, new insights into the phenomena of interest to nursing can be identified. Examining environmental aspects, such as light, noise, or warmth, can provide new insight into human response to health and illness. For example, when a client in an isolation room becomes disoriented, obvious things to consider would be

medical pathology and fluid and electrolyte balance. From Nightingale's perspective, the impact of the environment would be an initial concern. Thus, the nurse would examine patterns of light, noise, ventilation, and interaction with other humans as potential sources of environmental stress on the client. For example, stress can be caused by a lack of the usual cycle of light from day to night, or from disrupted sleep patterns caused by noise. Examining the phenomena, using Nightingale's Environmental Model as a guide, assists the nurse in identifying the relationship between various environmental factors and the client's disorientation.

2. Theories must be logical in nature. Nightingale's environmental model is logical. Although the environment is not defined in the broad manner that it is today, there are few gaps. Most notable is the scant information on the psychosocial environment when compared to the physical environment. There is nothing illogical in Nightingale's discussion of the physical or psychosocial environment. She built her conclusions from observations, she made her case, drew her conclusions, and then acted. Nightingale believed she used logic to come to her conclusions.

3. Theories must be relatively simple yet generalizable. Nightingale's writings are simple, as is the articulation of her model. In *Notes on nursing* she was writing to the woman who could read about caring for the home and family. At times she used words that are no longer in common use to describe aspects of her model. Yet, the beauty of her model is its generalizability, including its continued applicability today. Nightingale's model can be applied in the most complex hospital intensive care environment, the home, a work site, or the community at large. Concepts related to pure air, light, noise, and cleanliness can be applied across specific environments.

For example, noise, or noxious sound, can be found in any environment. The hospital has carts, monitors, and other machines that disrupt sleep and rest. The intensive care unit is noted for its number of staff members, machines, and alarms, adding to the noise of the environment. A home may be near an interstate highway with loud truck noises, or an airport with planes taking off and landing day and night, or a home may be isolated in the country, with outside manmade noises being rare. A work site may be filled with machine noises, computer whines, or large machine alarms. Finally, in our modern society a community may be involved in a war with shelling, bombing, and gunfire disrupting sleep, making it difficult to study or do other work.

4. Theories can be the bases for hypotheses that can be tested or for theory to be expanded. Nightingale has stimulated the development of nursing science with her work. She has had a profound effect on many of the other nursing theorists cited in this book. These individuals have indicated the influence of Nightingale by citing her in their work or commenting on her influence in a commemorative edition of *Notes on nursing*. For example, Leininger (1992) analyzed what Nightingale did and did not say about caring, noting that although Nightingale never defined human care she did make inferences about treating the sick. Levine (1992) first wrote about

Nightingale in 1962 and discussed the excitement she felt at holding notes written in Nightingale's own hand. Newman (1992) spoke of the timelessness of *Notes on nursing* and the impact it has had on her work. The research related to the impact of the environment on client health has been influenced by Nightingale. Hypotheses based on her work continue to be generated.

5. Theories contribute to and assist in increasing the general body of knowledge within the discipline through the research implemented to validate them. Nightingale's theory seems to have more relevance to practitioners today than ever before. More and more data are becoming available to indicate the critical nature of the impact of the environment on the health and well-being of individuals. This information is relevant in all environments, from the intensive care unit to the community.

6. Theories can be used by practitioners to guide and improve their practice. Nightingale's theory has broad applicability to the practitioner. Reading her work raises a consciousness in the nurse about how the environment influences client outcomes. Considering the effect of noise may make a staff more aware of sounds they can control. For example, the noise of placing a clipboard or other equipment on the top of an incubator is disruptive of an infant's sleep. Or, after reading Nightingale's discussion of the importance of light to the well-being of clients and examining the scientific information on light waves, the importance of light and darkness in sleep–rest cycles and the release of growth hormone, the neonatal intensive care nurse may begin to turn the lights down at night to encourage a normal sleep–wake cycle in the developing premature infant.

7. Theories must be consistent with other validated theories, laws, and principles but will leave open unanswered questions that need to be investigated. Although Nightingale did not believe in the germ theory, the practices she recommended were not inconsistent with the scientific knowledge we have today. In fact, many of her suggestions, which she based on observations of client responses to their environment, have been documented as scientifically sound when tested with rigorous application of modern research methods.

Nightingale's theory works well with ecological, systems, adaptation, and interpersonal theories. Systems theory discusses the relationships between various layers of the individual and his or her environment. This is precisely what Nightingale did in her discussions of the effects of the physical environment on the individual. She also discussed how individuals respond to their disease process and viewed nursing's role as putting the client in the best position possible for nature to act upon. This allows clients to adapt or change to their diseased state and maximize their state of health. While not as specific about the influence of the psychosocial environment on the client, Nightingale observed that conversations about clients within their hearing could cause distress. She viewed clients as important persons to communicate with concerning their illness. While this was not as well defined as Peplau or other interactionists, it was an important aspect of her organization of nursing care. Adaptation theory is another that can be synthesized with Nightingale's environmental model. As clients respond to the environment, they adapt by doing whatever they need to do to conserve energy and repair their body to their highest level of health.

SUMMARY

Nightingale has been called timeless by many of the individuals who have written about her. That Nightingale's writings are as meaningful in the late twentieth century as they were in the nineteenth century is an indication of her genius. The example in this chapter applies Nightingale's concepts to a child in an intensive care unit, but they can also be applied to the senior citizen in a nursing home, the family in their inner city home, or the child in the school. Although Nightingale spoke specifically to the health of human beings, she acknowledged that the health of the home and the community are critical components of the individual's health.

REFERENCES

Agnew, L. R. C. (1958). Florence Nightingale—Statistican. *American Journal of Nursing, 58,* 644–646.

American Nurses' Association. (1980). *Nursing: A social policy statement.* Kansas City: Author.

Cohen, I. B. (1984, March). Florence Nightingale. *Scientific American, 250,* 131–132.

Falco, S. M. (1989). Major concepts in the development of nursing theory. *Recent Advances in Nursing, 24.*

Hegge, M. (1990, April/May). In the footsteps of Florence Nightingale: Rediscovering the roots of nursing. *Imprint, 74–75.*

Leininger, M. M. (1992). Reflections on Nightingale with a focus on human care theory and leadership. In F. Nightingale. *Notes on nursing: What it is and what it is not* (Com. ed.) (pp. 28–38). Philadelphia: Lippincott.

Levine, M. (1992). Nightingale redux. In F. Nightingale. *Notes on nursing: What it is and what it is not* (Com. ed.) (pp. 39–43). Philadelphia: Lippincott.

Miller, J. G. (1978). *Living systems.* New York: McGraw-Hill.

Newman, M. A. (1992) Nightingale's vision of nursing theory and health. In F. Nightingale. *Notes on nursing: What it is and what it is not* (Com. ed.) (pp. 44–47). Philadelphia: Lippincott.

Nightingale, F. (1860). Vol. II, cited in Palmer, I. S. Florence Nightingale: Reformer, reactionary, researcher. *Nursing Research, 26,* 84–85.

Nightingale, F. N. (1871). *Introductory notes on lying-in institutions.* London: Longmans, Green.

Nightingale, F. N. (1992). *Notes on nursing: What it is and what it is not* (Com. ed.). Philadelphia: Lippincott. (Original publication 1859.)

Palmer, I. S. (1980). Florence Nightingale: Reformer, reactionary, researcher *Nursing Research, 26,* 84–85.

Vicinus, M., & Nergaard, B. (Eds.). (1990). *Ever yours, Florence Nightingale: Selected letters.* Cambridge, MA: Harvard University Press.

Webster's ninth new collegiate dictionary. (1991). Springfield, MA: Merriam.

C H A P T E R 4

HILDEGARD E. PEPLAU*

Janice Ryan Belcher
Lois J. Brittain Fish

■ ■ ■

*Throughout her career, Dr. Hildegard Peplau has been a pioneer in nursing.
Dr. Peplau (b. 1909) was born in Reading, Pennsylvania, and started her career
by graduating from a diploma nursing program in Pottstown, Pennsylvania, in
1931. Afterward, she graduated from Bennington College with a BA in Interpersonal Psychology in 1943, and from Columbia University in New York with
an MA in Psychiatric Nursing in 1947, and an EdD in Curriculum Development
in 1953. Dr. Peplau's nursing experience includes private and general duty
hospital nursing, the U.S. Army Nurse Corps, nursing research, and private
practice in psychiatric nursing. She taught graduate psychiatric nursing for many
years and is a Professor Emeritus from Rutgers University. Dr. Peplau influenced
the development of many nursing programs, including the creation of the first
postbaccalaureate nursing program in Belgium.*

Hildegard Peplau published the book Interpersonal relations in nursing *in
1952. She also published numerous articles in professional magazines on topics
ranging from interpersonal concepts to current issues in nursing. Her work on
anxiety, hallucinations, and the nurse as an individual therapist is especially
groundbreaking. Her pamphlet "Basic principles of patient counseling" was
derived from her research and workshops ("Profile," 1974).*

*Dr. Peplau has long had national and international recognition as a nurse and
leader in health care. She has served with many organizations, including the World
Health Organization, the National Institute of Mental Health, and the Nurse Corps.
She is past Executive Director and past President of the American Nurses' Association and a Fellow of the American Academy of Nursing. She has served as a nursing
consultant to various foreign countries and to the Surgeon General of the Air Force.
Although Dr. Peplau "retired" in 1974, she continues professional writing in journals and books. Her 1952 book was reissued in 1988 by Springer, New York.*

Hildegard Peplau (1952/1988) published *Interpersonal relations in nursing*,
referring to her book as a "partial theory for the practice of nursing"
(p. 261). It is quite remarkable that Peplau referred to her book as a partial

---

*Interpersonal relations in nursing, *Peplau, 1988, Springer Publishing Company, Inc., New
York. Used with permission*

theory for nursing in 1952 since this was before the thrust of nursing theory development. In this book, Peplau discussed the phases of the interpersonal process, roles for nursing, and methods for studying nursing as an interpersonal process. This chapter defines the crux of Peplau's nursing theory as the phases of the interpersonal process and links her other concepts to this central core.

According to Peplau (1952/1988), nursing is therapeutic because it is a healing art, assisting an individual who is sick or in need of health care. Nursing can be viewed as an interpersonal process because it involves interaction between two or more individuals with a common goal. In nursing, this common goal provides the incentive for the therapeutic process in which the nurse and patient* respect each other as individuals, both of them learning and growing as a result of the interaction. An individual learns when she or he selects stimuli in the environment and then reacts to these stimuli.

The attainment of this goal, or any goal, is achieved through a series of steps following a sequential pattern. As the relationship of the nurse and patient develops in these steps, the nurse can choose how she or he practices nursing by using different skills and technical abilities, and by assuming various roles.

When the nurse and patient first identify a problem, they begin to develop a course of action to solve the problem. Each of them approaches this course of action from diverse backgrounds and individual uniqueness. Each individual may be viewed as a unique biological-psychological-spiritual-sociological structure, one that will not react the same as any other individual. Both the nurse and the patient have learned their unique perceptions from different environments, mores, customs, and beliefs of that individual's given culture. Each person comes with preconceived ideas that influence perceptions, and it is these differences in perception that are so important in the interpersonal process. In addition, the nurse has a broad range of such nursing knowledge as stress–crisis management and developmental theories, which leads to a greater understanding of the nurse's professional role in the therapeutic process. As nurse and patient continue the relationship, they begin to understand one another's roles and the factors surrounding the problem. From this understanding, both the nurse and patient collaborate and share in mutual goals until the problem is resolved.

As the nurse and the patient work together, they become more knowledgeable and mature throughout the process. Peplau (1952/1988) views nursing as a "maturing force and an educative instrument" (p. 8). She believes nursing is a learning experience of oneself as well as of the other individual involved in the interpersonal action. This concept was supported by Genevieve Burton, another nursing author from the 1950s, who states, "Behavior of others must be understood in light of self understanding" (Burton, 1958, p. 7). Thus, persons who are aware of their own feelings, perceptions, and actions are also more likely to be aware of another individual's reactions.

---

*Patient will be used throughout this chapter since it is Peplau's definition of the individual who is in need of health care.

Each therapeutic encounter influences the nurse's and the patient's personal and professional development. As the nurse works with the patient to resolve problems in everyday life, the nurse's practice becomes increasingly more effective. Thus, the kind of person the nurse is and becomes has a direct influence on her or his skill in the therapeutic, interpersonal relationship.

Peplau identifies four sequential phases in interpersonal relationships: (1) *orientation,* (2) *identification,* (3) *exploitation,* and (4) *resolution.* Each of these phases overlaps, interrelates, and varies in duration as the process evolves toward a solution. Different nursing roles are assumed during the various phases. These roles can be broadly described as follows:

- **Teacher**   One who imparts knowledge concerning a need or interest
- **Resource**   One who provides specific, needed information that aids in understanding of a problem or a new situation
- **Counselor**   One who, through the use of certain skills and attitudes, aids another in recognizing, facing, accepting, and resolving problems that are interfering with the other person's ability to live happily and effectively
- **Leader**   One who carries out the process of initiation and maintenance of group goals through interaction
- **Technical expert**   One who provides physical care by displaying clinical skills and operating equipment in this care
- **Surrogate**   One who takes the place of another

PEPLAU'S PHASES IN NURSING

Orientation

In the initial phase of *orientation,* the nurse and patient meet as two strangers. The patient and/or the family has a "felt need" (Peplau, 1952/1988, p. 18); therefore, professional assistance is sought. However, this need may not be readily identified or understood by the individuals who are involved. For example, a 16-year-old girl may call the community mental health center just because she feels "very down." It is in this phase that the nurse needs to assist the patient and family to realize what is happening to the patient.

It is of the utmost importance that the nurse work collaboratively with the patient and family in analyzing the situation, so that they together can recognize, clarify, and define the existing problem. In the previous example the nurse, in the counselor's role, helps the teenaged girl who feels "very down" to realize that these feelings stem from an argument with her mother over last evening's date. As the nurse listens, a pattern evolves: The girl argues with her mother and then feels depressed. As these feelings are discussed, the girl recognizes that the arguing is the precipitating factor leading to the depression. Thus, the nurse and the patient have defined the problem. Later, the girl and her parents agree to discuss the issue with the nurse. Therefore, by mutually clarifying and defining the problem in the orientation phase, the patient can direct the accumulated energy from her anxiety about unmet needs and begin working with the presenting problem. Nurse–patient rapport is established and continues to be strengthened while concerns are being identified.

While the patient and family are talking to the nurse, a mutual decision needs to be made regarding what type of professional assistance the patient and family need. The nurse, as a resource person, may work with them. As an alternative, the nurse might, with the mutual agreement of all parties involved, refer the family to another source such as a psychologist, social worker, or psychiatrist. In the orientation phase, the nurse, patient, and family decide what types of services are needed.

The orientation phase is directly affected by the patient's and nurse's attitudes about giving or receiving aid from a reciprocal person. In this beginning phase, the nurse needs to be aware of her or his personal reactions to the patient. For example, the nurse may react differently to the 40-year-old man with abdominal pain who enters the emergency room quietly in contrast to the 40-year-old man with abdominal pain who enters the emergency room boisterously after a few alcoholic drinks. The nurse's, as well as the patient's, culture, religion, race, educational background, experiences, and preconceived ideas and expectations all influence the nurse's reaction to the patient. In addition, the same factors influence the patient's reaction to the nurse (see Fig. 4–1). For example, the patient may have stereotyped the nurse as being able to perform only technical skills, such as giving medications or

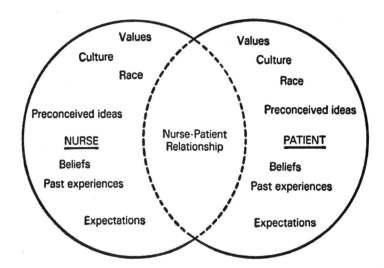

Figure 4–1. Factors influencing the blending of the nurse–patient relationship.

taking blood pressures, and therefore may not perceive the nurse as a resource person who can help define the problem. Nursing is an interpersonal process, and both the patient and nurse have an equally important part in the therapeutic interaction.

The nurse, the patient, and the family work together to recognize, clarify, and define the existing problem. This in turn decreases the tension and anxiety associated with the felt need and the fear of the unknown. Decreasing tension and anxiety prevents future problems that might arise as a result of repressing or not resolving significant events. Stressful situations are identified through therapeutic interaction. It is imperative that the patient recognize and begin to work through feelings connected with events before an illness.

In summary, in the beginning of the orientation phase, the nurse and the patient meet as strangers. At the end of the orientation phase, they are concurrently striving to identify the problem and are becoming more comfortable with one another. In addition, the patient becomes more comfortable in the helping environment. The nurse and the patient are now ready to logically progress to the next phase, identification.

Identification

In the next phase, *identification,* the patient responds selectively to people who can meet his or her needs. Each patient responds differently in this phase. For example, the patient might actively seek out the nurse or stoically wait until the nurse approaches. The response to the nurse is threefold: (1) participate with and be interdependent with the nurse, (2) be autonomous and independent from the nurse, or (3) be passive and dependent on the nurse (Peplau, 1952/1988). An example is that of a 70-year-old man who wants to plan his new 1,600 calorie diabetic diet. If the relationship is interdependent, the nurse and patient collaborate on the meal planning. Should the relationship be independent, the patient plans the diet himself with minimal input from the nurse. In a dependent relationship, the nurse does the meal planning for the patient.

Throughout the identification phase, both the patient and nurse must clarify each other's perceptions and expectations (Peplau, 1952/1988). Past experiences of both the patient and the nurse will influence their expectations during this interpersonal process. As mentioned in the orientation phase, the initial attitudes of the patient and nurse are important in building a working relationship for identifying the problem and choosing appropriate assistance.

In the identification phase, the perception and expectations of the patient and nurse are even more complex than in the orientation phase. The patient is now responding to the helper selectively. This requires a more intense therapeutic relationship.

To illustrate, a patient who has had a mastectomy may mention to the nurse her inability to understand the arm exercises that have been explained to her as being an important regimen following surgery. The nurse observes that the affected arm is edematous (swollen). While the nurse is exploring possible reasons for the edema, the patient admits she is not doing her arm exercises. The patient states that a friend told her that exercising after surgery delays healing. To facilitate the patient's understanding and subsequent resumption of the exercises, the nurse can identify professional people, such as the physical therapist, the nurse, and the physician, who will clarify the patient's misconceptions. Generally, it is best if the nurse objectively discusses each professional's role with the patient so that she will be aware of the advantages and disadvantages of consulting with each professional. However, in this case, the patient states that she does not care to discuss the exercises with the nurse or physical therapist because she perceives her physician to be the only one who has the appropriate information. Thus, previous perceptions of nursing and physical therapy can influence the patient's current decision on the selection of the professional person.

While working through the identification phase, the patient begins to have feelings of belonging and a capacity for dealing with the problem. These changes begin to decrease feelings of helplessness and hopelessness, creating an optimistic attitude from which inner strength ensues.

Exploitation

Following identification, the patient moves into the *exploitation* phase, in which the patient takes advantage of all services available. The degree to which these services are used is based upon the needs and interests of the patient. The individual begins to feel as though he or she is an integral part of the helping environment and begins to take control of the situation by extracting help from the services offered. In the previous example of the woman with an edematous arm, the patient, who is now in the exploitation phase, begins to understand the information regarding the arm exercises. She reads pamphlets and watches videotapes describing the exercises; she discusses concerns with the nurse; and she may inquire about joining an exercise group through the physical therapy department.

During this phase some patients may make more demands than they did when they were seriously ill. They may make many minor requests or may use other attention-getting techniques, depending on their individual needs. These actions may often be difficult, if not impossible, for the health care provider to completely understand. The nurse may need to deal with the subconscious forces causing the patient's actions, and may need to use interviewing techniques as tools to explore, understand, and adequately deal with underlying patient problems. So that the nurse–patient rapport established to this point is not damaged, a therapeutic relationship must be maintained by the nurse that conveys an attitude of acceptance, concern, and trust. The nurse must encourage the patient to recognize and explore feelings, thoughts, emotions, and behaviors by providing a nonjudgmental atmosphere and a therapeutic emotional climate.

Some patients may take an active interest in, and become involved in, self-care. Such patients become self-sufficient and demonstrate initiative by establishing appropriate behavior for goal attainment. Through self-determination, patients progressively develop responsibility for self, belief in potentialities, and adjustment toward self-reliance and independence. These patients realistically begin to establish their own goals toward improved health status. They strive to achieve a direction in their lives that promotes a feeling of well-being. Patients who develop self-care become productive, they trust and depend on their own capabilities, and they also become responsible for their own actions. As a result of this self-determination, they develop sources of inner strength that allow them to face new challenges.

While in impaired health, most patients fluctuate between dependence on others and independent functioning at an optimal health level. This point is illustrated by using the previous example of the woman who had an edematous arm after surgery. On some days she wants to actively exercise on schedule. Other days she states she is too tired to exercise at all. When the patient does not exercise, the nurse needs to intervene by reminding the patient of her scheduled exercises.

This type of inconsistent behavior can be compared to the adjustment reaction of the adolescent in a dependency–independency conflict. The patient may temporarily be in a dependent role while having the simultaneous need for independence. Various triggers create the onset of this psychological disequilibrium. The patient vacillates unpredictably between the two behaviors and appears confused and anxious, protesting dependence while fearing independence. In caring for patients who fluctuate between dependence and independence, the nurse must approach the specific behavior that is presented rather than trying to handle the composite problem of inconsistency. The nurse should provide an atmosphere of acceptance and support, one in which the person can become more self-aware and begin to use his or her strengths to minimize weaknesses.

In exploitation, the nurse uses communication tools such as clarifying, listening, accepting, teaching, and interpreting to offer services to the patient. The patient then takes advantage of the services offered based upon his or her needs and interests. Throughout this phase, the patient works collaboratively with the nurse to meet challenges and work toward maximum health. Thus, in the exploitation phase, the nurse aids the patient in using services to help solve the problem. Progress is made toward the final step—the resolution phase.

Resolution

The last phase in Peplau's interpersonal process is *resolution*. The patient's needs have already been met by the collaborative efforts between the patient and nurse. The patient and nurse now need to terminate their therapeutic relationship and dissolve the links between them.

Sometimes the nurse and patient have difficulty dissolving these links. Dependency needs in a therapeutic relationship often continue psychologically after the physiological needs have been met. The patient may feel that it "is just not time yet" to end the relationship. For example, a new mother has a desire to learn infant care. During the first home visit, the community health nurse and the new mother set their goal of having the mother properly

TABLE 4–1. PHASES OF THE NURSE–PATIENT RELATIONSHIP

Phase	Focus
Orientation	Problem-defining phase
Identification	Selection of appropriate professional assistance
Exploitation	Use of professional assistance for problem-solving alternatives
Resolution	Termination of the professional relationship

demonstrate various facets of infant care by the fourth visit. After instruction and demonstration by the community health nurse on the first visit, the mother demonstrates correctly all facets of infant care by the fourth visit. Their goal is met. The relationship is ended because the mother's problem was solved. However, one week after the resolution, the mother telephones the community health nurse five times with minor questions on infant care. The mother has not dissolved the dependency link with the community health nurse.

The final resolution may also be difficult for the nurse. In the previous example, the mother may be willing to terminate the relationship; however, the community health nurse may continue to visit the home to watch the baby develop. The nurse may be unable to free herself or himself from this bond in their relationship. In resolution, as in the other phases, anxiety and tension increase in the patient and the nurse if there is unsuccessful completion of the phase.

During successful resolution, the patient drifts away from identifying with the helping person, the nurse. The patient then becomes independent from the nurse as the nurse becomes independent from the patient. As a result of this process, both the patient and nurse become stronger maturing individuals. The patient's needs are met, and movement can be made toward new goals. Resolution occurs only with the successful completion of the previous phases. Table 4–1 indicates the focus of each phase.

PEPLAU'S THEORY AND NURSING'S METAPARADIGM

Nursing's metaparadigm includes the four concepts of human beings, health, society/environment, and nursing. Peplau (1952/1988) defines *man** as an organism that "strives in its own way to reduce tension generated by needs" (p. 82). *Health* is defined as "a word symbol that implies forward movement of personality and other ongoing human processes in the direction of creative, constructive, productive, personal, and community living" (p. 12).

---

*Peplau uses *man* and *he* in the generic sense.

Although Peplau (1952/1988) does not directly address *society/environment,* she does encourage the nurse to consider the patient's culture and mores when the patient adjusts to hospital routine. Currently, when a nurse considers the patient's environment, the nurse examines many more factors, such as cultural background and home and work environments, rather than considering only a patient's adjustment to the hospital. Peplau has a narrow perception of the environment, which is a major limitation of her theory. The theory does not examine the broad range of environmental influences on the person but focuses more on the psychological tasks "within the person" (Sills, 1977, p. 202), a view that was timely in 1949 when the book was written. In examining the historical trends within psychiatric nursing, this view is categorized as being "within the person," as later contrasted to views of "within the relationship" and "within the social system," both of which consider a broader range of environmental influences on the person (Sills, p. 202).

Hildegard Peplau (1952/1988) considers *nursing* to be a "significant, therapeutic, interpersonal process" (p. 16). She defines it as a "human relationship between an individual who is sick, or in need of health services, and a nurse especially educated to recognize and to respond to the need for help" (pp. 5–6). The nurse assists the patient in this interpersonal process. Major concepts within this process are nurse, patient, therapeutic relationship, goals, human needs, anxiety, tension, and frustration.

RELATIONSHIP BETWEEN PEPLAU'S PHASES AND THE NURSING PROCESS

Peplau's continuum of the four phases of *orientation, identification, exploitation,* and *resolution* can be compared to the nursing process as discussed in Chapter 2 (see Table 4–2). The nursing process in Chapter 2 is defined as "a deliberate, intellectual activity whereby the practice of nursing is approached in an orderly, systematic manner" (see p. 15).

There are similarities between the nursing process and Peplau's interpersonal phases. Both Peplau's phases and the nursing process are sequential and focus on therapeutic interactions. Both stress that the nurse and patient should use problem-solving techniques collaboratively, with the end purpose of meeting the patient's needs. Both emphasize assisting the patient to define general complaints more specifically so that specific patient needs can be identified. Both use observation, communication, and recording as basic tools for nursing practice.

The nursing process and Peplau's interpersonal phases are also different. When considering differences, it must be taken into account that Peplau's book *Interpersonal relations in nursing* was first published in 1952. Professional nursing today has more defined goals and more specialty areas of practice. Nursing has moved away from the role of physician's helper and toward consumer advocacy. The American Nurses' Association, in the 1973

TABLE 4–2. COMPARISON OF NURSING PROCESS AND PEPLAU'S PHASES

Nursing Process	Peplau's Phases
Assessment Data collection and analysis. Need not necessarily be a "felt need"; may be nurse-initiated.	*Orientation* Nurse and patient come together as strangers; meeting initiated by patient who expresses a "felt need"; work together to recognize, clarify, and define facts related to need. (*Note:* Data collection is continuous.)
Nursing Diagnosis Summary statement based on nurse analysis.	Patient clarifies "felt need."
Planning Mutually set goals.	*Identification* Interdependent goal setting. Patient has feeling of belonging and selectively responds to those who can meet his or her needs. Patient-initiated.
Implementation Plans initiated that move toward achievement of mutually set goals. May be accomplished by patient, health care professional, or patient's family.	*Exploitation* Patient actively seeking and drawing on knowledge and expertise of those who can help. Patient-initiated.
Evaluation Based on mutually established expected behaviors. May lead to termination of relationship or initiation of new plans.	*Resolution* Occurs after other phases are successfully completed. Leads to termination of relationship.

Standards of nursing practice, states: "Nursing diagnoses are derived from health status data" (p. 2). Peplau (1952/1988), however, wrote that the physician's primary function was "recognizing the full import of the nuclear problem and the kind of professional assistance that is needed," which results, for the physician, in "the task of evaluating and diagnosing the emergent problem" (p. 23). Peplau's 1952 view opposes the current viewpoint of independent functioning by nurses.

Nursing functions, according to Peplau (1952/1988), include clarification of the information the physician gives the patient as well as collection of data about the patient that may point out other problem areas. In contrast, given today's expanded roles in nursing, independent nurse practitioners may or may not refer the patient to the physician, depending on the patient's needs. Through expanded roles, nursing is becoming more accountable and responsible, giving professional nursing greater legal independence than previously. The nursing process provides a mode for evaluating the quality of nursing care. Such evaluation is the core of legal accountability.

Peplau identifies needs, frustration, conflict, and anxiety as important concepts in nursing situations. Furthermore, she states that these concepts must be addressed for patient and nurse growth to occur. These concepts can readily be identified as having been influenced by some theories of the time, especially Harry S. Sullivan's (1947) interpersonal theory and Sigmund Freud's (1936) theory of psychodynamics.

Today's nurse evaluates many concepts such as intrafamily dynamics, socioeconomic forces (eg, financial resources), personal space considerations, and community social service resources for each patient. These concepts provide a broader perspective for viewing the patient in his or her environment than do Peplau's concepts of needs, frustration, conflict, and anxiety. Today, even a family, a group, or a community may be collectively defined as the patient in the nursing process.

Nursing has also broadened its perspective from that represented in Peplau's original 1952 publication. Nursing now assists the patient to reach a fuller health potential through health maintenance and promotion. As long ago as 1970, Martha Rogers wrote, "Maintenance and promotion of health, prevention of disease, nursing diagnosis, intervention, and rehabilitation encompass the scope of nursing's goals" (p. 86). Today, nurses actively seek to identify health problems in a variety of community and institutional settings.

The specific components of the nursing process and Peplau's phases are now discussed. Peplau's orientation phase parallels the beginning of the *assessment phase* in that both the nurse and patient come together as strangers. This meeting is initiated by the patient, who expresses a need, although the need is not always understood. Conjointly, the nurse and patient begin to work through recognizing, clarifying, and gathering facts important to this need. This step is presently referred to as data collection in the assessment phase of the nursing process.

In the nursing process the patient's need is not necessarily a felt need. For example, the nurse may be currently working in the community by assessing people who perceive themselves to be healthy. A school nurse screens hearing for school children. If a hearing deficit is found, a referral is initiated by the nurse. Children do not usually seek out the nurse for this deficit. In this situation, the need must be identified for the child and for the parents to persuade them to seek assistance for the hearing deficit. For example, the nurse sends home a note about the hearing deficit so that the parents and child become aware of the problem. The nurse may also have to follow up the note with a telephone call or home visit. The nurse is actively helping the child and family to identify a need.

Orientation and assessment are not synonymous and must not be confused. Collecting data is continuous throughout Peplau's phases. In the nursing process, the initial collection of data is the nursing assessment, and further collection of data becomes an integral part of reassessment.

In the nursing process, the *nursing diagnosis* evolves once the health problems or deficits are identified. The nursing diagnosis is a summary statement of the data collected and analyzed. Peplau (1952/1988) writes that "during the period of orientation the patient clarifies his first, whole impression of his problem" (p. 30); whereas in the nursing process, the nurse's judgment forms the diagnosis from the data collected.

Mutually set goals evolve from the nursing diagnosis. These goals give direction to the plan and indicate the appropriate helping resources. When the nurse and patient discuss helping resources, the patient can selectively identify with the resource persons. According to Peplau, the patient is then viewed as being in the identification phase.

While collaborating on mutual goals, the nurse and patient may have conflicts based on preconceptions and expectations of each person, as described earlier in Peplau's identification phase. The nurse and patient must resolve any discrepancies before mutual goals can be set. Goal setting should be an interdependent activity between the patient and nurse.

The next phase in the nursing process is the *planning* phase. In the planning phase, the nurse must specifically formulate how the patient is going to achieve the mutually set goals. The nurse actively seeks patient input so that the patient feels like an integral part of the plan. When the patient feels involved in the plan, compliance is more likely to occur. In the planning phase, the nurse considers the patient's own skills for handling his or her problems. Peplau (1952/1988) stresses that the nurse wants to develop a therapeutic relationship so that the patient's anxiety will be constructively channeled into seeking resources, so that feelings of hopelessness will decrease. Planning can still be considered to be within Peplau's identification phase.

The patient also begins to have a feeling of belonging within the therapeutic relationship because both patient and nurse must have mutual respect, communication, and interest. This feeling of belonging must be analyzed and should assist the patient to develop a healthier personality rather than imitative behavior. Peplau (1952/1988) states, "Some patients identify too readily with nurses, expecting that all of their wants will be taken care of and nothing will be expected of them" (p. 32). In Peplau's identification phase, the patient selectively responds to people who can meet his or her personal needs. Therefore, the identification phase is initiated by the patient.

The planning stage of the nursing process gives direction and meaning to the nursing actions to be taken toward resolving the patient's problems. Using nursing education, the nurse bases the nursing plan on scientific knowledge. In addition, the nurse incorporates the patient's individual strengths and weaknesses into the plan.

In the *implementation* phase, as in Peplau's exploitation, the patient is finally reaping benefits from the therapeutic relationship by drawing on the nurse's knowledge and expertise. In both the implementation and exploitation phases, the individualized plans have already been formed, based on the patient's interest and needs. Similarly, in both phases the plans are geared toward completion of desired goals. However, there is a difference between exploitation and implementation. In exploitation, the patient is the one who actively seeks varying types of services to obtain the maximum benefits available, whereas in implementation there is a prescribed plan or procedure, holistic in nature, used to achieve predetermined goals or objectives based on nursing assessment. Thus, exploitation is oriented to the patient. In contrast implementation can be accomplished by the patient or by other persons, including health professionals and the patient's family.

In Peplau's resolution phase, all other phases have been successfully accomplished, the needs have been met, and resolution and termination are the end result. Although Peplau does not discuss *evaluation* per se, evaluation is an inherent factor in determining the readiness of the patient to proceed through the resolution phase.

In the nursing process, evaluation is a separate step, and mutually established expected end behaviors (goals) are used as evaluation tools. Time limits on attaining the goals are set for evaluation purposes, although these limits may change with reassessment. In evaluation, if the situation is clear-cut, the problem moves toward termination. If the problem is unresolved, goals and objectives are not met; if nursing care is ineffective, a reassessment must be done. New goals, planning, implementation, and evaluation are then established.

PEPLAU'S WORK AND THE CHARACTERISTICS OF A THEORY

Peplau's (1952/1988) book is now compared to the characteristics of a theory introduced in this book's first chapter. Generally, Peplau's work is a theory of nursing.

1. Theories can interrelate concepts in such a way as to create a different way of looking at a particular phenomenon. The phases of orientation, identification, exploitation, and resolution interrelate the various components of each phase. This interrelationship creates a different perspective from which to view the nurse–patient interaction and the transaction of health care. The nurse–patient interaction can apply the concepts of human being, health, society/environment, and nursing. For example, in the phase of orientation there are components of nurse, patient, strangers, problem, and anxiety.

2. Theories must be logical in nature. Peplau's theory provides a logical, systematic way of viewing nursing situations. The four progressive phases in the nurse–patient relationship are logical, beginning with initial contact in the phase of orientation and ending with termination in the phase of resolution. Key concepts in the theory, such an anxiety, tension, goals, and frustration, are clearly defined with explicit relationships between them and the progressive phases.

3. Theories should be relatively simple yet generalizable. The phases provide simplicity regarding the natural progression of the nurse–patient relationship. This simplicity leads to adaptability in any nurse–patient interaction, thus providing generalizability. The basic nature of nursing is still considered an interpersonal process.

4. Theories can be the bases for hypotheses that can be tested or for theory to be expanded. Peplau's theory has generated testable hypotheses. Most of the research has centered on the concept of anxiety, not the nurse–patient relationship that is the core of her work. However, in 1989, Forchuk and Brown created an instrument to assess Peplau's nurse–client relationship and tested the instrument on 132 clients. Generally, nursing research has been scant and mostly descriptive (see Table 4–3). Much of the research has used very small sample sizes. For example, one study examined teaching the concept of anxiety to six female patients in a group setting (Hays, 1966). Another study used Peplau's work on anxiety to develop a framework and to conduct a study of 25 nursing students who worked with anxious patients (Burd, 1963).

In examining Peplau's theory, one limitation is that some areas are not specific enough to generate hypotheses. One reason for this limitation may be that her theory was written in 1949, before a more organized thrust in

TABLE 4–3. NURSING RESEARCH USING PEPLAU'S WORK AS A FRAMEWORK

Date and Author	Research	Findings
1989 Forchuk, C. & Brown, B.	Created an instrument to test Peplau's nurse–client relationship. Sample was 58 case management clients and 74 counseling/treatment clients.	The instrument provided an assessment of the nurse–patient relationship. Chronic schizophrenic clients had a long orientation phase.
1963 Burd, S. F.	Developed and tested a nursing intervention framework for working with anxious patients. Sample was 25 psychiatric nursing students consisting of 15 freshman and 10 graduate students.	Freshman students can develop beginning competency in interpersonal relationships. The earlier the students gains theoretical knowledge, the more the student is aware of his or her own anxiety. As students work with patients, patients respond by going through sequential phases including denial, ambivalence, and awareness of anxiety.
1961 Hays, D.	Provided a description of phases and steps of experiential teaching about anxiety to a patient group. Sample was 6 female psychiatric patients.	Verbal analysis of the group revealed that, when taught by the experiential method, the patients were able to apply the concepts of anxiety after the group was terminated.

nursing research began in the 1950s. In general, in analyzing Peplau's theory, more concept development and concrete descriptions need to be made before the theory can be empirically tested. For example, the nurse–patient relationship describes a certain progressive relationship, but otherwise more explicit relationships among the phases should be defined.

5. Theories contribute to and assist in increasing the general body of knowledge within the discipline through the research implemented to validate them. Peplau's work has contributed greatly to nursing's body of knowledge, not only in psychiatric–mental health nursing but also in nursing in general, such as her work on anxiety. With regard to her contribution to research in psychiatric–mental health nursing, in the 1950s two thirds of the nursing research concentrated on the nurse–patient relationship (Sills, 1977). At Teachers College, Columbia University, Peplau's 1952 work influenced the interpersonal nature and direction of clinical work and studies (Sills). Presently, as in the past, researchers continue to test her theory (H. E. Peplau, personal communication, November 4, 1987).

6. Theories can be used by practitioners to guide and improve their practice. Nursing is still defined as an interpersonal process built upon the progressive nurse–patient phases. As Peplau proposed, communication and interviewing skills remain fundamental nursing tools. Also, Peplau's anxiety continuum is still used for nursing interventions in working with anxious patients.

In applying Peplau's theory in clinical practice, one limitation is in working with the unconscious patient. A major assumption in the theory is that the nurse and patient can interact. For example, the phase of orientation begins when the patient has a felt need and initiates interaction between the nurse and the patient. This interaction is extremely limited in working with the unconscious patient.

7. Theories must be consistent with other validated theories, laws, and principles but will leave open unanswered questions that need to be investigated. In general, this theory is consistent with current theories and research. Interpersonal theories, including Sullivan's (1947) and Fromme's (1947), are foundations in the theory. Peplau's concepts and phases are consistent with other theories, such as Maslow's (1954) need theory and Selye's (1956) stress theory. General system theory can also be broadly applied to the four phases of the nurse–patient relationship (von Bertalanffy, 1968). For example, the nurse and patient can each be defined as a system. Both nurse and patient systems interact with each other, processing inputs, throughputs, and outputs so a specific goal can be met.

In summary, a theory has seven characteristics. In examining these, Peplau's 1952 work has the characteristics of a theory. Strengths include creating a unique way of viewing nursing and increasing nursing's body of knowledge. Limitations of this theory include the facts that some areas need to be further developed to be able to generate testable hypotheses, and that the theory is weak in application to the unconscious patient. Nursing research should focus on testing this theory's hypotheses for validation.

SUMMARY

Peplau's (1952/1988) book *Interpersonal relations in nursing* is still applicable in theory and practice. The core of Peplau's theory of nursing is the interpersonal process, which is an integral part of present-day nursing. This process consists of the sequential phases of orientation, identification, exploitation, and resolution. These phases overlap, interrelate, and vary in duration. The nurse and patient first clarify the patient's problems, and mutual expectations and goals are explored while deciding on appropriate plans for improving health status. This process is influenced by both the nurse's and patient's perceptions and preconceived ideas emerging from their individual uniqueness.

Peplau stresses that both the patient and nurse mature as the result of the therapeutic interaction. When two persons meet in a creative relationship, there is a continuing sense of mutuality and togetherness throughout the experience. Both individuals are involved in a process of self-fulfillment, which becomes a growth experience.

Peplau's phases can be compared with the nursing process. Both are sequential and focus on therapeutic interactions. Both processes focus on mutual exploration of the patient's problem. While involved in Peplau's phases and the nursing process, the patient and nurse begin to understand the patient's problem, uncover alternative approaches to the problem, and finally reach a solution.

Peplau's phases are also different from the nursing process. Peplau focuses on a specific nurse and patient relationship. In contrast, the nursing process may also view the patient collectively as a group, family, or community. Thus, today's nursing process includes more of the total environment than do Peplau's phases.

Peplau's nursing theory, the interpersonal process, has as its foundation theories of interaction. It has contributed to nursing in the areas of clinical practice, theory, and research, adding to today's base of nursing knowledge. Thus, Peplau's theory creates a unique view for understanding the nurse–patient relationship.

REFERENCES

American Nurses' Association. (1973). *Standards of nursing practice.* Kansas City: Author.

Burd, S. (1963). Effects of nursing interventions in anxiety of patients. In S. F. Burd, & M. A. Marshall (Eds.), *Some clinical approaches to psychiatric nursing* (pp. 307–320). London: Macmillan. [out of print]

Burton, G. (1958). *Personal, impersonal, and interpersonal: A guide for nurses.* New York: Springer. [out of print]

Forchuk, C., & Brown, B. (1989). Establishing a nurse–client relationship. *Journal of Psychosocial Nursing, 27,* 30–34.

Freud, S. (1936). *The problem of anxiety.* New York: Norton.

Fromme, E. (1947). *Man for himself.* New York: Rinehart.

Hays, D. (1966). Teaching a concept of anxiety. *Nursing Research, 10,* 108–113.

Maslow, A. (1954). *Motivation and personality.* New York: Harper & Row.

Peplau, H. E. (n.d.). *Basic principles of patient counseling.*

Peplau, H. E. (1988). *Interpersonal relations in nursing.* NY: Springer. (Original work published 1952, New York: G. P. Putnam's Sons.)

Profile: Hildegard E. Peplau, R.N., Ed.D (1974). *Nursing '74, 4,* 13.

Rogers, M. E. (1970). *An introduction to the theoretical basis of nursing.* Philadelphia: Davis. [out of print]

Selye, H. (1956). *The stress of life.* New York: McGraw-Hill.

Sills, G. (1977). Research in the field of psychiatric nursing, 1952–1977. *Nursing Research, 26,* 201–207.

Sullivan, H. S. (1947). *Conceptions of modern psychiatry.* Washington, D. C.: William Alanson White Psychiatric Foundation.

von Bertalanffy, L. (1968). *General system theory.* New York: Braziller.

BIBLIOGRAPHY

Beeber, L., Anderson, C. A., & Sills, G. M. (1990). Peplau's theory in practice, *Nursing Science Quarterly, 3,* 6–8.

Forchuk, C. (1991). Peplau's theory: Concepts and their relations. *Nursing Science Quarterly, 4,* 54–60.

Forchuk, C., Beaton, S., Crawford, L., Ide, L., Voorberg, N., & Bethune, J. (1989). Incorporating Peplau's theory and case management. *Journal of Psychosocial Nursing, 2,* 35–38.

Peplau, H. E. (1969, March). Theory: The professional dimension. In *Proceedings from the First Nursing Theory Conference.* University of Kansas Medical Center. (Reprinted 1986 in L. H. Nicholl (Ed.), *Perspectives on nursing theory,* (pp. 455–466). Boston: Little, Brown.)

Peplau, H. E. (1978). Psychiatric nursing: Role of nurses and psychiatric nurses. *International Nursing Review, 25,* 41–47.

Peplau, H. E. (1982). Some reflections on earlier days in psychiatric nursing. *Journal of Psychosocial Nursing and Mental Health Services, 20,* 17–24.

Peplau, H. E. (1985). Is nursing's self-regulatory power being eroded? *American Journal of Nursing, 85,* 140–143.

Peplau, H. E. (1985). The power of the dissociative state. *Journal of Psychosocial Nursing and Mental Health Services, 8,* 31–33.

Peplau, H. E. (1986). The nurse as counselor. *Journal of American College of Health, 35,* 11–14.

Peplau, H. E. (1987). Psychiatric skills, Tomorrow's world. *Nursing Times, 83,* 29–33.

Peplau, H. E. (1988). The art and science of nursing: Similarities, differences, and relations. *Nursing Science Quarterly, 1,* 8–15.

Peplau, H. E. (1989). Future directions in psychiatric nursing from the history. *Journal of Psychosocial Nursing, 2,* 18–21, 25–28.

Peplau, H. E. (1990). Evolution of nursing in psychiatric settings. In E. M. Varcarolis (Ed.), *Foundations of psychiatric mental health nursing.* Philadelphia, PA: Saunders.

Peplau, H. E. (1992). Interpersonal relations: A theoretical framework for application in nursing practice. *Nursing Science Quarterly, 5,* 13–18.

Thompson, L. (1980). Peplau's theory: An application to short-term individual therapy. *Journal of Psychosocial Nursing, 24,* 26–31.

Trench, A. S. (Executive producer), Wallace, D. (Producer), & Coberg, T. (Director). (1988). *Hildegard Peplau—The nurse theorists: Portraits of excellence* [Videotape]. Oakland, CA: Studio Three Production, Samuel Merritt College of Nursing.

C H A P T E R 5

VIRGINIA HENDERSON

Chiyoko Yamamoto Furukawa
Joan K. Howe

■ ■ ■

Virginia Henderson was born in Kansas City, Missouri, in 1897, the fifth child of a family of eight children. Most of her formative years were spent in Virginia, where the family lived during the period her father practiced law in Washington.

Henderson's interest in nursing evolved during World War I from her desire to help the sick and wounded military personnel. She enrolled in the Army School of Nursing in Washington, DC and graduated in 1921. In 1926, Henderson began the continuation of her education at Columbia University Teachers College and completed her BS and MA degrees in nursing education. She taught clinical nursing courses with a strong emphasis on the use of the analytical process at Teachers College from 1930 to 1948. In 1953, she was appointed Research Associate at Yale University School of Nursing. Now retired, she continues as Senior Research Associate Emeritus.

Henderson is the recipient of numerous recognitions for her outstanding contributions to nursing. She has received honorary doctoral degrees from the Catholic University of America, Pace University, University of Rochester, University of Western Ontario, and Yale University.

Her writings are far-reaching and have made an impact on nursing throughout the world. The publications The nature of nursing *(1966) and* Basic principles of nursing care *(1960) are widely known, and the latter has been translated into many languages for the benefit of non–English-speaking nurses. Although Henderson is in her tenth decade of life, she continues to contribute to the nursing literature. She has clarified her beliefs about nursing, nursing education, and nursing practice in view of recent technological and societal advances in publications, interviews, and personal appearances (Henderson, 1978, 1979a, 1979b, 1982a, 1985, 1987). Her most recent publication, in 1991, is* The nature of nursing—Reflections after 25 years. *The addendum to each chapter contains changes in her views and opinions relative to the 1966 first edition on the nature of nursing.*

Questions about the exclusive functions of nurses provided the impetus for Virginia Henderson to devote her career to defining nursing practice. Some of these questions were: What is the practice of nursing? What specific functions do nurses perform? What are nursing's unique activities? The development of her definition of nursing communicated her thoughts on these questions. She believed that an occupation that affects human life must outline its functions, particularly if it is to be regarded as a profession (Henderson, 1966, 1991). Her ideas about the definition of nursing were influenced by her nursing education and practice, by her students and colleagues at Columbia University School of Nursing, and by distinguished nursing leaders of her time. All these experiences and nursing practice were the dominating forces that gave her insight into nursing—what is it and what are its functions? A review of Henderson's educational preparation and nursing practice furnish the basis on which to examine her definition of nursing.

EDUCATIONAL AND PRACTICE BACKGROUND

Henderson's (1966) interpretation of the nurse's function is the synthesis of many positive and negative influences. A major influence was her basic nursing education in a general hospital affiliated with the Army School of Nursing. Her education emphasized learning by doing, speedy performance, technical competence, and successful mastery of nursing procedures (eg, catheterization, making beds, changing dressings). As a result, an impersonal approach to care emerged and was interpreted as professional behavior. Although the importance of ethics in nursing and a compassionate attitude toward humanity were stressed, these were not given as high a priority as the nursing procedures were.

Physician lectures were the major portion of classroom learning for the nursing students. The lectures used a cut-and-dried approach to learning and were a simplified version of medical education. The focus was disease, diagnosis, and treatment regimens. Henderson was discontented with the regimentalized care based on medical teaching. She recognized that this kind of nursing was merely an extension of medical practice (Henderson, 1966, 1991). Her dean, Annie W. Goodrich, agreed with this evaluation of nursing education.

Another educational concern for Henderson was a lack of an appropriate role model to emulate in giving nursing care. She yearned to observe patient care given by either her teacher or graduate nurses, which was impossible because students staffed the hospital in return for their nursing education. Thus, clinical practice was viewed as a self-learned process while students cared for the sick and wounded soldiers. She perceived this atmosphere to be one of indebtedness to the patients for having served the country in time of war. The nurse–patient relationship was described as warm and generous. The soldiers asked for little, and the nurses wanted to do all they could. This experience was believed to be unique and special, for the opportunity to express indebtedness to military patients did not exist in a civilian hospital.

Henderson's next educational experience, psychiatric nursing, was disappointing because the human relations skills that could have been learned in this setting failed to materialize. As in her previous experiences, the approach to psychiatric patient care continued to focus on disease entities and treatment. There was a lack of understanding about the nurse's role in the prevention of mental illness or in the curative aspects of care for the psychiatric patient. Her experience resulted in a sense of failure as a nurse. The only value of the psychiatric affiliation was the opportunity to gain some appreciation of mental illness.

The pediatric nursing experience at the Boston Floating Hospital was more positive and introduced three concepts of care: patient-centered, continuity of, and tender, loving care. The task-oriented and regimented approach to care was discarded in this setting. However, other shortcomings were identified, such as the failure to use family-centered care. Parents were not allowed to visit a sick child. Therefore, the child was isolated from parental support when it was most needed. Furthermore, Henderson saw little or no effort to assess the home environment to identify the needs of the child and family.

The final student experience at the Henry Street Visiting Nurse Agency in New York introduced her to community nursing care. The formal approach to patient care learned earlier was replaced with care that considered the sick person's life style. Henderson was concerned about discharging patients to the same environment that originally led them to hospitalization. She believed that the hospital care only served as a stopgap measure without getting to the cause of the problem. She recognized that this type of care failed to consider the person living outside the behavioral controls of the institutional setting.

As a graduate nurse, Henderson worked for several years at the Instructive Visiting Nursing Agency in Washington, DC, because she deplored the hospital system of nursing and did not want to be in it. This experience was rewarding and offered the opportunity to try out her ideas about nursing.

Her next position was teaching nursing students at the Norfolk Protestant Hospital diploma program in Virginia. She accepted this five-year responsibility without further education, a situation that was not uncommon because many diploma schools at that time did not require academic credentials for teaching. Despite this, she recognized the need for more knowledge and for clarification of the functions of nursing. Subsequently, she enrolled at Columbia University Teachers College to learn about the sciences and humanities relevant to nursing. These courses enabled Henderson to develop an inquiring and analytical approach to nursing.

After graduation, she briefly accepted the position of teaching supervisor at Strong Memorial Hospital's clinics in Rochester, New York. Next, she returned to Columbia, where her distinguished teaching career continued until 1948. While at this university, Henderson implemented several ideas about nursing in her medical-surgical nursing courses. The concepts taught were a patient-centered approach, the nursing problem method replacing the medical model, field experience, family follow-up care, and chronic illness care. She also established nursing clinics and encouraged coordinated multidisciplinary care.

THE DEVELOPMENT OF HENDERSON'S DEFINITION OF NURSING

Two events are the basis for Henderson's development of a definition of nursing. First, she participated in the revision of a nursing textbook. Second, she was concerned that many states had no provision for nursing licensure to ensure safe and competent care for the consumer.

In the revision of the *Textbook of the principles and practice of nursing,* written with Bertha Harmer, a Canadian nurse, Henderson recognized the need to be clear about the functions of the nurse (Harmer & Henderson, 1939; Safier, 1977). She believed a textbook that serves as a main learning source for nursing practice should present a sound and definitive description of nursing. Furthermore, the principles and practice of nursing must be built upon and derived from the definition of the profession.

Henderson was committed to the process of regulating nursing practice through licensure by each state. She believed that to accomplish this, nursing must be explicitly defined in Nurse Practice Acts that would provide the legal parameters for the nurse's functions in caring for consumers and safeguard the public from unprepared and incompetent practitioners.

Although official statements on the nursing function were published by the American Nurses' Association (ANA) in 1932 and 1937, Henderson (1966, 1991) viewed these statements as nonspecific and unsatisfactory definitions of nursing practice. Then, in 1955 the earlier ANA (1962) definition was modified to read as follows:

> The practice of professional nursing means the performance for compensation of any act in the observation, care, and counsel of the ill, injured, or infirm, or in the maintenance of health or prevention of illness of others, or in the supervision and teaching of other personnel, or the administration of medications and treatment as prescribed by a licensed physician or dentist; requiring substantial specialized judgment and skill and based on knowledge and application of the principles of biological, physical, and social science. The foregoing shall not be deemed to include acts of diagnosis or prescription of therapeutic or corrective measures (p. 7).

This statement was seen as an improvement because nursing functions were identified, but the definition still was thought to be very general and too vague. In the new statement, the nurse could observe, care for, and counsel the patient and could supervise other health personnel without herself or himself being supervised by the physician. The nurse was to give medications and do treatments ordered by the physician but was prohibited from diagnosing, prescribing treatment for, or correcting nursing care problems. Thus, Henderson viewed the statement as another unsatisfactory definition of nursing.

Henderson's extensive experiences as a student, teacher, practitioner, author, and participant in conferences on the nurse's function contributed to the development of her definition of nursing. She regretted that publications of conference debates and investigations were not widely circulated. Only a few nurses were privy to the information published about the outcomes of these conferences.

In 1955, Henderson's first definition of nursing was published in Bertha Harmer's revised nursing textbook (Harmer & Henderson, 1955). It reads as follows:

Henderson's First (1955) Definition

Nursing is primarily assisting the individual (sick or well) in the performance of those activities contributing to health, or its recovery (or peaceful death) that he would perform unaided if he had the necessary strength, will, or knowledge. It is likewise the unique contribution of nursing to help the individual to be independent of such assistance as soon as possible (p. 4).

This statement on nursing conveys the essence of Henderson's definition of nursing as it is known today. Since there was collaboration, it is instructive to compare Henderson's definition with Harmer's 1922 definition, which follows:

Harmer's 1922 Definition

Nursing is rooted in the needs of humanity and is founded on the ideal of service. Its object is not only to cure the sick and heal the wounded but to bring health and ease, rest and comfort to mind and body, to shelter, nourish, and protect and to minister to all those who are helpless or handicapped, young, aged or immature. Its object is to prevent disease and to preserve health. Nursing is, therefore, linked with every other social agency which strives for the prevention of disease and the preservation of health. The nurse finds herself not only concerned with the care of the individual but with the health of a people (p. 3).

Some similarities can be seen between the two definitions of nursing. Henderson's definition abbreviated and consolidated portions of Harmer's beliefs about nursing. Harmer's definition highlighted disease prevention, health preservation, and the need for linkages with other social agencies to strive for preventive care. Harmer stressed that nursing's role in society was oriented toward the community and wellness. Henderson placed more emphasis on the care of sick and well individuals and did not mention nursing's concern for the health and welfare of the aggregate. However, a one-line statement in *Basic principles of nursing* acknowledges that some nurses do function with groups rather than individuals (Henderson, 1960).

Henderson's focus on individual care is evident in that she stressed assisting individuals with essential activities to maintain health, to recover, or to achieve peaceful death. She proposed 14 components of basic nursing care to augment her definition (Henderson, 1966, 1991), as follows:

[The individual can]
1. Breathe normally.
2. Eat and drink adequately.
3. Eliminate body wastes.
4. Move and maintain desirable postures.
5. Sleep and rest.
6. Select suitable clothes—dress and undress.
7. Maintain body temperature within normal range by adjusting clothing and modifying the environment.
8. Keep the body clean and well groomed and protect the integument.
9. Avoid dangers in the environment and avoid injuring others.
10. Communicate with others in expressing emotions, needs, fears, or opinions.
11. Worship according to one's faith.
12. Work in such a way that there is a sense of accomplishment.
13. Play or participate in various forms of recreation.
14. Learn, discover, or satisfy the curiosity that leads to normal development and health and use the available health facilities (pp. 16–17).

In 1966, Henderson's ultimate statement on the definition of nursing was published in *The nature of nursing.* This statement was viewed as "the crystallization of my ideas" (p. 15):

The unique function of the nurse is to assist the individual, sick or well, in the performance of those activities contributing to health or its recovery (or to peaceful death) that he would perform unaided if he had the necessary strength, will or knowledge. And to do this in such a way as to help him gain independence as rapidly as possible (p. 15).

Except for slight wording changes, the 1955, 1966, and more recent 1978 definitions are quite similar, indicating that her definition of nursing, conceived earlier, remains intact (Harmer & Henderson, 1955; Henderson, 1966; Henderson & Nite, 1978). Henderson's definition of nursing in itself fails to fully explain her main ideas and views. To appreciate the breadth of her thoughts about nursing functions and the 14 components of basic nursing care, it is necessary to study *Basic principles of nursing care,* a publication of the International Council of Nurses (Henderson, 1960). This textbook eloquently describes each of the basic nursing care components so that they can be used as a guide to delineate the unique nursing functions. The definition of nursing and the fourteen components together outline the functions the nurse can initiate and control.

Henderson (1966, 1991) expects nurses to carry out the therapeutic plan of the physician as a member of the medical team. The nurse is the prime helper to the ill person in assuring that the medical prescriptions are instituted. This nursing function is believed to foster the therapeutic nurse–client relationship. As a member of an interdisciplinary health team, the nurse assists the individual to recovery or provides support in dying. The ideal situation for a nurse is full participation as a team member with no interference with the nurse's unique functions. The nurse serves as a substitute for whatever the patient lacks in order to make him or her "complete," "whole," or "independent," considering his or her available physical strength, will, or knowledge to attain good health.

The nurse is cautioned about tasks that detract from the professional role and the need to give priority to the nurse's unique functions. However, Henderson encourages the nurse to assume the role and functions of other health workers if the need is apparent and the nurse has expertise. On a worldwide basis, nursing functions differ from country to country, or even within countries. The ratio of nurses to physicians and to other health care providers affects what nurses do. Consequently, the public is confused about the nurse's role, particularly since the creation of nurse practitioners.

In her most recent publication, Henderson (1991) acknowledges that defining nursing has been unsuccessful: "In spite of the fact that generations of nurses have tried to define it, 'the nature of nursing' remains a question" (p. 7). In her opinion, nurses are no closer to consensus on the official definition of nursing than in 1966. She states the only difference now is that nursing education offers courses on nursing theory and nursing process. If *The nature of nursing* were to be written today, she feels she would be obliged to include a discussion of both nursing theory and the nursing process.

Furthermore, with respect to a universal definition of nursing, Henderson (1991) concludes that there is difficulty in promoting the notion of universality. She bases her view upon her numerous visits to countries worldwide where she observed the variations in nursing education coupled with differing nursing practices used to serve the needs of various populations.

HENDERSON'S THEORY AND NURSING'S METAPARADIGM

In viewing the concept of the *human* or individual, Henderson considers the biological, psychological, sociological, and spiritual components. Her 14 components of nursing functions can be categorized in the following manner: The first nine components are physiological; the tenth and fourteenth are psychological aspects of communicating and learning; the eleventh component is spiritual and moral; and the twelfth and thirteenth components are sociologically oriented to occupation and recreation. She refers to humans as having basic needs that are included in the 14 components. However, she goes on to state, "It is equally important to realize that these needs are satisfied by infinitely varied patterns of living, no two of which are alike" (Henderson, 1960, p. 3). Henderson (1966, 1991) also believes that mind and body are inseparable. It is implied that the mind and body are interrelated.

Henderson emphasizes some aspects of the concept of *society/environment*. In her writing, she primarily discusses individuals. She sees individuals in relation to their families but minimally discusses the impact of the community on the individual and family. In the book co-written with Harmer (Harmer & Henderson, 1955), she supports the tasks of private and public agencies in keeping people healthy. She believes that society wants and expects the nurse's service of acting for individuals who are unable to function independently (Henderson, 1966, 1991). In return, she expects society to contribute to nursing education:

> The nurse needs the kind of education that, in our society, is available only in colleges and universities. Training programs operated on funds pinched from the budgets of service agencies cannot provide the preparation the nurse needs (p. 69).

This generalized education gives the nurse a better understanding of the consumers of nursing care and the various environmental facts that influence people.

Henderson's beliefs about *health* are related to human functioning. Her definition of health is based on the individual's ability to function independently, as outlined in the 14 components. Because good health is a challenging goal for individuals, she argues that it is difficult for the nurse to help the person reach it (Henderson, 1960). She also refers to nurses stressing promotion of health and prevention and cure of disease (Henderson, 1966). Henderson (1960) explains how the factors of age, cultural background, physical and intellectual capacities, and emotional balance affect one's health. These conditions are always present and affect basic needs. Because of her concern for the welfare of people, Henderson (1989) believes that nurses "should be in the forefront of those who work for social justice, for a healthful environment, for access to adequate food, shelter, and clothing, and universal opportunities for education and employment, realizing that all of these as well as preventive and creative health care are essential to the well-being of citizens" (p. 82). By working on various social issues, nurses can have an impact on people's health.

Henderson's concept of nursing is interesting from the perspective of time. She was one of the earlier leaders who believed nurses need a liberal education, including knowledge of sciences, social sciences, and humanities. Aside from using the definition of nursing and the 14 components of basic nursing care, the nurse is expected to carry out the physician's therapeutic plan. Individualized care is the result of the nurse's creativity in planning for care. Furthermore, the nurse is expected to improve patient care by using the results of nursing research:

> The nurse who operates under a definition that specifies an area of independent practice, or an area of expertise, must assume responsibility for identifying problems, for continually validating her function, for improving the methods she uses, and for measuring

the effect of nursing care. In this era research is the name we attach to the most reliable type of analysis (Henderson, 1966, p. 38).

For Henderson, the nurse must be knowledgeable, have some base for practicing individualized and humane care, and be a scientific problem solver. In her update of *The nature of nursing*, Henderson (1991) sees "research in nursing as *essential* to the validation and improvement of practice" (p. 58). Even though she believes that caring for patients "is an important, really essential element of nurses' service," she also emphasizes that "nursing practice and nursing education should nevertheless be based on research" (p. 58). It's important that nursing care be improved by implementing valid research results.

HENDERSON AND THE NURSING PROCESS

Henderson (1980) views the nursing process as "really the application of the logical approach to the solution of a problem. The steps are those of the scientific method" (p. 906). With this approach, each person can receive individualized care. Likewise, with the nursing process, individualized care is the outcome.

In Henderson's more recent writings, she raises some issues regarding the nursing process. One of the issues asks if the problem-solving approach of the nursing process is peculiar to nursing. She compares the nursing process to the traditional steps of the medical process: "the nursing history parallels the medical history; the nurse's health assessment, the physician's medical examination; the nursing diagnosis corresponds to the physician's diagnosis; nursing orders to the plan of medical management; and nursing evaluation to medical evaluation" (Henderson, 1980, p. 907). It looks as if the language has been changed to fit nursing's purpose. Could other health care workers use the steps of the nursing process to fit their practice? If so, then what makes the nursing process peculiar to nursing?

Another issue Henderson raises also deals with problem solving. But now she asks if problem solving is all there is to nursing. Henderson (1987) states, " 'the' makes it so specific that activities outside those in the problem solving steps of the process cannot be peculiar to or characteristic of nursing" (p. 8). She questions where intuition, experience, authority, and expert opinion fit into the nursing process since they are not stressed. She further comments, "Expert opinion or authority is also, by implication, discredited as a basis for practice" (Henderson, 1982a, p. 108). Does the "the" in the nursing process make it too limiting for effective practice?

A third issue Henderson raises flows from the problem-solving approach. She asks where the art of nursing fits into the nursing process. If one views science as objective with little left undefined and art as subjective with some parts hard to define, then where does intuition fit? Henderson (1987) argues that "The nursing process now weighted so heavily on the scientific side, seems to belittle the intuitive, artistic side of nursing" (p. 8). She also claims, "nursing process stresses the science of nursing rather than the mixture of science *and art* on which it seems effective health care services of any kind is based" (Henderson, 1987, p. 9). Does the nursing process disregard the subjective and intuitive qualities used in nursing?

The fourth concern Henderson raises about the nursing process deals with the lack of collaboration among health care workers, the patient, and the family. She states, "As currently defined, nursing process does not seem to suggest a collaborative approach on diagnosis, treatment, *or* care by health care workers, nor does it suggest the essential rights of patients and their families in all of these questions" (Henderson, 1982a, p. 109). Henderson (1987) thinks the nursing process stresses an independent function for the nurse rather than a collaborative one with other health professionals, the patient, and the patient's family. Does the nursing process focus more on independent nursing functions than on interdependent functions?

Perhaps it is semantics that are a problem with the nursing process. The real value of the nursing process depends on one's understanding, interpretation, integration, and use of it. The nursing process discussed in Chapter 2 is now examined with Henderson's definition of nursing.

Even though Henderson's definition and explanation of nursing do not directly fit with the steps of the nursing process, a relationship between the two can be demonstrated. Although Henderson does not refer directly to assessment, she implies it in her description of the 14 components of basic nursing care. The nurse uses the 14 components to assess the individual's needs. For example, in assessing the first component, "breathe normally," the nurse gathers all pertinent data about the person's respiratory status. The nurse then moves to the next component and gathers data in that area. The gathering of data about the person continues until all components have been assessed.

To complete the assessment phase of the nursing process, the nurse needs to analyze the data. According to Henderson, the nurse must have knowledge about what is normal in health and disease. Using this knowledge base, then, the nurse compares the assessment data with what was known about that area. For example, if respirations were observed to be 40 per minute in an adult aged 40, the nurse would conclude that this person's respiratory rate is faster than normal. Or if a laboratory report showed that the urine was highly concentrated, the nurse would know this "means that the patient's fluid intake is inadequate, unless he is losing body fluids by other routes" (Henderson, 1960, p. 19). With a scientific knowledge base, the nurse can draw conclusions from the assessment data. Henderson (1960) states the following:

> The nursing needed by the individual is affected by age, cultural background, emotional balance, and his physical and intellectual capacities. All of these should be considered in the nurse's evaluation of the patient's needs for help (p. 7).

Following the analysis of the data according to these factors, the nurse then determines the nursing diagnosis. Henderson does not specifically discuss nursing diagnoses. She believes the physician makes the diagnosis, and the nurse acts upon that diagnosis. However, if one looks at Henderson's definition, the nursing diagnosis deals with identifying the individual's ability to meet human needs with or without assistance, taking into account that person's strength, will, and knowledge. Given the assessment data and its analysis, the nurse *can* identify actual problems such as abnormal respirations. In addition, potential problems may be identified. For example, with Component 11, about one's faith, a potential problem could develop because of hospitalization and a change in the person's normal activities of daily living. If, based on the nurse's assessment and analysis of the data, a person was unable to meet this need, then a nursing diagnosis regarding an actual problem would be made.

Once the nursing diagnosis is made, the nurse proceeds to the planning phase of the nursing process, about which Henderson (1960) states:

> All effective nursing care is planned to some extent. A written plan forces those who make it to give some thought to the individual's needs—unless they simply fit the person's regimen into the institution's routines (p. 11).

She also contends that *discharge planning* is influenced by the other members of the family (Henderson, 1960). Furthermore, plans need continuing modification that is based on the individual's needs. Henderson advocates written nursing care plans so others giving care can follow the planned sequence. She emphasizes that "nursing care is always arranged around, or fitted into, the physician's therapeutic plan" (p. 11). Henderson outlines the planning phase as making the plan fit the individual's needs, updating the plan as necessary on the basis of those needs, being specific so others can implement it, and fitting with the physician's prescribed plan. Written nursing care plans, in essence, identify the nursing needs of the person. Even though Henderson does not apply the current terminology about nursing plans, she uses the same ideas.

Implementation follows the planning of nursing care. For Henderson (1966, 1991), nursing implementation is based on helping the patient meet the 14 components. For example, in helping the individual with sleep and rest, the nurse tries known methods of inducing sleep and rest before giving drugs. Henderson summarizes, "I see nursing as primarily complementing the patient by supplying what he needs in knowledge, will, or strength to perform his daily activities and to carry out the treatment prescribed for him by the physician" (p. 21). Henderson also states, "This primary function of the practicing nurse, of course, must be performed in such a way that it promotes the physician's therapeutic plan" (p. 27). So the nurse needs to carry out the physician's orders of treatment along with her nursing care.

Another important aspect of implementation that Henderson (1966, 1991) discusses is the relationship between nurse and patient. The nurse gets "inside the skin" to better understand the patient's needs and carry out measures to meet those needs. Henderson (1960) also speaks about the quality of nursing care:

> The danger of turning over the physical care of the patient to relatively unqualified nurses is two-fold. They may fail to assess the patient's needs adequately but, perhaps more important, the qualified nurse, being deprived of the opportunity while giving physical care to assess his needs, may not find any other chance to do so. In this connection it should also be pointed out that it is easier for any person to develop an emotional supportive role with another if he can perform a tangible service (pp. 10–11).

This statement clearly supports the idea that the competent nurse uses both the interpersonal process and assessment while giving care.

Henderson (1966) bases the evaluation of each person "according to the speed with which, or the degree to which, he performs independently the activities that make, for him, a normal day" (p. 27). This notion is outlined in the definition of and the unique function of the nurse. For evaluation purposes, changes in a person's level of functioning need to be observed and recorded. A comparison of the data about the person's functional abilities is done pre- and post-nursing care. All changes are noted for evaluation.

To summarize the stages of the nursing process as applied to Henderson's definition of nursing and to the 14 components of basic nursing care, refer to Table 5–1.

HENDERSON'S WORK AND THE CHARACTERISTICS OF A THEORY

Henderson wrote her definition of nursing before the development of concepts and theories about nursing. Her intent was to identify the specific functions the nurse performs rather than to describe the theoretical basis for nursing practice. Nevertheless, some characteristics of a theory as discussed in Chapter 1 can be applied to Henderson's work.

1. Theories can interrelate concepts in such a way as to create a different way of looking at a particular phenomenon. Henderson uses the concepts of fundamental human needs, biophysiology, culture, and interaction-communication. These concepts are borrowed from other disciplines rather than being unique to nursing. In a way, one might view the collection of these concepts as middle-level theory since delineating nursing practice was a major goal of Henderson's.

Maslow's (1970) hierarchy of human needs fits well with the 14 basic components. The first nine components are physiological and safety needs. The remaining five components deal with love and belonging, social esteem, and self-actualization needs. Henderson uses the biophysiological concept when she stresses the importance of physiology and physiological balances in making decisions about nursing care. The concept of culture as it affects

TABLE 5–1. A SUMMARY OF THE NURSING PROCESS AND OF HENDERSON'S FOURTEEN COMPONENTS AND DEFINITION OF NURSING

Nursing Process	Henderson's Fourteen Components and Definition of Nursing
Nursing assessment	Assess needs of human being based on the 14 components of basic nursing care:
	1. Breathe normally 8. Keep body clean and well-groomed
	2. Eat and drink adequately
	3. Eliminate body wastes 9. Avoid dangers in environment
	4. Move and maintain posture 10. Communicate
	5. Sleep and rest 11. Worship according to one's faith
	6. Suitable clothing, dress or undress 12. Work accomplishment
	13. Recreation
	7. Maintain body temperature 14. Learn, discover, or satisfy curiosity
	Analysis: Compare data to knowledge base of health and disease.
Nursing diagnosis	Identify individual's ability to meet own needs with or without assistance, taking into consideration strength, will, or knowledge.
Nursing plan	Document how the nurse can assist the individual, sick or well.
Nursing implementation	Assist the sick or well individual in the performance of activities in meeting human needs to maintain health, recover from illness, or to aid in peaceful death. Implementation based on physiological principles, age, cultural background, emotional balance, and physical and intellectual capacities. Carry out treatment prescribed by the physician.
Nursing evaluation	Use the acceptable definition of nursing and appropriate laws related to the practice of nursing. The quality of care is drastically affected by the preparation and native ability of the nursing personnel rather than the amount of hours of care. Successful outcomes of nursing care are based on the speed with which or degree to which the patient performs independently the activities of daily living.

human needs is learned from the family and other social groups. Because of this, Henderson suggests that a nurse is unable to fully interpret or supply all the requirements for the individual's well-being. At best the nurse can merely assist the individual in meeting human needs.

The concept of interaction–communication can be seen in Henderson's writings. She believes sensitivity to nonverbal communication is essential to encourage the expression of feelings (Henderson, 1966). Furthermore, a prerequisite to validate a patient's needs is a constructive nurse–patient relationship. As mentioned earlier, several concepts can be identified from the definition of nursing and the 14 components of nursing care. Each of the concepts can be interrelated to describe nursing as it is viewed by Henderson. How the concepts interrelate remains to be tested.

2. Theories must be logical in nature. Henderson's definition and components are logical. The nurse assists the individual to perform those activities contributing to health or its recovery, or peaceful death, and encourages independence as quickly as possible. The 14 components are a guide for the individual and nurse in reaching the chosen goals. The components start with physiological functioning and move to the psychosocial aspects, which conveys the idea that bodily operation is a priority to emotional or cognitive status.

3. Theories should be relatively simple yet generalizable. Henderson's work is relatively simple yet generalizable with some limitations. Her work can be applied to the health of individuals of all ages. Nurses functioning at various levels and in diverse cultures have used Henderson's definition and components in their practice. An important shortcoming is the lack of empirical testing to determine the generalizability of the definition and the 14 components.

4. Theories can be the bases for hypotheses that can be tested or for theory to be expanded. Henderson's definition of nursing cannot be viewed as a theory; therefore, it is impossible to generate testable hypotheses from it. However, some questions that investigate the definition of nursing and the 14 components may be useful. Some examples of these questions follow:

1. Is the sequence of the 14 components followed by nurses in the United States and other countries?
2. What priorities are evident in the use of the basic nursing functions?
3. Do nurses give care to presenting medical problems initially and then use the unique functions?
4. Which clinical specialty areas of nursing practice include or exclude Components 10 through 14?

Henderson (1977) is an advocate of conducting research in nursing. She favors studies directed to improving practice rather than those conducted as an academic or theoretical endeavor.

In a recent publication, support for the application of research in nursing practice is emphasized and encouraged (Henderson, 1991). Henderson acknowledges that, "research is identified as one of the right processes nurses use in arriving at a valid reason for their actions" (p. 56). However, there are no suggestions made regarding the empirical testing of her concepts that underlie her 1966 definition of nursing. The reason for this may be that Henderson views the research process as time-consuming and inappropriate to use for minute-by-minute life decisions. She believes that research is not a substitute for instinctive and intuitive reactions to situations but that these reactions are influenced by the nurse's knowledge of sciences that guide human behavior in the society of which nursing is a integral part.

5. Theories contribute to and assist in increasing the general body of knowledge within the discipline through the research implemented to validate them. Henderson's ideas of nursing practice are well accepted throughout the world as a basis for nursing care. However, the impact of the definition and components have not been established through research. Well-designed empirical studies are needed to determine Henderson's contribution to world-wide knowledge about nursing practice and patient outcomes. This would help validate Henderson's beliefs about the unique function of nursing.

Henderson (1991) acknowledges that currently nurses try to base their practice on scientific knowledge that guides other health care providers as well. She hopes that all providers of care are lifelong learners who study and recognize the need for change that is based upon research findings.

6. Theories can be used by practitioners to guide and improve their practice. Ideally, the nurse would improve nursing practice by using Henderson's definition and 14 components to improve the health of individuals and thus reduce illness. The final desirable outcome would be a measure of recovery rate, health promotion, and maintenance, or a peaceful death.

With respect to Henderson's (1991) most recent thoughts on the use of theories, she states, "application of general principles should be part of any effort to improve or advance a profession" (p. 98). However, she disagrees with the current nursing education practice that encourages students to adopt and practice the theory of others. If she were to write *The nature of nursing* today, she would stress to students not only the need to study the existing theories but also the need to recognize that the guiding concept should be their own, for the reason that the mixture of concepts studied may differ from those concepts uniquely suited to that individual nurse.

7. Theories must be consistent with other validated theories, laws, and principles but will leave open unanswered questions that need to be investigated. There is a potential for comparison of Henderson's definition and components with validated theories, laws, and principles. The concepts of fundamental human needs, culture, independence, and interaction–communication are widely investigated by nurse researchers as well as by those in the social and psychological disciplines. In the 1980s, Henderson (1982b) supported the idea that nursing must accept the responsibility for conducting investigations on nursing practice. Furthermore, she said the focus ought to be on measures of consumer welfare, satisfaction, and cost-effectiveness.

In the 1990s, Henderson (1991) continues to believe in nursing practice based upon psychological and biological research. Unlike the past, when many nurses relied upon custom, tradition, or authority to be responsible for their practice, she believes today's nurses explore to find reasons for ineffective or effective therapeutic interventions which use scientific rationale.

LIMITATIONS

Henderson based her ideas about nursing care on fundamental human needs and the physical and emotional aspects of the individual. A major shortcoming in her work is the lack of a conceptual linkage between physiological and other human characteristics. The concept of the holistic nature of human beings does not clearly emerge from her publications. However, it must be kept in mind that Henderson wrote her ideas about nursing before the emergence of the holism concept. If the assumption is made that the 14 components are stated in their order of priority, the relationship among the components is unclear. Each component does affect the next one on the list. In 1985, however, Henderson did state some beliefs about her acceptance of the holistic approach to nursing.

If priority according to individual needs is implied in the listing of the components, does a presenting emotional problem take a backseat to physical care? Is the emotional area of care deferred until the physiological needs have been given proper attention? Henderson specifies that the nurse must consider such factors as age, temperament, social or cultural status, and physical and intellectual capacity in the use of the components, thus emphasizing differences among individuals. How these factors interrelate and influence nursing care is vague, except individualized care must emerge when all factors of a person are taken into account in the process of nursing.

In a critique of a major international conference on primary care, Henderson (1989) offered some conclusions about the weaknesses of today's nurses. She thought that the basic sciences (eg, biophysical sciences) as well as the scientific method and its application to nursing were neglected in the presentations. Other areas in which a lack of knowledge by the presenters was of concern to Henderson included budgeting and financial management, holistic family-centered and community-based approaches to health care, policy making and planning processes, roles of leaders as change agents, taking risks with unpopular actions, and being assertive. These concerns underscore the currency of Henderson's thinking and views about nursing; many of these concerns were not reflected in her earlier writings.

In fairness to Henderson, her effort to define nursing evolved before the discussions of a theoretical basis for the profession emerged. Therefore, the lack of theory in her definition of nursing should not lessen her contribution to nurses and nursing. Her pioneering spirit to lead nursing toward a profession and accountability to the public for competent care were enormous contributions to society as well as to nursing.

Last, in assisting the individual in the dying process, Henderson contends that the nurse helps, but she gives little explanation of what the nurse does. In her definition of nursing, the placing of a parenthesis around the words "peaceful death" is curious. It leads one to wonder why the parentheses were used—perhaps it was merely to single out this event as an important one in which nursing has a significant role.

CONCLUSIONS

The concept of nursing formulated by Henderson in her definition of nursing and the 14 components of basic nursing is uncomplicated and self-explanatory. Therefore, it could be used without difficulty as a guide for nursing practice by most nurses. Many of the ideas she presented continue to be used worldwide in both developed and undeveloped countries to guide nursing curricula and practice, which is validated by the demand for her ICN publication that in 1972 was in its seventh printing.

If a suggestion can be made to improve Henderson's concept of nursing, it is the incorporation of theory. For example, it would be interesting to see how holism or general systems theory might explain the relationship of the components of basic nursing care. Confirmation of whether or not the list of components are prioritized is needed to clarify what the nurse ought to do if the presenting problem is other than a physical one.

In view of the time in which Henderson published her definition of nursing, she deserves much credit as a leader in the development of nursing practice, education, and licensure. Her work ought to be considered a beginning and impetus for nurses to pursue the highest academic degree. This is critical for analyses of nursing practice and for identifying and testing the theoretical bases for patient care.

SUMMARY

In conclusion, Henderson provides the essence of what she believes is a definition of nursing as follows:

> I believe that the function the nurse performs is primarily an independent one—that of acting for the patient when he lacks knowledge, physical strength, or the will to act for himself as he would ordinarily act in health, or in carrying out prescribed therapy. This function is seen as complex and creative, as offering unlimited opportunity for the application of the physical, biological, and social sciences, and the development of skills based on them (Henderson, 1960, p. 7).

REFERENCES

ANA Statement on Auxiliary Personnel in Nursing Service. (1962). *The American Journal of Nursing, 62,* 7.

Harmer, B. (1922). *Textbook of the principles and practice of nursing.* New York: Macmillan. [out of print]

Harmer, B., & Henderson, V. (1939). *Textbook of the principles and practice of nursing* (4th ed.). New York: Macmillan. [out of print]

Harmer, B., & Henderson, V. (1955). *Textbook of the principles and practice of nursing* (5th ed.). New York: Macmillan. [out of print]

Henderson, V. (1960). *Basic principles of nursing care.* Geneva: International Council of Nurses.

Henderson, V. (1966). *The nature of nursing.* New York: Macmillan. [out of print]

Henderson, V. (1977). We've come a long way but what of the direction? *Nursing Research, 26,* 163–164.

Henderson, V. (1978). The concept of nursing. *Journal of Advanced Nursing, 3,* 16–17.

Henderson, V. (1979a). Preserving the essence of nursing in a technological age, Part I. *Nursing Times, 75,* 2012–2013.

Henderson, V. (1979b). Preserving the essence of nursing in a technological age, Part II. *Nursing Times, 75,* 2056–2058.

Henderson, V. (1980) Nursing—Yesterday and tomorrow. *Nursing Times, 76,* 905–907.

Henderson, V. (1982a). The nursing process—Is the title right? *Journal of Advanced Nursing, 7,* 103–109.

Henderson, V. (1982b). Speech at History of Nursing Museum, Philadelphia, May, 1982.

Henderson, V. (1985). The essence of nursing in high technology. *Nursing Administration Quarterly, 9,* 1–9.

Henderson, V. (1987). Nursing process—A critique. *Holistic Nursing Practice, 1,* 7–18.

Henderson, V. (1989). Countdown to 2000: A major international conference for the primary health care team, 21–23 September 1987, London. *Journal of Advanced Nursing, 14,* 81–85.

Henderson, V. (1991). *The nature of nursing—Reflections after 25 years.* New York: National League for Nursing.

Henderson, V., & Nite, G. (1978). *Principles and practice of nursing* (6th ed.). New York: Macmillan.

Maslow, A. (1970). *Motivation and personality* (2nd ed.). New York: Harper & Row.

Safier, G. (1977). *Contemporary American leaders in nursing.* New York: McGraw-Hill.

BIBLIOGRAPHY

Campbell, C. (1985). Virginia Henderson: The definitive nurse. *Nursing Mirror, 160,* 12.

Fulton, J. S. (1987). Virginia Henderson: Theorist, prophet, poet. *Advances in Nursing Science, 10,* 1–9.

Henderson, V. (1985). Health records and nursing. *Connecticut Nursing News, 54,* 1, 4.

Henderson, V. (1982). Is the study of history rewarding for nurses? *Society for Nursing History Gazette, 2,* 1–2.

Henderson, V. (1986). Some observations on health care by health services or health industries (editorial). *Journal of Advanced Nursing, 1,* 1–2.

Henderson, V., & Watt, S. (1983). Epidermolysis bullosa. *Nursing Times, 79,* 43–46.

Henderson, V., & Watt, S. (1983). 70+ and going strong. Virginia Henderson: A nurse for all ages. *Geriatric Nursing, 4,* 58–59.

Henderson, V., and others. (1977). *Reference resource for research and continuing education in nursing.* Kansas City: American Nurses Association Publication No. 6125.

McCarty, P. (1987). How can nurses prepare for year 2000? (A response from Virginia Henderson). *The American Nurse, 19,* 3, 6.

Shamansky, S. L. (1964). CHN revisited: A conversation with Virginia Henderson. *Public Health Nursing, 1,* 193–201.

Shamansky, S. L. (1984). Virginia Henderson: A national treasure. *Focus Critical Care, 11,* 60–61.

EVELYN ADAM'S EXTENSION
OF VIRGINIA HENDERSON'S WORK

Julia B. George

Evelyn Adam (b. 1929), a Canadian nurse, received her undergraduate nursing education in Canada. She earned her MS in nursing from the University of California at Los Angeles. While at UCLA, she met Dorothy Johnson, who served as a strong influence on her professional life (Creekmur, DeFelice, Doub, Hodel, & Petty, 1989). Adam (1985) differentiates between a theory and a conceptual model in part by indicating that a theory may be useful to more than one discipline but a conceptual model is discipline specific. Therefore, Adam (1980) developed concepts from the work of Virginia Henderson into a conceptual model.

There are six major units in Adam's conceptual model (Adam, 1980). The first is the *goal of the profession,* that which members of the profession seek to achieve. Adam defines the goal of nursing as seeking to maintain or restore the client's independence in meeting 14 fundamental needs. Each need has dimensions that are biological, psychological, and sociocultural. The second unit is the *beneficiary,* that person or group of persons toward whom professional activity is directed. For nursing, this is the client or patient. The third unit is *role,* the part played by the professional. Nurses have a unique role, although they share certain functions with other health professionals. It is this unique role that society expects nurses to perform. This role is complementary-supplementary to the client's strength, will, knowledge, or all three.

The fourth unit is *source of difficulty,* the probable source of problems being experienced by the beneficiary. These problems may occur in any one or more of the 14 fundamental needs. When needs are not met, the person is not whole. The fifth unit is *intervention,* the *focus,* or area on which the professional's attention is centered, and *modes,* the means or methods of intervention that are available to the professional. These may be associated with the implementation phase of the nursing process. The sixth unit is the *consequences,* the results of the professional's efforts toward the goal. Information for this unit may be found in the evaluation phase of the nursing process.

REFERENCES

Adam, E. (1980). *To be a nurse.* Philadelphia: Saunders.

Adam, E. (1985). Toward more clarity in terminology—Frameworks, theories and models. *Journal of Nursing Education, 24,* 151–155.

Creekmur, T., DeFelice, J., Doub, M., Hodel, A., Marriner-Tomey, A., & Petty, C. Y. (1994). Evelyn Adam: Conceptual model for nursing. In A. Marriner-Tomey. *Nursing theorists and their work* (3rd ed.) (pp. 493–506). St. Louis: Mosby.

LYDIA E. HALL

*Julia B. George**

■ ■ ■

Lydia E. Hall received her basic nursing education at York Hospital School of Nursing in York, Pennsylvania. Both her BS in Public Health Nursing and MA in teaching Natural Sciences are from Teachers College, Columbia University, New York.

Lydia Hall was the first director of the Loeb Center for Nursing and Rehabilitation and continued in that position until her death in 1969. Her experience in nursing spans the clinical, educational, research, and supervisory components. Her publications include several articles on the definition of nursing and quality of care. Lydia Hall put forth what she considered a basic philosophy of nursing upon which the nurse may base patient care.

LOEB CENTER FOR NURSING AND REHABILITATION

As a nurse theorist Lydia Hall is unique in that her beliefs about nursing were demonstrated in practice with relatively little documentation in the literature. Hall originated the philosophy of care of Loeb Center at Montefiore Hospital, Bronx, New York. Loeb Center opened in January 1963 to provide professional nursing care to persons past the acute stage of illness. The center's functioning concept was that the need for professional nursing care increases as the need for medical care decreases.

Those in need of continued professional care who were 16 years of age or older and who were no longer experiencing an acute biological disturbance were transferred from the acute care hospital to Loeb Center. Good candidates for care at Loeb were those who had a desire to come to Loeb, were recommended by their physicians, and possessed a favorable potential for recovery and return to the community.

Physically, Loeb Center has a capacity of 80 beds and is attached to Montefiore Hospital. The rooms are arranged with patient comfort and maneuverability as the first priority. The patients also have access to a large

*Gratitude is expressed to Kathleen Hale for her contributions to this chapter in the first edition.

communal dining room. The primary care givers are registered professional nurses. Nonpatient care activities are supplied by messenger–attendants and ward secretaries. The center's philosophy, as stated by Bowar-Ferres (1975), is as follows:

> Loeb's primary purpose was and is to demonstrate that high quality nursing care given by registered nurses, in a non-directive setting, offers a supportive setting to people in the post-acute phase of their illness that enables them to recover sooner, and to leave the center able to cope with themselves and what they must face in the future (p. 810).

To create a nondirective setting, there are very few rules or routines, no schedules, and no dictated mealtimes or specified visiting hours (Bower-Ferres, 1975). The nurses at Loeb strive to help the patient determine and clarify goals and, with the patient, work out ways to achieve the goals at the individual's pace, consistent with the medical treatment plan and congruent with the patient's sense of self.

LYDIA HALL'S THEORY OF NURSING

Lydia Hall presented her theory of nursing visually by drawing three interlocking circles, each circle presenting a particular aspect of nursing. The circles represent *care, core,* and *cure.*

The Care Circle

The care circle (Fig. 6–1) represents the nurturing component of nursing and is exclusive to nursing. Nurturing involves using the factors that make up

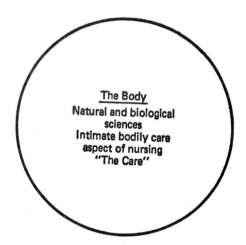

The Body
Natural and biological sciences
Intimate bodily care aspect of nursing
"The Care"

Figure 6–1. The care circle of patient care. *(From Hall, L. Nursing—What is it? p. 1. Publication of the Virginia State Nurses' Assocation, Winter 1959. Used with permission.)*

the concept of mothering (care and comfort of the person) and provide for teaching–learning activities.

The professional nurse provides bodily care for the patient and helps the patient to complete such basic daily biological functions as eating, bathing, elimination, and dressing. When providing this care, the nurse's goal is the comfort of the patient.

Providing care for a patient at the basic needs level presents the nurse and patient with an opportunity for closeness. As closeness develops, the patient can share and explore feelings with the nurse. This opportunity to explore feelings represents the teaching–learning aspect of nurturing.

When functioning in the care circle, the nurse applies knowledge of the natural and biological sciences to provide a strong theoretical base for nursing implementations. In interactions with the patient the nurse's role needs to be clearly defined. A strong theory base allows the nurse to maintain a professional status rather than a mothering status, while at the same time incorporating closeness and nurturance in giving care. The patient views the nurse as a potential comforter, one who provides care and comfort through the laying on of hands.

The Core Circle

The core circle (Fig. 6–2) of patient care is based in the social sciences, involves the therapeutic use of self, and is shared with other members of the health team. The professional nurse, by developing an interpersonal relationship with the patient, is able to help the patient verbally express feelings regarding the disease process and its effects. Through such expression the patient is able to gain self-identity and further develop maturity. As Hall (1965) says:

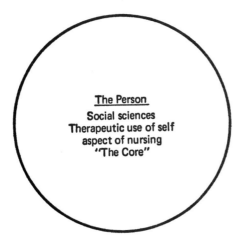

The Person
Social sciences
Therapeutic use of self
aspect of nursing
"The Core"

Figure 6–2. The core circle of patient care. *(From Hall, L. Nursing—What is it? p. 1. Used with permission.)*

To look at and listen to self is often too difficult without the help of a significant figure (nurturer) who has learned how to hold up a mirror and sounding board to invite the behaver to look and listen to himself. If he accepts the invitation, he will explore the concerns in his acts and as he listens to his exploration through the reflection of the nurse, he may uncover in sequence his difficulties, the problem area, his problem, and eventually the threat which is dictating his out-of-control behavior.

The professional nurse, by use of the reflective technique (acting as a mirror for the patient), helps the patient look at and explore feelings regarding his or her current health status and related potential changes in life style. The nurse uses a freely offered closeness to help the patient bring into awareness the verbal and nonverbal messages being sent to others. Motivations are discovered through the process of bringing into awareness the feelings being experienced. With this awareness the patient is now able to make conscious decisions based on understood and accepted feelings and motivations. The motivation and energy necessary for healing exist within the patient, rather than in the health care team.

The Cure Circle

The cure circle of patient care (Fig. 6–3) is based in the pathological and therapeutic sciences and is shared with other members of the health team. The professional nurse helps the patient and family through the medical, surgical, and rehabilitative prescriptions made by the physician. During this aspect of nursing care, the nurse is an active advocate of the patient.

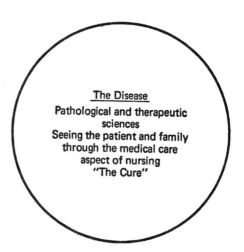

Figure 6–3. The cure circle of patient care. *(From Hall, L. Nursing—What is it? p. 1. Used with permission.)*

The nurse's role during the cure aspect is different from the care circle because many of the nurse's actions take on a negative quality of avoidance of pain rather than a positive quality of comforting. This is negative in the sense that the patient views the nurse as a potential cause of pain, one who is involved in such actions as administering injections, versus the potential comforter who provides care and comfort.

Interaction of the Three Aspects of Nursing

Because Hall emphasizes the importance of a total person approach, it is important that the three aspects of nursing (see Fig. 6–4) not be viewed as functioning independently but as interrelated. The three aspects interact, and the circles representing them change size, depending on the patient's total course of progress.

In the philosophy of Loeb Center, the professional nurse functions most therapeutically when patients have entered the second stage of their hospital stay (ie, they are recuperating and are past the acute stage of illness). During this recuperation stage, the care and core aspects are the most prominent, and the cure aspect is less prominent (see Fig. 6–5). The size of the circles represents the degree to which the patient is progressing in each of the three areas. The professional nurse at this time is able to help the patient reach the core of his problem through the closeness provided by the care aspect of nursing.

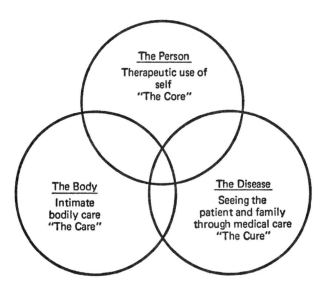

Figure 6–4. Hall's three aspects of nursing.

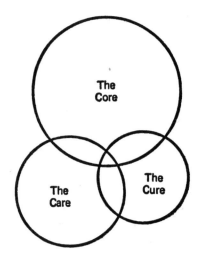

Figure 6-5. Care and core predominate.

HALL'S THEORY AND NURSING'S METAPARADIGM

Although the concept of nursing is identified by Hall, she does not speak directly to the other three concepts of human, health, and society/environment. However, inferences can be made from her work, as noted below.

The *individual* human who is 16 years of age or older and past the acute stage of a long-term illness is the focus of nursing care in Hall's work. The source of energy and motivation for healing is the individual care recipient, not the health care provider. Hall emphasizes the importance of the individual as unique, capable of growth and learning, and requiring a total person approach.

Health can be inferred to be a state of self-awareness with conscious selection of behaviors that are optimal for that individual. Hall stresses the need to help the person explore the meaning of his or her behavior to identify and overcome problems through developing self-identity and maturity.

The concept of *society/environment* is dealt with in relation to the individual. Hall is credited with developing the concept of Loeb Center because she assumed that the hospital environment during treatment of acute illness creates a difficult psychological experience for the ill individual (Bowar-Ferres, 1975). Loeb Center focuses on providing an environment that is conducive to self-development. In such a setting, the focus of the action of nurses is the individual, so that any actions taken in relation to society or environment are for the purpose of assisting the individual in attaining a personal goal.

Nursing is identified as consisting of participation in the care, core, and cure aspects of patient care. Care is the sole function of nurses, whereas core and cure are shared with other members of the health care team. However, the major purpose of care is to achieve an interpersonal relationship with the individual that will facilitate the development of core (ie, the development of self-identity and self-direction by the patient).

HALL'S THEORY AND THE NURSING PROCESS

Hall places the motivation and energy needed for healing within the patient. This aspect of her theory influences the nurse's total approach to the five phases of the nursing process: assessment, diagnosis, planning, implementation, and evaluation.

The *assessment* phase involves collection of data about the health status of the individual. According to Hall, the process of data collection is directed for the benefit of the patient rather than for the benefit of the nurse. Data collection should be directed toward increasing the patient's self-awareness. Through use of observation and reflection, the nurse is able to assist the patient in becoming aware of both verbal and nonverbal behaviors. In the individual, increased awareness of feelings and needs in relation to health status increases the ability for self-healing.

The assessment phase also pertains to guiding the patient through the cure aspect of nursing. The health team collects biological data (physical and laboratory) to help the patient and family understand and progress through the medical regimen.

The second phase is the *nursing diagnosis*, or statement of the patient's need or problem area. How a nurse envisions the nursing role influences the interpretation of assessment data and conclusions reached. Viewing the patient as the power for self-healing directs conclusions differently than if the healing power rests in the physician or nurse. The patient is the one in control, the one who identifies the need.

Planning involves setting priorities and mutually establishing patient-centered goals. The patient decides what is of highest priority and also what goals are desirable.

The core is involved in planning. The role of the nurse is to use reflection to help the patient become aware of and understand needs, feelings, and motivations. Once motivations are clarified, Hall indicates that the patient is the best person to set goals and arrange priorities. The nurse seeks to increase patient awareness and to support decision making based on the patient's new level of awareness. The nurse works with the patient to help keep the goals consistent with the medical prescription. The nurse needs to draw on a knowledge base in the social and scientific areas to present the patient with creative alternatives from which to choose.

Implementation involves the actual institution of the plan of care. This phase is the actual giving of nursing care. In the care and core circles, the nurse works with the patient, helping with bathing, dressing, eating, and other care and comfort needs. The professional nurse uses a "permissive non-directive teaching–learning approach" to implement nursing care, thus helping the patient reach the established goals (Bowar-Ferres, 1975, p. 813). This includes "helping the patient with his feelings, providing requested information and supporting patient-made decisions" (Brown, 1970, p. 159). The nurse also helps the patient and family through the cure aspect of nursing, working with the patient and family to help them understand and implement the medical plan.

Evaluation is the process of assessing the patient's progress toward the health goals. The evaluation phase of the process is directed toward deciding whether or not the patient is successful in reaching the established goals. The following questions apply to the use of Hall's theory in the evaluation phase:

1. Is the patient learning "who he is, where he wants to go, and how he wants to get there?" (Bowar-Ferres, 1975, p. 813.)
2. Is the patient learning to understand and explore the feelings that underlie behavior?
3. Is the nurse helping the patient see motivations more clearly?
4. Are the patient's goals congruent with the medical regime? Is the patient successful in meeting the goals?
5. Is the patient physically more comfortable?

Whether or not a person is growing in self-awareness regarding his or her feelings and motivations can be recognized through changes in his or her outward behavior.

HALL'S WORK AND THE CHARACTERISTICS OF A THEORY

Hall's work can be compared to the characteristics of a theory as presented in Chapter 1.

1. Theories can interrelate concepts in such a way as to create a different way of looking at a particular phenomenon. The use of the terms *care, core,* and *cure* is unique to Hall. She interrelated these concepts and in 1963 provided a different way of looking at the phenomenon of care of the individual with a long-term illness, which was an acute social problem of the time. Although other developments in health care have altered the need to some extent, her ideas are still relevant and useful, particularly if some of the limitations she imposed are removed. For example, care, core, and cure needs exist in acute and ambulatory settings and in individuals younger than 16.

2. Theories must be logical in nature. On first reading, Hall's work appears to be completely and simply logical. However, closer scrutiny reveals that although Hall indicates that care, the bodily laying on of hands, is the only aspect that is solely nursing—implying that it is the major focus for nursing—her major emphasis is on core. The care aspect is a means for achieving core rather than an end in itself (Barnum, 1994). Although this is not illogical, the initial impression is not the true logic of the work.

3. Theories should be relatively simple yet generalizable. Hall's work is simple in its presentation. However, the openness and flexibility required for its application may not be so simple for nurses whose personality, educational preparation, and experience have not prepared them to function with minimal structure. This and the self-imposed age and illness requirements limit the generalizability. Although the need for structure is a personal characteristic of the nurse, the limitations of age and stage of illness do not necessarily apply outside of Loeb Center.

4. Theories are the bases for hypotheses that can be tested or for theory to be expanded, and 5. Theories contribute to and assist in increasing the general body of knowledge within the discipline through the research implemented to validate them. These two characteristics are certainly true for Hall's work and have been demonstrated in the research conducted to evaluate the effectiveness of Loeb Center. This research was conducted at Hall's insistence, in spite of the enthusiastic acceptance of her philosophy by those in the Montefiore health care community (Brown, 1970). This research is evidence that hypotheses can be developed and tested. In addition, the sharing of a report about the Loeb Center in a Congressional hearing is evidence of an increase in the general body of knowledge (Loeb Center, 1963).

6. Theories can be used by practitioners to guide and improve their practice. If no other characteristic of a theory was met by Hall's work, the Loeb Center is an ideal demonstration of this characteristic. Hall's work was designed for practice and has been implemented successfully.

7. Theories must be consistent with other validated theories, laws, and principles but will leave open unanswered questions that need to be investigated. Hall recognized the importance of knowledge of validated theories, laws, and principles. She indicated the theoretical base for each of the aspects of patient care. The care aspect is based in the natural and biological sciences, core in the social sciences, and cure in the pathological and therapeutic sciences. The specific applications of these sciences provide a source of unanswered questions to be investigated.

Hall's work presents interrelated concepts in a way that provides a new view of a particular phenomenon. It is logical in nature, simpler in presentation than application but capable of being generalized, can be the basis of testable hypotheses, has led to research, is used by practitioners to guide practice, and is consistent with other validated theories, laws, and principles. Thus, her work may be considered a theory.

APPLICATION AND LIMITATIONS OF THE THEORY

Hall's theory of nursing has several areas that limit its application to patient care. The first of these areas is the stage of illness. Hall applies her ideas of nursing to a patient who has passed the acute stage of biological stress—that is, the patient who is experiencing the acute stage of illness is not included in Hall's approach to nursing care. However, it is possible to apply the care, core, and cure ideas to the care of those who are acutely ill. The acutely ill individual often needs care in relation to basic needs, as well as core awareness of what is going on and, in cure, understanding of the plan of medical care.

A second limiting factor is age. Hall refers only to adult patients in the second stage of their illness, thus eliminating all younger patients. On the basis of this theory, Loeb Center admits only patients 16 years of age and older. However, it would be possible to apply Hall's theory with younger individuals. Certainly adolescents younger than 16 are capable of seeking self-identity.

A third limiting factor is the description of how to help a person toward self-awareness. The only tool of therapeutic communication Hall discusses is reflection. By inference, all other techniques of therapeutic communication are eliminated. This emphasis on reflection arises from the belief that both the problem and the solution lie in the individual and that the nurse's function is to help the individual find them. But reflection is not always the most effective technique to be used. Other techniques, such as active listening and nonverbal support, may be used to facilitate the development of self-identity.

Fourth, the family is mentioned only in the cure circle. This means that the nursing contact with families is used only in regard to the patient's own medical care. It does not allow for helping a family increase awareness of the family's self.

Finally, Hall's theory relates only to those who are ill. This would indicate no nursing contact with healthy individuals, families, or communities, and it negates the concept of health maintenance and health care to prevent illness.

Basically, Hall's theory can be readily applied within the confines of the definition of adults past the acute stage of illness. However, this is too confining for a total view of nursing, which includes working with individuals, families, and communities throughout the life cycle and in varying states of health.

However, it should be noted that the nurse who uses Hall's theory functions in a manner similar to the method of assignment known as primary nursing. Considering that Hall instituted Loeb Center in the early 1960s, her ideas certainly provided leadership and innovation in nursing practice. She also deserves praise for having the courage to create a new environment in which to put her ideas into practice.

SUMMARY

Hall's theory of nursing involves three interlocking circles, each representing one aspect of nursing. The care aspect represents intimate bodily care of the patient. The core aspect deals with the innermost feelings and motivations of the patient. The cure aspect tells how the nurse helps the patient and family through the medical aspect of care. The main tool the nurse uses to help the patient realize his or her motivations and to grow in self-awareness is that of reflection.

Of the major concepts in nursing's metaparadigm, only nursing is defined as the function necessary to carry out care, core, and cure. Hall presents a philosophical view of humans as having the energy and motivation for self-awareness and growth. Definitions of health and society or environment must be inferred. Her work may be considered a theory because it meets each of the characteristics of theories presented in Chapter 1.

Lydia Hall's theory may be used in the nursing process. The core, care, and cure aspects are all applicable to each phase of the nursing process. The limitations of Hall's theory—illness orientation, age, restrictions on family contact, and use of reflection only—can be overcome by taking a broader view of care, core, and cure and by emphasizing the aspect that is most appropriate for a particular situation.

REFERENCES

Barnum, B. J. S. (1994). *Nursing theory: Analysis, application, evaluation* (4th ed.). Philadelphia: Lippincott.

Bowar-Ferres, S. (1975). Loeb Center and its philosophy of nursing. *The American Journal of Nursing, 75,* 810–815.

Brown, E. L. (1970). *Nursing reconsidered: A study of change, Part 1: The professional role in institutional nursing.* Philadelphia: Lippincott.

Hall, L. (1959). *Nursing—What is it?* Publication of the Virginia State Nurses Association.

Hall, L. (1965). Another view of nursing care and quality. Address given at Catholic University Workshop, Washington, D.C.

Loeb Center for Nursing and Rehabilitation Project Report, Congressional Record, May–June 1963, pp. 1515–1562.

BIBLIOGRAPHY

Alfano, G. (1984). Administration means working with nurses. *American Journal of Nursing, 64,* 83–85.

Alfano, G. (1969). Loeb Center. *Nursing Clinics of North America, 4,* 3.

Bernardin, E. (1964). Loeb Center—As the staff nurse sees it. *American Journal of Nursing, 64,* 85–86.

Hall, L. (1955). Quality of nursing care. *Public Health News, New Jersey State Department of Health, 36,* 212–215.

Hall, L. (1963). A center for nursing. *Nursing Outlook, 2,* 805–806.

Hall, L. (1964). Can nursing care hasten recovery? *American Journal of Nursing, 64,* 6.

Hall, L. (1969). The Loeb Center for Nursing and Rehabilitation at Montefiore Hospital and Medical Center. *International Journal of Nursing Studies, 6,* 81–95.

Isler, C. (1964). New concepts in nursing therapy: More care as the patient improves. *RN, 27,* 58–70.

DOROTHEA E. OREM

Peggy Coldwell Foster
Agnes M. Bennett*

■ ■ ■

Dorothea E. Orem, MSNEd, DSc, RN was born in 1914 in Baltimore, Maryland. She began her nursing education at Providence Hospital School of Nursing in Washington, DC. After receiving her diploma in the early 1930s, she earned her Bachelor of Science in nursing education in 1939 and her Master of Science in nursing education in 1945 from the Catholic University of America.

She has received several honorary degrees including a Doctor of Science from Georgetown University in 1976; Doctor of Science from the Incarnate Word College, San Antonio, Texas, in 1980; and Doctor of Humane Letters from Illinois Western University, Bloomington, Illinois, in 1988. Orem is a member of Sigma Theta Tau and Pi Gamma Mu. She has received several national awards, including the Catholic University of America's Alumni Achievement Award for Nursing Theory in 1980, and the Linda Richards Award from the National League for Nursing in 1991. Orem was named an Honorary Fellow of the American Academy of Nursing in 1992.

During her professional nursing career, she has worked as a staff nurse, private duty nurse, nurse educator, nurse administrator, and consultant. Orem continues to work as a nurse consultant and to develop her nursing theory.

> *If you give a man a fish he will have a single meal; If you teach him how to fish he will eat all his life.* —Kuan Tzer

During 1958–1959, as a consultant to the Office of Education, Department of Health, Education, and Welfare, Dorothea E. Orem participated in a project to improve practical (vocational) nurse training. This work stimulated her to consider the question, "What condition exists in a person when that person or others determine that that person should be under nursing care?" Her answer encompassed the idea that a nurse is "another self." This idea evolved into her nursing concept of "self-care" (Orem, 1991, p. 3). That is,

*Gratitude is expressed to Nancy Janssens for her contributions to this chapter in previous editions.

when they are able, individuals care for themselves. When the person is unable to provide self-care, then the nurse provides the assistance needed. For children, nursing care is needed when the parents or guardians are unable to provide the amount and quality of care needed.

In 1959, Orem's concept of nursing as the provision of self-care was first published. In 1965, she joined with several faculty members from the Catholic University of America to form a Nursing Model Committee. In 1968, a portion of the Nursing Model Committee, including Orem, continued their work through the Nursing Development Conference Group (NDCG). This group was formed to produce a conceptual framework for nursing and to establish the discipline of nursing. The NDCG published *Concept formalization in nursing: Process and product* in 1973 and 1979.

Orem further developed her nursing concepts of self-care and in 1971 published *Nursing: Concepts of practice*. The second, third and fourth editions of this book were published in 1980, 1985, and 1991. The first edition focused on the individual. The second edition was expanded to include multiperson units (families, groups, and communities). The third edition presented Orem's general theory of nursing as it is constituted from three related theoretical constructs: self-care, self-care deficits, and nursing systems. In the fourth edition (1991) her writing incorporates a greater emphasis on the child, groups, and society.

OREM'S GENERAL THEORY OF NURSING

Orem (1991) states her general theory as follows:

> The condition that validates the existence of a requirement for nursing in an adult is *the absence of the ability to maintain continuously that amount and quality of self-care which is therapeutic in sustaining life and health, in recovering from disease or injury, or in coping with their effects*. With children, the condition is the *inability of the parent (or guardian) to maintain continuously for the child the amount and quality of care that is therapeutic* (p. 41).

Orem developed the Self-Care Deficit Theory of Nursing (her general theory), which is composed of three interrelated theories: (1) the theory of self-care, (2) the self-care deficit theory, and (3) the theory of nursing systems. Incorporated within these three theories are six central concepts and one peripheral concept. Understanding these central concepts of self-care, self-care agency, therapeutic self-care demand, self-care deficit, nursing agency, and nursing system, as well as the peripheral concept of basic conditioning factors, is essential to understanding her general theory.

The Theory of Self-Care

To understand the theory of self-care it is important to understand the concepts of self-care, self-care agency, basic conditioning factors, and therapeutic self-care demand. *Self-care* is the performance or practice of activities that individuals initiate and perform on their own behalf to maintain life, health, and well-being. When self-care is effectively performed, it helps to maintain structural integrity and human functioning, and it contributes to human development (Orem, 1991).

Self-care agency is the human's ability or power to engage in self-care. The individual's ability to engage in self-care is affected by basic conditioning factors. These *basic conditioning factors* are age, gender, developmental state, health state, sociocultural orientation, health care system factors (i.e., diagnostic and treatment modalities), family system factors, patterns of living (eg, activities regularly engaged in), environmental factors, and resource adequacy and availability. "Normally, adults voluntarily care for themselves. Infants, children, the aged, the ill, and the disabled require complete care or assistance with self-care activities" (Orem, 1991, p. 117). The *therapeutic self-care demand* is the totality of "self-care actions to be performed for some duration in order to meet known self-care requisites by using valid methods and related sets of operations and actions" (p. 123). The therapeutic self-care demand is modeled on deliberate action—that is, "action deliberately performed by some members of a social group to bring about events and results that benefit others in specified ways" (p. 79).

An additional concept incorporated within the theory of self-care is self-care requisites. Orem (1991) presents three categories of *self-care requisites,* or requirements, as: (1) universal, (2) developmental, and (3) health deviation. Self-care requisites can be defined as actions directed toward the provision of self-care. *Universal self-care requisites* are associated with life processes and the maintenance of the integrity of human structure and functioning. They are common to all human beings during all stages of the life cycle and should be viewed as interrelated factors, each affecting the others. A common term for these requisites is the activities of daily living. Orem (1991) identifies self-care requisites as follows:

1. The maintenance of a sufficient intake of air.
2. The maintenance of a sufficient intake of water.
3. The maintenance of a sufficient intake of food . . .
4. The provision of care associated with elimination processes and excrements.
5. The maintenance of a balance between activity and rest.
6. The maintenance of a balance between solitude and social interaction.
7. The prevention of hazards to human life, human functioning, and human well-being.
8. The promotion of human functioning and development within social groups in accord with human potential, known human

limitations, and the human desire to be normal. *Normalcy* is used in the sense of that which is essentially human and that which is in accord with the genetic and constitutional characteristics and the talents of individuals (p. 126).

Developmental self-care requisites are "either specialized expressions of universal self-care requisites that have been particularized for developmental processes or they are new requisites derived from a condition . . . or associated with an event" (Orem, 1991, p. 130). Examples are adjusting to a new job or adjusting to body changes such as facial lines or hair loss.

Health deviation self-care is required in conditions of illness, injury, or disease or may result from medical measures required to diagnose and correct the condition (eg, right upper quadrant abdominal pain when foods with a high fat content are eaten, or learning to walk using crutches following the casting of a fractured leg.) The health deviation self-care requisites are as follows:

1. Seeking and securing appropriate medical assistance . . .
2. Being aware of and attending to the effects and results of pathologic conditions and states . . .
3. Effectively carrying out medically prescribed diagnostic, therapeutic, and rehabilitative measures . . .
4. Being aware of and attending to or regulating the discomforting or deleterious effects of prescribed medical care measures . . .
5. Modifying the self-concept (and self-image) in accepting oneself as being in a particular state of health and in need of specific forms of health care
6. Learning to live with the effects of pathologic conditions and states and the effects of medical diagnostic and treatment measures in a life-style that promotes continued personal development (Orem, 1991, p. 134).

In the theory of self-care, Orem explains *what* is meant by self-care and lists the various factors that affect its provision. In the self-care deficit theory, she specifies *when* nursing is needed to assist the individual in the provision of self-care.

The Theory of Self-Care Deficit

The theory of self-care deficit is the core of Orem's (1991) general theory of nursing because it delineates when nursing is needed. Nursing is required when an adult (or in the case of a dependent, the parent or guardian) is incapable of or limited in the provision of continuous effective self-care. Nursing may be provided if the "care abilities are less than those required for meeting a known self-care demand . . . [or] self-care or dependent-care abilities exceed or are equal to those required for meeting the current self-care demand, but a future deficit relationship can be foreseen because of predictable decreases in care abilities, qualitative or quantitative increases in the care demand, or both" (p. 71); when individuals need "to incorporate newly prescribed, complex self-care measures into their self-care systems, the performance of which requires specialized knowledge and skills to be acquired through training and experience" (p. 174); or the individual needs help "in recovering from disease or injury, or in coping with their effects" (p. 41). It is important to note that the first category includes universal, developmental, and health-deviation self-care needs whereas the other categories focus on health-deviation self-care.

Orem (1991) identifies the following five methods of helping:

1. Acting for or doing for another
2. Guiding and directing
3. Providing physical or psychological support
4. Providing and maintaining an environment that supports personal development
5. Teaching (p. 9).

The nurse may help the individual by using any or all of these methods to provide assistance with self-care.

Orem presents a model to show the relationship between her concepts (Fig. 7–1). From this model it can be seen that at any given time an individual

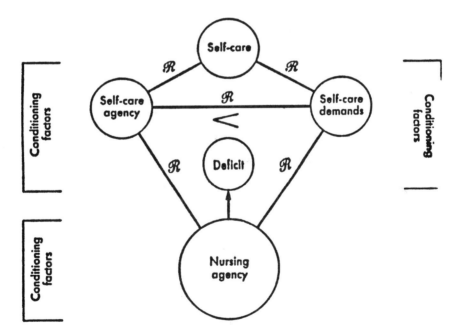

Figure 7–1. A conceptual framework for nursing. (R = relationship; < = deficit relationship, current or projected.) *(Used with permission from Orem, D. E. (1991).* Nursing: Concepts of practice *(4th ed.). St. Louis: Mosby, p. 64.)*

has specific self-care abilities as well as therapeutic self-care demands. If there are more demands than abilities, nursing is needed. The activities in which nurses engage when they provide nursing care can be used to describe the domain of nursing. Orem (1991) has identified five areas of activity for nursing practice:

- Entering into and maintaining nurse–patient relationships with individuals, families, or groups until patients can legitimately be discharged from nursing
- Determining if and how patients can be helped through nursing
- Responding to patients' requests, desires, and needs for nurse contacts and assistance
- Prescribing, providing, and regulating direct help to patients (and their significant others) in the form of nursing
- Coordinating and integrating nursing with the patient's daily living, other health care needed or being received, and social and educational services needed or being received (p. 340).

Self-care has been defined and the need for nursing explained in the first and second theories. In Orem's third theory of nursing systems, she outlines *how* the patient's self-care needs will be met by the nurse, the patient, or both.

The Theory of Nursing Systems

The nursing system, designed by the nurse, is based on the self-care needs *and* abilities of the patient to perform self-care activities. If there is a self-care deficit, that is, if there is a deficit between what the individual can do (self-care agency) and what needs to be done to maintain optimum functioning (self-care demand), then nursing is required.

Nursing agency is a complex property or attribute of people educated and trained as nurses that enables them to act, to know, and to help others meet their therapeutic self-care demands by exercising or developing their own self-care agency (Orem, 1991). Nursing agency is analogous to self-care agency in that both symbolize characteristics and abilities for specific types of deliberate action. They differ in that nursing agency is exercised for the benefit and well-being of others, and self-care agency is developed and exercised for the benefit of oneself.

Orem (1991) has identified three classifications of nursing systems to meet the self-care requisites of the patient (see Fig. 7–2). These systems are the wholly compensatory system, the partly compensatory system, and the supportive-educative system.

The design and elements of the nursing system define "(1) the scope of the nursing responsibility in health care situations; (2) the general and specific roles of nurses, patients, and others; (3) reasons for nurses' relationships with patients; and (4) the kinds of actions to be performed and the performance patterns and nurses' and patients' actions in regulating patients' self-care

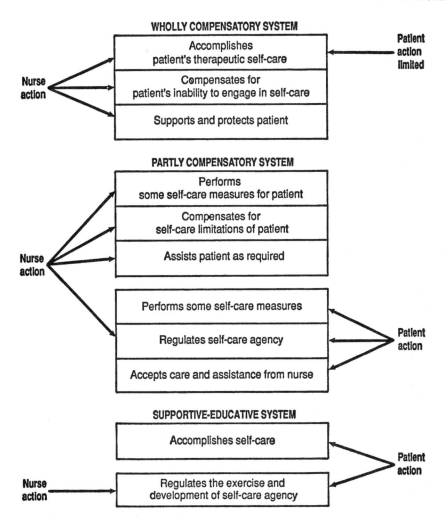

Figure 7–2. Basic nursing systems. *(Adapted with permission from Orem, D. E. (1991).* Nursing: Concepts of practice *(4th ed.), St. Louis: Mosby, p. 288.)*

agency and in meeting their therapeutic self-care demand" (Orem, 1991, pp. 285, 287).

The *wholly compensatory nursing system* is represented by a situation in which the individual is unable "to engage in those self-care actions requiring self-directed and controlled ambulation and manipulative movement or the medical prescription to refrain from such activity. . . . Persons with these limitations are socially dependent on others for their continued existence and well-being" (Orem, 1991, p. 289). Subtypes of the wholly compensatory system are nursing systems for people who are: "[1] unable to engage in any form of deliberate action, for example, persons in a coma, . . . [2] aware and who may be able to make observations, judgments, and decisions about self-care and other matters but cannot or should not perform actions requiring ambulation and manipulative movements, . . . [3] unable to attend to themselves and make reasoned judgments and decisions about self-care and other matters but who can be ambulatory and may be able to perform some measures of self-care with continuous guidance and supervision" (p. 289). Examples of persons in the second subtype could include those with C3–C4 vertebral fractures, and those in the third subtype, persons who are severely mentally retarded.

The *partly compensatory nursing system* is represented by a situation in which "both nurse and patient perform care measures or other actions involving manipulative tasks or ambulation. . . . [Either] the patient or the nurse may have the major role in the performance of care measures" (Orem, 1991, p. 291). An example of a person needing nursing care in the partly compensatory system would be an individual who has had recent abdominal surgery. This patient might be able to wash his or her face and brush his or her teeth but needs the nurse for help in ambulating and in changing the surgical dressing.

The third nursing system is the *supportive-educative system*. In this system, the person "is able to perform or can and should learn to perform required measures of externally or internally oriented therapeutic self-care but cannot do so without assistance" (Orem, 1991, p. 291). This is also known as a supportive-developmental system. In this system the patient is doing all of the self-care. The "patient's requirements for help are confined to decision making, behavior control, and acquiring knowledge and skills" (p. 291). The nurse's role, then, is to promote the patient as a self-care agent. An example of a person in this system would be a 16-year-old who is requesting birth control information. The nurse's role in this system is primarily that of a teacher or consultant.

One or more of the three types of systems may be used with a single patient. For example, a woman in labor may move from a supportive-educative system while she is in early labor to a partly compensatory system as her labor advances. If she requires a cesarean delivery, her care might require her to be in a wholly compensatory system. She would then progress to a partly compensatory system as she recovers from the anesthetic. Later, as she prepares to go home, a supportive-educative system would again be appropriate.

OREM'S THEORY AND NURSING'S METAPARADIGM

Orem discusses each of the four major concepts of human beings, health, society, and nursing in her work. "*Human beings* are distinguished from other living things by their capacity (1) to reflect upon themselves and their environment, (2) to symbolize what they experience, and (3) to use symbolic creations (ideas, words) in thinking, in communicating, and in guiding efforts to do and to make things that are beneficial for themselves or others" (Orem,

1991, p. 180). Integrated human functioning includes physical, psychological, interpersonal, and social aspects. Orem believes that individuals have the potential for learning and developing. The way an individual meets self-care needs is not instinctual but is a learned behavior. Factors that affect learning include age, mental capacity, culture, society, and the emotional state of the individual. If the individual cannot learn self-care measures, others must learn the care and provide it.

In the fourth edition of *Nursing: Concepts of practice*, Orem (1991) considers human beings from two different perspectives. The first is as persons viewed as moving "toward maturation and achievement of the individual's human potential. . . . *Self-realization* and *personality development* are terms used at times to refer to the process of personalization" (p. 185). The second perspective "focuses on structural and functional differentiations within the unity that is a human being . . . developed by various human and life sciences . . . [including] biochemistry, biophysics, human anatomy, and human physiology, . . . psychology, psychophysiology and social psychology" (p. 186). Orem emphasizes, however, that both perspectives need to be integrated for effective nursing.

Orem (1991) supports the World Health Organization's definition of *health* as the state of physical, mental, and social well-being and not merely the absence of disease or infirmity. She states that "the physical, psychological, interpersonal and social aspects of health are inseparable in the individual" (p. 180). Orem also presents health based on the concept of preventive health care. This health care includes the promotion and maintenance of health (primary prevention), the treatment of disease or injury (secondary prevention), and the prevention of complications (tertiary prevention).

About *nursing,* Orem (1991) states:

> In modern society, adults are expected to be self-reliant and responsible for themselves and for the well-being of their dependents. Most social groups further accept that persons who are helpless, sick, aged, handicapped, or otherwise deprived should be helped in their immediate distress and helped to attain or regain responsibility within their existing capacities. Thus, both self-help and help to others are valued by society as desirable activities. Nursing as a specific type of human service is based on both values. In most communities people see nursing as a desirable and necessary service (p. 41).

Orem speaks to several factors related to the concept of nursing. These are the art and prudence of nursing, nursing as a service, role theory related to nursing, and technologies in nursing. The art of nursing is "the quality of individual nurses that allows them to make creative investigations and analyses and syntheses of the variables and conditioning factors within nursing situations in order to work toward the goal of the production of effective systems of nursing assistance for individual or multiperson units" (p. 256).

These decisions require a theoretical base in the discipline of nursing and in the sciences, arts, and humanities. This base directs decisions when designing nursing systems within the nursing process. "*Nursing prudence* is the quality of nurses that enables them (1) to seek and take counsel in new or difficult nursing situations, (2) to make correct judgments . . . , (3) to decide to act in a particular way, and (4) to take action" (p. 256). The development of the individual nurse's art and prudence is affected by unique life and nursing experiences.

Orem (1991) further defines nursing as a human service. Nursing is distinguished from other human services by its focus on persons with inabilities to maintain the continuous provision of health care (pp. 4–5). Nursing is needed when the adult is unable "to maintain continuously that amount and quality of self-care which is therapeutic in sustaining life and health, in recovering from disease or injury, or in coping with their effects" (p. 41). With children, nursing is needed when the parent or guardian is unable to "maintain continuously for the child the amount and quality of care that is therapeutic" (p. 41). For children, nursing may be needed to assist with development or maturation.

The nurse's and the patient's roles define the expected behaviors for each in the specific nursing situation. Various factors that influence the expected role behaviors are culture, environment, age, sex, the health setting, and finances. The roles of nurse and patient are complementary. That is, a certain behavior of the patient elicits a certain response in the nurse, and vice versa. Both work together to accomplish the goal of self-care.

In the nurse–patient relationship, the nurse or patient may experience role conflict because each is performing concurrent roles; for example, the patient also has expected behaviors from his roles as father, husband, Cub Scout leader, soccer coach, and librarian. Thus, the conflict in the behaviors required for the various roles may affect the performance of self-care.

It is important to note that although Orem (1991) recognizes that specialized technologies are usually developed by members of the health professions, she emphasizes the need for social and interpersonal dimensions in nursing. The effective integration of social and interpersonal technologies with regulatory technologies promotes quality professional nursing. She states, "Treatment or regulatory operations are the practical activities through which what is prescribed is executed and through which the diagnosed condition or problem is treated in order to remove it[,] to control it or to keep it within boundaries compatible with human life, health, and well-being" (p. 266).

OREM'S THEORY AND THE NURSING PROCESS

According to Orem (1991), "Nursing process is a term used by nurses to refer to the professional-technologic operations of nursing practice and to associated planning and evaluative operations" (p. 269). Process is a continuous and regular action or succession of actions taking place or carried out in a definite manner.

TABLE 7-1. COMPARISON OF OREM'S NURSING PROCESS AND THE NURSING PROCESS

Nursing Process[a]	Orem's Nursing Process
1. Assessment 2. Nursing diagnosis	Step 1. Diagnosis and prescription; Determine why nursing is needed. Analyze and interpret–make judgments regarding care.
3. Plans with scientific rationale	Step 2. Design of a nursing system and plan for delivery of care.
4. Implementation 5. Evaluation	Step 3. Production and management of nursing systems.

[a]Five-step process outlined in Chapter 2 of this text.

Orem (1991) discusses a three-step nursing process which she labels the technologic process operations of nursing practice. These steps are shown in Table 7–1 as:

- Step 1. Nursing diagnosis and prescription—that is, determining why nursing is needed; analysis and interpretation—making judgments regarding care, also labeled case management operations.
- Step 2. Designing the nursing system and planning for delivery of care.
- Step 3. The production and management of nursing systems, also labeled planning and controlling.

Nursing Diagnosis and Prescription (Step 1)

"Nursing diagnosis necessitates investigation and the accumulation of facts about patients' self-care agency and their therapeutic self-care demand and the existent or projected relationships between them" (Orem, 1991, p. 270). The goal defines the direction and nature of the actions. Prescriptive operations specify the means (course of actions, care measures) to be used to meet particular self-care requisites, or to meet all components of the therapeutic self-care demand. Orem emphasizes that, in nursing diagnostic and prescriptive operations and in the regulatory or treatment operations, patients' and families' abilities and interests in collaboration affect what nurses can do.

Designs for Regulatory Operation (Step 2)

Designing an effective and efficient system of nursing involves selecting valid ways of assisting the patient. This design includes nurse and patient roles in relation to which self-care tasks will be performed when adjusting the therapeutic self-care demands, regulating the exercise of self-care agency, protecting the already developed powers of self-care agency, and assisting with the new developments in self-care agency (Orem, 1991).

Planning is the movement from the design of nursing systems to ways and means of their production. A plan sets forth the organization of essential tasks to be performed in accordance with role responsibilities (Orem, 1991). The planning for implementation of the design and related procurement activities determines when nurses should be with patients and when essential materials and equipment will be available and ready for use.

Production and Management of Nursing Systems (Step 3)

Regulatory nursing systems are produced when nurses interact with patients and take consistent action to meet their prescribed therapeutic self-care demands and regulate the exercise or development of their capabilities for self-care. In this, the third step of the technologic nursing process, nurses act to produce and manage nursing systems (Orem, 1991).

During the interactions of nurses and patients, nurses do the following:

1. Perform and regulate the self-care tasks for patients or assist patients with their performance of self-care tasks
2. Coordinate self-care task performance so that a unified system of care is produced and coordinated with other components of health care
3. Help patients, their families, and others bring about systems of daily living for patients that support the accomplishment of self-care and are, at the same time, satisfying in relation to patients' interests, talents, and goals
4. Guide, direct, and support patients in their exercise of, or in withholding the exercise of, their self-care agency
5. Stimulate patients' interest in self-care by raising questions and promoting discussions of care problems and issues when conditions permit
6. Support and guide patients in learning activities and provide cues for learning as well as instructional sessions
7. Support and guide patients as they experience illness or disability and the effects of medical care measures and as they experience the need to engage in new measures of self-care or change their ways of meeting ongoing self-care requisites
8. Monitor patients and assist patients to monitor themselves to determine if self-care measures were performed and to determine the effects of self-care, the results of efforts to regulate the exercise or development of self-care agency, and the sufficiency and efficiency of nursing action direction to these ends
9. Make characterizing judgments about the sufficiency and efficiency of self-care, the regulation of the exercise or development of self-care agency, and nursing assistance
10. Make judgments about the meaning of the results derived from nurses' performance of the preceding two operations for

the well-being of patients and make or recommend adjustments in the nursing care system through changes in nurse and patient roles (Orem, 1991, pp. 280–281).

The first seven operations constitute direct nursing care. The last three are for the purpose of deciding if the care provided should be continued in the present form or changed. This comprises the evaluation component of the nursing process.

The following example demonstrates the use of Orem's theory and the nursing process (see Tables 7–2 and 7–3):

Situation. Ms. M., a well-groomed university faculty member of Italian Catholic descent, is 48 years old, 5 feet 2 inches, and weighs 175 pounds. She smokes one and a half packs of cigarettes per day. She was very happily married for 25 years and has been widowed for six months. She and her husband enjoyed social activities, including playing bridge, gourmet cooking, and collecting antiques. She has not participated in any of these activities since her husband's death because of lack of interest and energy. Currently, she engages in no regular exercise, eats mainly fast foods during her 12-hour working day, and eats a late evening meal before retiring.

Ms. M.'s mother died of a stroke and her father had a heart attack at age 50. During her annual physical two weeks ago, her vital signs were 138/86, P 92, R 30, T 98.4 (F). Her laboratory values were all within normal limits except a blood cholesterol of 280 mg. Her physician advised her to lose 40 pounds but recognized that Ms. M. has inadequate knowledge of basic nutrition and has not been motivated to lose weight. He foresees potential problems related to cardiovascular disease.

Step 1. Orem defines Step 1 as the diagnosis and prescription phase, determining if nursing is needed. In this assessment phase, the nurse collects data in six areas:

1. The person's health status
2. The physician's perspective of the person's health
3. The person's perspective of his or her health
4. The health goals within the context of life history, life style, and health status
5. The person's requirements for self-care
6. The person's capacity to perform self-care

Specific data are gathered in the areas of the individual's universal, developmental, and health-deviation self-care needs and their interrelationship. Data are also collected about the individual's knowledge, skills, motivation, and orientation.

Within Step 1, the nurse seeks answers to the following questions:

TABLE 7–2. APPLICATION OF OREM'S THEORY TO NURSING PROCESS

	Assessment				
Personal Factors	Universal Self-Care	Developmental Self-Care	Health Deviations	Medical Problem and Plan	Self-Care Deficits
Age	Air, water, food	Specialized needs for developmental process	Conditions of illness or injury	Physician's perspective of condition	Difference between self-care needs and self-care capabilities
Sex	Excrements	New requisites from a condition	Treatments to correct the condition	Medical diagnosis	
Height	Activity and rest	Requisites associated with an event		Medical treatment	
Weight	Solitude and social interaction				
Culture	Hazards to life and well-being				
Race	Promotion of human functioning and development				
Marital Status					
Religion					
Occupation					

Nursing Diagnosis	Plan	Implementation	Evaluation
Based on self-care deficits	Nursing goals and objectives: a. Congruent with nursing diagnosis b. Based on self-care demands c. Promote patient as self-care agent Designing the Nursing System: a. Wholly compensatory b. Partly compensatory c. Supportive-educative Appropriate methods of helping: a. Guidance b. Support c. Teaching d. Acting or doing for e. Providing developmental environment	Nurse–patient actions to: a. Promote patient as self-care agent b. Meet self-care needs c. Decrease self-care deficits	Effectiveness of nurse–patient actions to: a. Promote patient as self-care agent b. Meet self-care needs c. Decrease self-care deficits

Adapted from Pinnell, N. N. & de Meneses, M. (1986). *The nursing process—Theory, application and related processes*, Norwalk, Conn.: Appleton-Century-Crofts, p. 66. Used with permission.

TABLE 7–3. APPLICATION OF OREM'S THEORY USING MS. M.'S CASE STUDY WITHIN THE NURSING PROCESS

Personal Factors	Universal Self-Care	Developmental Self-Care	Health Deviations	Medical Problem and Plan	Self-Care Deficits
48 yr	Smokes 1.5 ppd	Loss of husband	Potential for cardiac disease related to obesity, smoking, cholesterol, lack of exercise, family history	Diagnoses of obesity with potential for cardiac disease and low motivation for weight loss	Difference between Ms. M.'s knowledge base and life style which increases risk for heart attack or stroke
Female	Fast foods	Loss of social activity		Prescription to:	
5'2"	Late pm meal			Monitor cholesterol levels and vital signs	
175 lb	No data			Decrease cholesterol and fat intake	
Italian	No exercise			Increase exercise	
White	Decreased social interaction × 6 mo				
Catholic	Family history:				
University faculty	F—heart attack age 50				
	M—stroke				
	Cholesterol 280 mg				
	High-fat diet				
	Lacks knowledge of risk factors and cardiovascular functioning				
	T = 98.4				
	138/96				
	P = 92				
	R = 30				
	Works 12 hour days				
	Well groomed				

Nursing Diagnosis	Plan	Implementation	Evaluation
Potential for impaired cardiovascular functioning related to her lack of knowledge about relationship between current life style and risk of heart attack or stroke	Nursing goals and objectives: *Goal:* To decrease risk for cardiac impairment *Objective:* Ms. M. will state that high cholesterol levels increase her risk for cardiac impairment Design of Nursing System: Supportive-educative Methods of helping: Guidance, support, teaching, and provision of a developmental environment	Jointly develop contract related to goal of cholesterol reduction Ms. M. will keep a 3-day food diary Ms. M. will learn about cholesterol and its effects on cardiovascular functioning Ms. M. will request or obtain cholesterol and fat content of fast foods Ms. M. will learn about low cholesterol and fat foods, foods which decrease cholesterol, and restaurants which serve low cholesterol and fat foods Jointly analyze food diary and decide how to decrease choles-terol and fat intake Jointly determine Italian foods which are low in cholesterol and fat, or recipes which may be adapted Ms. M.'s accomplish-ments will be reinforced	Does Ms. M. understand that with her present life style her risk of heart attack or stroke is high? Did Ms. M. select low-cholesterol foods? Is Ms. M.'s cholesterol level lower? Did Ms. M.'s self-care deficit decrease? Was the supportive-educative system effective in promoting Ms. M. as a self-care agent?

1. What is the patient's therapeutic care demand? Now? At a future time?
2. Does the patient have a deficit for engaging in self-care to meet the therapeutic self-care demand?
3. If so, what is its nature and the reasons for its existence?
4. Should the patient be helped to refrain from engagement in self-care or to protect already developed self-care capabilities for therapeutic purposes?
5. What is the patient's potential for engaging in self-care at a future time period? Increasing or deepening self-care knowledge? Learning techniques of self-care? Fostering willingness to engage in self-care? Effectively and consistently incorporating essential self-care measures (including new ones) into the systems of self-care and daily living? (Orem, 1985, pp. 225–226).

Once the assessment data have been gathered, they must be analyzed. In the category of universal self-care needs, Ms. M. demonstrates a deficit in adequate air, water, and food intake because she is 5 feet 2 inches, weighs 175 pounds, and consumes excessive calories, fat, and cholesterol from fast food and late-night meals. Ms. M. shows an imbalance between activity and rest because she has minimal exercise. There is also an imbalance between her solitude and social interaction since her husband's death, which is a significant loss for her in the mid-life developmental needs category. Ms. M.'s elevated cholesterol levels, when interrelated with her family history of stroke and heart attack, present a hazard to her life, functioning, and well-being. The physician's perspective is that Ms. M. needs to lose 40 pounds because of her family history and elevated blood cholesterol but that she has limited nutritional knowledge. However, Ms. M. has a motivational deficit to lose weight because her Italian cultural tradition associates food with family and love.

Based on the analysis of Ms. M.'s data, she has potential hazards to her health related to obesity, high cholesterol, smoking, social isolation, and decreased exercise. The analysis of the collected data leads to the nursing diagnosis, enabling the nurse to prioritize self-care deficits. The nursing diagnosis must include the response and etiology pattern. Within Orem's framework, the nursing diagnosis would be stated as an inability to meet the self-care demand (the response) related to the self-care deficit (etiology) (Ziegler, Vaughn-Wrobel, & Erlen, 1986). For Ms. M. the response pattern would be "potential for impaired cardiovascular functioning," and the etiology would be "lack of knowledge about how her current life style increases her risk for heart attack and stroke." Therefore, for Ms. M. the nursing diagnosis could be stated: "Potential for impaired cardiovascular functioning related to lack of knowledge about how her current life style increases her risk for heart attack and stroke."

Step 2. Orem defines Step 2 as designing the nursing systems and planning for the delivery of nursing. The nurse designs a system that is wholly compensatory, partly compensatory, or supportive-educative. "The actual design of a concrete nursing system emerges as nurses and patients interact and take action in order to calculate and meet patient's therapeutic self-care demands, to compensate for or overcome the identified action limitations of patients, and to regulate the development and exercise of patients' self-care abilities" (Orem, 1991, p. 285).

Using Orem's model, the goals are congruent with the nursing diagnosis to enable the patient to become an effective self-care agent. Goals are directed by the response statement of the nursing diagnosis and are focused on health. The goal for Ms. M. would be: Decrease her risk of cardiovascular impairment.

Once the goals have been determined, the objectives can be stated. An example of an objective for Ms. M. would be: Ms. M. will state that high cholesterol levels increase her risk for cardiac impairment. Other objectives might relate to the risk factors of obesity, lack of exercise, smoking, and family history. The designed nursing system for Ms. M. would be the supportive-educative nursing system.

Step 3. Within Orem's (1991) nursing process, Step 3 includes the production and management of the nursing system. In this step, the nurse performs and regulates the patient's self-care tasks, or assists the patient in doing so; coordinates the performance of self-care with other components of health care; helps patients, families and others create and use systems of daily living that meet self-care needs in a satisfying way; guides, directs, and supports patients in exercising, or not exercising, self-care agency; stimulates patient's interest in care problems; supports learning activities; supports and guides the patient in adapting the needs arising from medical measures; monitors and assists in self-monitoring the performance and effects of self-care measures; judges the sufficiency and efficiency of self-care, self-care agency, and nursing agency; adjusts the nursing care system as needed.

The nurse and patient actions are directed by the etiology component of the nursing diagnosis. "Lack of knowledge about how her current life style increases her risk for heart attack and stroke" is the etiology component of Ms. M.'s nursing diagnosis. When the nurse and patient implement this supportive-educative system, each has specific roles. Examples of these roles might be: Together they would develop a contract relating to the goal of blood cholesterol reduction. Ms. M. would keep a three-day food diary. The nurse would provide information about cholesterol and its effects on cardiovascular function. Ms. M. would request and obtain the fat and cholesterol content of the fast-food menu items from the restaurants she frequents. The nurse would provide information about specific foods that are low in fat and cholesterol, those food items that help reduce cholesterol, and a list of fast-food restaurants that offer low-fat and low-cholesterol food items. Together they would analyze the three-day food diary and decide how Ms. M. might modify her diet to reduce her fat and cholesterol intake. They would determine which Italian dishes are low in fat and cholesterol or how these recipes can be adapted. As her blood cholesterol levels decrease, Ms. M. would be praised for her accomplishments. During this implementation, the nurse would teach, guide, and support Ms. M. while providing a developmental environment.

Step 3 includes evaluation. The nurse and patient together do the evaluation. Questions they might ask are: When evaluating some of Ms. M.'s plans, does she understand that her present life style may increase her risk of developing a heart attack or stroke? Did she select low-fat and low-cholesterol fast foods? Did she attain her goal of reducing her blood cholesterol levels? Were the plans effective in decreasing the self-care deficit? Was the nursing system effective in promoting the patient as a self-care agent?

Evaluation is an ongoing process. It is essential that the nurse and patient continually evaluate any changes in the data that would affect the self-care deficit, the self-care agent, and the nursing system.

OREM'S WORK AND THE CHARACTERISTICS OF A THEORY

Orem presented a conceptual framework in 1959. Since then her work has continued to evolve. Orem's general theory of nursing was formulated and expressed in 1979–1980. This Self-Care Deficit Theory of Nursing is comprised of three interrelated theories: the theory of self-care, the theory of self-care deficit, and the theory of nursing systems. In the following seven paragraphs, Orem's general theory is compared with the characteristics of a theory from Chapter 1 of this text.

1. **Theories can interrelate concepts in such a way as to create a different way of looking at a particular phenomenon.** Orem's theoretical constructs of self-care, self-care deficits, and nursing systems are interrelated in her general comprehensive theory of nursing. This interrelationship provides a view of the practice of nursing (a particular phenomenon) that is unique.

2. **Theories must be logical in nature.** Orem's theory follows a logical thought process. She states her general theory, then presents the central idea of each of the three interrelated theories. In her discussion of each interrelated theory, she presents presuppositions that express larger contexts within which the theory or its parts can be understood. She also presents propositions or statements that describe a concept or explain and predict the relationship between concepts.

3. **Theories should be relatively simple yet generalizable.** Orem's theory has been used in both nursing education and practice. The theory is used by several schools of nursing as a theoretical foundation for a student's basic preparation for practice. Orem's concept of self-care with its proposition of universal self-care needs is easily understood by beginning and advanced nursing practitioners as the activities of daily living. The theories of self-care deficits and nursing systems can be comprehended and applied to all individual patients and, with further adaptation, to multiperson units.

4. **Theories are the bases for hypotheses that can be tested or for theory to be expanded.** Orem's theory of self-care has been used to generate testable hypotheses in a variety of settings. Several researchers have tested

Orem's theory in the area of self-care agency, including studies focused on the development of tools to measure aspects of self-care (see Bibliography at end of chapter).

5. Theories contribute to and assist in increasing the general body of knowledge within the discipline through the research implemented to validate them. Orem focuses on nursing as a helping art that assists an individual to meet self-care needs and that is the foundation for nursing practice. Research on self-care needs and the assistance to meet them adds to nursing's body of knowledge. Orem's theory is being tested by several nursing researchers.

6. Theories can be used by the practitioners to guide and improve their practice. Orem's theory is used by nurses in a variety of settings. These settings include that of an independent practitioner of nursing, rehabilitation, hemodialysis, bone marrow transplant, psychiatric care, and public and community health. Others have documented self-care in relation to children in pain and with leukemia, women with gestational diabetes, persons receiving enterostomal therapy, adult diabetics, the elderly, and the terminally ill (see Bibliography at end of chapter).

7. Theories must be consistent with other validated theories, laws, and principles but will leave open unanswered questions that need to be investigated. Orem's theory is consistent with role theory, need theory, field theory, and health promotion concepts. For example, she discusses the importance of an understanding of the roles of nurse and patient while determining the patient's need for nursing care.

STRENGTHS AND LIMITATIONS

In the preface to the fourth edition of *Nursing: Concepts of practice,* Orem (1991) outlines the following five broad divisions: contextual and process features of nursing practice, the self-care deficit theory of nursing, the characteristics of nursing as a practical science, nursing administration, and nursing education. In the text she describes her general theory, which is supported by three interrelated theories. Within these theories, six central concepts and one peripheral concept are identified. These provide the reader with a blueprint for the structure of Orem's Self-Care Deficit Theory of Nursing.

Orem's theory is derived from a clinical base. She states that, "in working on the components of [her] theory [she] needs to work with other people—utilizing data from clinicians" (Trench, Wallace, & Coberg, 1988). She cites Susan Taylor's work, which includes the position of family involvement within the self-care deficit nursing theory (Orem, 1991). Also, the Self-Care Deficit Theory of Nursing has been supported by clinical case-study data (Orem & Taylor, 1986).

Orem's theory of nursing provides a comprehensive base for nursing practice. It has utility for professional nursing in the areas of education, clinical practice, administration, research, and nursing information systems. A major strength of Orem's theory is that it is applicable for nursing by the beginning practitioner as well as the advanced clinician. The terms *self-care, nursing systems,* and *self-care deficit* are easily understood by the beginning nursing student and can be explored in greater depth as the nurse gains more knowledge and experience.

A major strength of Orem's (1991) theory is that she specifically defines when nursing is needed: Nursing is needed when the individual cannot maintain continuously that amount and quality of self-care necessary to sustain life and health, recover from disease or injury, or cope with their effects.

Orem (1991) promotes the concepts of professional nursing. She defines the roles of vocational, technical, and professional nurses, and recognizes the importance of each. She indicates that thinking nursing and conceptualizing the dynamics and structure of nursing situations is distinct from viewing nursing as skilled performance of tasks.

Her self-care premise is contemporary with the concepts of health promotion and health maintenance. Self-care in Orem's theory is comparable to holistic health in that both promote the individual's responsibility for health care. This is especially relevant with today's emphasis on early hospital discharge, home care, and outpatient services. Orem (1991) recognizes the term *client* as a regular seeker of services but prefers the term *patient* for one who is "under the care of nurses, physicians, or other direct health care providers" (p. 30).

According to Orem (1991), "nursing should select the type of nursing system or sequential combination of nursing systems that will have an optimum effect in achieving the desired regulation of patients' self-care agency and the meeting of their self-care requisites" (p. 292). Some practitioners have found Orem's theory to be more clinically applicable when more than one system is used concurrently (Knust & Quarn, 1983).

Another strength is Orem's delineation of three identifiable nursing systems. These are easily understood by the beginning nursing student. However, Orem's use of the term *system* is different from that used in general system theory. She defines a system as a "single, whole thing" (Orem, 1991, p. 269). In general system theory, a system is viewed as a dynamic, flowing process.

Orem (1991) has expanded her initial focus of individual self-care to include multiperson units (families, groups, and communities). She notes that when multiperson units are served by nurses, the resulting nursing systems combine the features of partly compensatory and supportive-educative nursing systems. However, an incongruence is present because she suggests that "it is advisable at this stage of the development of nursing knowledge to confine the use of the three nursing systems to situations where individuals are the units of care or service" (p. 289).

Orem's elaboration on self-care requisites seem to be essential to her theory and emerge as a core concept. Her theory would be more readily understood if the term *peripheral concept* were eliminated when she defines basic conditioning factors.

Orem's theory is simple yet complex. However, the essence is clouded by ancillary descriptions. The term *self-care* is used with numerous configurations.

This multitude of terms, such as self-care agency, self-care demand, self-care premise, self-care deficit, self-care requisites, and universal self-care, can be very confusing to the reader.

Other limitations include her discussion of health. Health is often viewed as dynamic and ever changing. Orem's model of the boxed nursing systems (see Fig. 7–2) implies three static conditions of health. She refers to a "concrete nursing system," which connotes rigidity. Another impression from the model of nursing systems is that a major determining factor for placement of a patient in a system is the individual's capacity for physical movement. Throughout her work there is limited acknowledgment of the individual's emotional needs.

SUMMARY

Orem presents her general theory of nursing, The Self-Care Deficit Theory of Nursing, which is composed of the three interrelated theories of self-care, self-care deficit, and nursing systems. Incorporated within and supportive of these theories are the six central concepts of self-care, self-care agency, therapeutic self-care demand, self-care deficit, nursing agency, and nursing system, as well as the peripheral concept of basic conditioning factors.

Nursing is needed when the self-care demands are greater than the self-care abilities. Nursing systems are designed by the nurse when it has been determined that nursing care is needed. The systems of wholly compensatory, partly compensatory, and supportive-educative specify the roles of the nurse and the patient.

Throughout Orem's work, she interprets nursing's metaparadigm of human beings, health, nursing, and society. She defines three steps of nursing process as (1) diagnosis and prescription, (2) design of a nursing system and planning for the delivery of care, and (3) production and management of nursing systems. This process parallels the nursing process of assessment, diagnosis, planning, implementation, and evaluation.

Orem's theory of self-care has pragmatic application to nursing practice. It has been applied by nursing clinicians in a variety of settings. The theory has been used as the basis for nursing school curricula and the base for a nursing information system.

Orem's Self-Care Deficit Theory of Nursing continues to evolve; its impact is international. Its widespread use reflects its utility for professional nursing. This theory offers a unique way of looking at the phenomenon of nursing. Orem's work contributes significantly to the development of nursing theories.

REFERENCES

Knust, S. J., & Quarn, J. M. (1983). Integration of self-care theory with rehabilitation nursing. *Rehabilitation Nursing,* 26–28.

Nursing Development Conference Group. (1973). *Concept formalization in nursing: Process and product.* Boston: Little, Brown.

Nursing Development Conference Group. (1979). *Concept formalization in nursing: Process and product* (2nd ed.). Boston: Little, Brown.

Orem, D. E. (1959). *Guides for developing curricula for the education of practical nurses.* Washington, DC: Government Printing Office.

Orem, D. E. (1971). *Nursing: Concepts of practice.* New York: McGraw-Hill. [out of print]

Orem, D. E. (1980). *Nursing: Concepts of practice* (2nd ed.). New York: McGraw-Hill. [out of print]

Orem, D. E. (1985). *Nursing: Concepts of practice* (3rd ed.). New York: McGraw-Hill. [out of print]

Orem, D. E. (1991). *Nursing: Concepts of practice* (4th ed.). St. Louis: Mosby.

Orem, D. E., & Taylor, S. G. (1986). Orem's General Theory of Nursing. In P. Winstead-Fry (Ed.), *Case studies in nursing theory* (pp. 37–71). New York: National League for Nursing.

Trench, A. S. (Executive producer), Wallace, D. (Producer), & Coberg, T. (Director). (1988). *Dorothea E. Orem—The nurse theorists: Portraits of excellence.* Oakland, CA: Studio Three Production, Samuel Merritt College of Nursing.

Ziegler, S. M., Vaughn-Wrobel, B. C., & Erlen, J. A. (1986). *Nursing process, nursing diagnosis, nursing knowledge—Avenues to autonomy.* Norwalk, CT: Appleton-Century-Crofts.

BIBLIOGRAPHY

Allan, J. D. (1990). Focusing on living, not dying: A naturalistic study of self-care among seropositive gay men. *Holistic Nursing Practice, 4*(2), 56–63.

Brock, A. M., & O'Sullivan, P. (1985). A study to determine what variables predict institutionalization of the elderly. *Journal of Advanced Nursing, 10,* 533–537.

Bromley, B. (1980). Applying Orem's Self-Care Theory in enterostomal therapy. *American Journal of Nursing, 80,* 245–249.

Chang, B. L., Cuman, G., Linn, L. S., Ware, J. E., & Kane, R. L. (1985). Adherence to health care regimens among elderly women. *Nursing Research, 34,* 27–31.

Denyes, M. J. (1982). Measurement of self-care agency in adolescents. *Nursing Research, 31,* 63.

Fitzgerald, S. (1980). Utilizing Orem's Self-Care Model in designing an educational program for the diabetic. *Topics in Clinical Nursing, 2,* 57–65.

Foote, A., Holcombe, J., Piazza, D., & Wright, P. (1993). Orem's theory used as a guide for the nursing care of an eight-year-old child with leukemia. *Journal of Pediatric Oncology Nursing, 10*(1), 26–32.

Frey, M. A., & Denyes, M. J. (1989). Health and illness self-care in adolescents with IDDM: A test of Orem's theory. *Advances in Nursing Science, 12*(1), 67–75.

Gulick, E. E. (1987). Parsimony and model confirmation of the ADL Self-Care Scale for Multiple Sclerosis persons. *Nursing Research, 36,* 278–283.

Jirovec, M. M., & Kasno, J. (1993). Predictors of self-care abilities among the institutionalized elderly. *Western Journal of Nursing Research, 15,* 314–326.

Kearney, B. Y., & Fleischer, B. J. (1979). Development of an instrument to measure the exercise of self-care agency. *Research in Nursing and Health, 2,* 25–34.

Keohane, N. S., & Lacey, L. A. (1991). Preparing the woman with gestational diabetes for self-care. *Journal of Obstetric, Gynecologic and Neonatal Nursing, 20,* 189–193.

Kinlein, M. L. (1977). *Independent nursing practice with clients,* Philadelphia: Lippincott.

Kubricht, D. W. (1984). Therapeutic self-care demands expressed by outpatients receiving external radiation therapy. *Cancer Nursing, 7,* 43–52.

Mack, C. J. (1992). Assessment of the autologous bone marrow transplant patient according to Orem's self-care model. *Cancer Nursing, 15,* 429–436.

McDermott, M. A. N. (1993). Learned helplessness as an interacting variable with self-care agency: Testing a theoretical model. *Nursing Science Quarterly, 6,* 28–38.

Murphy, P. (1981). A hospice model and self-care theory. *Oncology Nursing Forum, 8,* 19–21.

Patterson, E. T., & Hale, E. S. (1985). Making sure: Integrating menstrual care practices into activities of daily living. *Advances in Nursing Science, 7*(3), 18–31.

Reed, P. G. (1986). Developmental resources and depression in the elderly. *Nursing Research, 35,* 368–374.

Scrak, B. M., Zimmerman, J., Wilson, M., & Greenstein, R. (1987). Moving from the gas station to a nurse-managed psych clinic. *American Journal of Nursing, 87,* 188–190.

Stollenwerk, R. (1985). An emphysema client: Self-care. *Home Healthcare Nurse, 3*(2), 36–40.

Taylor, S. G., & McLaughlin, K. (1991). Orem's General Theory of Nursing and community nursing. *Nursing Science Quarterly, 4,* 153–160.

Villarruel, A. M., & Denyes, M. J. (1991). Pain assessment in children: Theoretical and empirical validity. *Advances in Nursing Science, 14,* 32–41.

Weaver, M. T. (1983). Perceived self-care agency: A LISREL factor analysis of Bickel and Hanson's questionnaire. *Nursing Research, 36,* 381–387.

Woods, N. F. (1985). Self-care practices among young adult married women. *Research in Nursing and Health, 8,* 21–31.

Wyatt, G. K., & Omar, M. A. (1985). Interventions useful to the public health nurse: Improving health behaviors. *Journal of Nursing Education, 24,* 168–170.

Zinn, A. (1986). A self-care program for hemodialysis patients based on Dorothea Orem's concepts. *Journal of Nephrology Nursing, 3*(2), 65–77.

DOROTHY E. JOHNSON

Marie L. Lobo

■ ■ ■

Dorothy Johnson was born in Savannah, Georgia, in 1919, the last of seven children. Her Bachelor of Science in Nursing was from Vanderbilt University, Nashville, Tennessee, and her Masters in Public Health from Harvard. She began publishing her ideas about nursing soon after graduation from Vanderbilt. Most of her teaching career was in pediatric nursing at the University of California, Los Angeles. She retired as Professor Emeritus, January 1, 1978, and currently lives in Florida.

Dorothy Johnson has influenced nursing through her publications since the 1950s. Throughout her career, Johnson has stressed the importance of research-based knowledge about the effect of nursing care on clients. Johnson was an early proponent of nursing as a science as well as an art. She also believed nursing had a body of knowledge reflecting both the science and the art. From the beginning, Johnson (1959) proposed that the knowledge of the science of nursing necessary for effective nursing care included a synthesis of key concepts drawn from basic and applied sciences.

In 1961, Johnson proposed that nursing care facilitated the client's maintenance of a state of equilibrium. Johnson proposed that clients were "stressed" by a stimulus of either an internal or external nature. These stressful stimuli created such disturbances, or "tensions," in the patient that a state of disequilibrium occurred. Johnson identified two areas of foci for nursing care that are based on returning the client to a state of equilibrium. First, nursing care should reduce stimuli that are stressors, and second, "nursing care should provide support of the client's 'natural' defenses and adaptive processes" (p. 66).

In 1992, Johnson articulated that much of her thinking was influenced by Florence Nightingale. Johnson related that she was first exposed to Nightingale in the mid-1940s.

While reading Nightingale's (1859/1992) *Notes on nursing* she found that Nightingale focused on the "fundamental needs" of people rather than on the disease process. She also noted that Nightingale focused on the relationship of the person to the environment rather than the disease to the person. In the 1950s and 1960s, as Johnson developed her model, an increasing number of observational studies on child and adult behavior patterns were published. During these same years, general system theory was also discussed frequently. All these experiences influenced Johnson (1992) in the development of her Behavioral Systems Model.

In 1968, Johnson first proposed her model of nursing care as the fostering of "the efficient and effective behavioral functioning in the patient to prevent illness" (Johnson, 1968, April, p. 2). The patient is identified as a behavioral system with multiple subsystems. At this point Johnson began to integrate concepts related to systems models into her work. Johnson's (1968) integration of systems concepts into her work was further illustrated by her statement of belief that nursing was "concerned with man as an integrated whole and this is the specific knowledge of order we require" (p. 207). Not only did nurses need to care for the "whole" client, but the generation of nursing knowledge needed to take a course in the direction of concern with the entire needs of the client.

In the mid- to late-1970s, several nurses published conceptualizations of nursing based on Johnson's behavioral systems model. Some of these were revised in the 1980s. Auger (1976), Damus (1980), Grubbs (1980), Holaday (1980), and Skolny and Riehl (1974) are authors who have interpreted Johnson. Roy (1989), Wu (1973), and others were sharing their beliefs about nursing at the same time, and Johnson's influence, as their professor, is clearly reflected in their works. In 1980, Johnson published her conceptualization of the Behavioral System Model for Nursing. This is the first work published by Johnson that explicates her definitions of the Behavioral System Model. The evolution of this complex model is clearly demonstrated in the progression of Johnson's ideas from works published in the 1950s to her latest available work published in 1980.

DEFINITION OF NURSING

Johnson (1980) developed her Behavioral System Model for nursing from a philosophical perspective "supported by a rich, sound, and rapidly expanding body of empirical and theoretical knowledge" (p. 207). From her early beliefs, which focused on the impaired individual, Johnson evolved a much broader definition of nursing. By 1980, she defined nursing as "an external regulatory force which acts to preserve the organization and integration of the patient's behavior at an optimal level under those conditions in which the behavior constitutes a threat to physical or social health, or in which illness is found" (p. 214). Based on this definition, the following four goals of nursing are to assist the patient to become a person:

1. Whose behavior is commensurate with social demands
2. Who is able to modify his behavior in ways that support biologic imperatives

3. Who is able to benefit to the fullest extent during illness from the physician's knowledge and skill
4. Whose behavior does not give evidence of unnecessary trauma as a consequence of illness (p. 207).

ASSUMPTIONS OF THE BEHAVIORAL SYSTEM MODEL

Johnson makes several layers of assumptions in the development of her conceptualization of the Behavioral System Model. Assumptions are made about the system as a whole as well as about the subsystems. Another set of assumptions deals with the knowledge base necessary to practice nursing.

As with Rogers (1970) and Roy (1989), Johnson believes that nurses need to be well grounded in the physical and social sciences. Particular emphasis should be placed on knowledge from both the physical and social sciences that is found to influence behavior. Thus, Johnson believes it would be of equal importance to have information available about endocrine influences on behavior as well as about psychological influences on behavior.

In developing assumptions about behavioral systems, Johnson was influenced by Buckley, Chin, and Rapport, early leaders in the development of systems concepts. Johnson (1980) cites Chin (1961) as the source for her first assumption about systems. In constructing a behavioral system, the assumption is made that there is " 'organization, interaction, interdependency, and integration of the parts and elements' (Chin, 1961) of behavior that go to make up the system" (p. 208). It is the interrelated parts that contribute to the development of the whole.

The second assumption about systems also evolves from the work of Chin. A system " 'tends to achieve a balance among the various forces operating within and upon it' (1961), and that man strives continually to maintain a behavioral system balance and steady states by more or less automatic adjustments and adaptations to the 'natural' forces impinging upon him" (p. 208). The individual is continually presented with situations in everyday life that require adaptation and adjustment. These adjustments are so natural that they occur without conscious effort by the individual. Johnson (1980) says:

> The third assumption about a behavioral system is that a behavioral system, which both requires and results in some degree of regularity and constancy in behavior, is essential to man; that is to say, it is functionally significant in that it serves a useful purpose both in social life and for the individual (p. 208).

The patterns of behavior characteristic of the individual have a purpose in the maintenance of homeostasis by the individual. The development of behavioral patterns that are acceptable to both society and the individual foster the individual's ability to adapt to minor changes in the environment.

The final assumption about the behavioral system is that the "system balance reflects adjustments and adaptations that are successful in some way and to some degree" (Johnson, 1980, p. 208). Johnson acknowledges that the achievement of this balance may and will vary from individual to individual. At times this balance may *not* be exhibited as behaviors that are acceptable or meet society's norms. What may be adaptive for the individual in coping with impinging forces may be disruptive to society as a whole. Most individuals are flexible enough, however, to be in some state of balance that is "functionally efficient and effective" for them (p. 209).

The integration of these assumptions by the individual provides the behavioral system with the patterns of action to form "an organized and integrated functional unit that determines and limits the interaction between the person and his environment and establishes the relationship of the person to the objects, events, and situations in his environment" (Johnson, 1980, p. 209). The function of the behavioral system, then, is to regulate the individual's response to input from the environment so that the balance of the system can be maintained.

Four assumptions are made about the structure and function of each subsystem. These four assumptions are the "structural elements" common to each of the seven subsystems. The first assumption is "from the form the behavior takes and the consequences it achieves can be inferred what *drive* has been stimulated or what *goal* is being sought" (Johnson, 1980, p. 210). The ultimate goal for each subsystem is expected to be the same for all individuals. However, the methods of achieving the goal may vary depending on culture or other individual variations.

The second assumption is that each individual has a "predisposition to act, with reference to the goal, in certain ways rather than in other ways" (Johnson, 1980, pp. 210–211). This predisposition to act is labeled "set" by Johnson. The concept of "set" implies that despite having only a few alternatives from which to select a behavioral response, the individual will rank those options and choose the option considered most desirable.

The third assumption is that each subsystem has available a repertoire of choices or "scope of action" alternatives from which choices can be made Johnson (1980) subsumes under this assumption that larger behavioral repertoires are available to more adaptable individuals. As life experiences occur, individuals add to the number of alternative actions available to them. At some point, however, the acquisition of new alternatives of behavior decreases as the individual becomes comfortable with the available repertoire. The point at which the individual loses the desire or ability to acquire new options is not identified by Johnson.

The fourth assumption about the behavioral subsystems is that they produce observable outcomes—that is, the individual's behavior (Johnson, 1980). The observable behaviors allow an outsider—in this case the nurse— to note the actions the individual is taking to reach a goal related to a specified subsystem. The nurse can then evaluate the effectiveness and efficiency of these behaviors in assisting the individual in reaching one of these goals.

In addition, each of the subsystems has three functional requirements. First, each subsystem must be "*protected* from noxious influences with which the system cannot cope" (Johnson, 1980, p. 212). Second, each subsystem must be "*nurtured* through the input of appropriate supplies from the environment" (p. 212). Finally, each subsystem must be "*stimulated* for use to enhance growth and prevent stagnation" (p. 212). As long as the subsystems are meeting these functional requirements, the system and the subsystems are viewed as self-maintaining and self-perpetuating. The internal and external environments of the system need to remain orderly and predictable for the system to maintain homeostasis or remain in balance. The interrelationships of the structural elements of the subsystem are critical for each subsystem to function at a maximum state. The interaction of the structural elements allows the subsystem to maintain a balance that is adaptive to that individual's needs.

An imbalance in a behavioral subsystem produces tension, which results in disequilibrium. The presence of tension resulting in an unbalanced behavioral system requires the system to increase energy use to return the system to a state of balance (Johnson, 1968, April). Nursing is viewed as a part of the external environment that can assist the client to return to a state of equilibrium or balance.

Johnson's Behavioral System Model

Johnson (1980) believes each individual has patterned, purposeful, repetitive ways of acting that comprise a behavioral system specific to that individual. These actions or behaviors form an "organized and integrated functional unit that determines and limits the interaction between the person and his environment and establishes the relationship of the person to the objects, events, and situations in his environment" (p. 209). These behaviors are "orderly, purposeful and predictable . . . [and] sufficiently stable and recurrent to be amenable to description and explanation" (p. 209). Johnson identifies seven subsystems within the Behavioral System Model, an identification that is at variance with others who have published interpretations of Johnson's model. Johnson (1980) states that the seven subsystems identified in her 1980 publication are the only ones to which she subscribes, and she recognizes they are at variance with Grubbs. These seven subsystems were originally identified in Johnson's 1968 paper presented at Vanderbilt University. The seven subsystems are considered to be interrelated, and changes in one subsystem affect all the subsystems.

Johnson has never produced a schematic representation of her system. Conner, Harbour, Magers and Watt (1994); Loveland-Cherry and Wilkerson (1989); and Torres (1986) have produced similar schematic representations of Johnson's model (see Fig. 8–1).

Johnson's Seven Behavioral Subsystems

The *attachment* or *affiliative* subsystem is identified as the first response system to develop in the individual. The optimal functioning of the affiliative

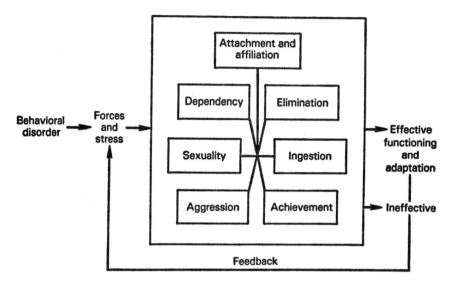

Figure 8–1. Jonson's model. *(From Torres, G. (1986).* Theoretical foundations of nursing. *Norwalk, CT: Appleton-Century-Crofts, p. 121. Used with permission.)*

subsystem allows "social inclusion, intimacy, and the formation and maintenance of a strong social bond" (Johnson, 1980, p. 212). Attachment to a significant caregiver has been found to be critical for the survival of an infant. As the individual matures, the attachment to the caretaker continues and there are additional attachments to other significant individuals as they enter both the child's and the adult's network. These "significant others" provide the individual with a sense of security.

The second subsystem identified by Johnson is the *dependency* subsystem. Johnson (1980) distinguishes the dependency subsystem from the attachment or affiliative subsystem. Dependency behaviors are "succoring" behaviors that precipitate nurturing behaviors from other individuals in the environment. The result of dependency behavior is "approval, attention or recognition, and physical assistance" (p. 213). It is difficult to separate the dependency subsystem from the affiliative or attachment subsystem because without someone invested in or attached to the individual to respond to that individual's dependency behaviors, the dependency subsystem has no animate environment in which to function.

The *ingestive* subsystem relates to the behaviors surrounding the intake of food. It is related to the biological system. However, the emphasis for nursing, from Johnson's (1980) perspective, is the meanings and structures of the social events surrounding the occasions when food is eaten. Behaviors related to the ingestion of food may relate more to what is socially acceptable in a given culture than to the biological needs of the individual.

The *eliminative* subsystem relates to behaviors surrounding the excretion of waste products from the body. Johnson (1980) admits this may be difficult to separate from a biological system perspective. However, as with behaviors surrounding the ingestion of food, there are socially acceptable behaviors for the time and place for humans to excrete waste. Human cultures have defined different socially acceptable behaviors for excretion of waste, but the existence of such a pattern remains from culture to culture. Individuals who have gained physical control over the eliminative subsystem control those subsystems rather than behave in a socially unacceptable manner. For example, biological cues are often ignored if the social situation dictates that it is objectionable to eliminate wastes at a given time.

The *sexual* subsystem reflects behaviors related to procreation (Johnson, 1980). Both biological and social factors affect behaviors in the sexual subsystem. Again, the behaviors are related to culture and vary from culture to culture. Behaviors also vary according to the gender of the individual. The key is that the goal in all societies has the same outcome—behaviors acceptable to society at large.

The *aggressive* subsystem relates to behaviors concerned with protection and self-preservation. Johnson (1980) views the aggressive subsystem as one that generates defensive responses from the individual when life or territory is threatened. The aggressive subsystem does not include those behaviors with a primary purpose of injuring other individuals, but rather those whose purpose is to protect and preserve self and society.

Finally, the *achievement* subsystem provokes behaviors that attempt to control the environment. Intellectual, physical, creative, mechanical, and social skills are some of the areas that Johnson (1980) recognizes. Other areas of personal accomplishment or success may also be included in this subsystem.

JOHNSON'S BEHAVIORAL SYSTEM MODEL AND NURSING'S METAPARADIGM

Johnson views *human beings* as having two major systems: the biological system and the behavioral system. It is the role of medicine to focus on the biological system, whereas nursing's focus is the behavioral system. There is recognition of the reciprocal actions that occur between the biological and behavioral systems when some type of dysfunction occurs in one or the other of the systems.

Society relates to the environment in which an individual exists. According to Johnson, an individual's behavior is influenced by all the events in the environment. Cultural influences on the individual's behavior are viewed as profound. However, it is felt that there are many paths, varying from culture to culture, that influence specific behaviors in a group of people, although the outcome for all the groups or individuals is the same.

Health is an elusive state that is determined by psychological, social, biological, and physiological factors (Johnson, 1978). Johnson's behavioral model supports the idea that the individual is attempting to maintain some balance or equilibrium. The individual's goal is to maintain the entire behavioral system efficiently and effectively but with enough flexibility to return to an acceptable balance if a malfunction disrupts the original balance.

Nursing's primary goal is to foster equilibrium within the individual, which allows for the practice of nursing with individuals at any point in the health–illness continuum. Nursing implementations may focus on alterations of a behavior that is not supportive to maintaining equilibrium for the individual. In earlier works, Johnson focused nursing on impaired individuals. By 1980, she stated that nursing is concerned with the organized and integrated whole, but that the major focus is on maintaining a balance in the behavioral system when illness occurs in the individual.

JOHNSON'S BEHAVIORAL SYSTEM AND THE NURSING PROCESS

Johnson's Behavioral System Model easily fits the nursing process model. Grubbs (1980) developed an assessment tool based on Johnson's seven subsystems, plus a subsystem she labeled "restorative," which focused on activities of daily living. Activities of daily living are considered to include such areas as patterns of rest, hygiene, and recreation. A diagnosis can be made related to insufficiencies or discrepancies within a subsystem or between subsystems. Planning for the implementation of nursing care should start at the subsystem level with the ultimate goal of effective behavioral functioning of the entire system. Implementations by the nurse present to the client an external force for the manipulation of the subsystem back to the state of equilibrium. Evaluation of the result of this implementation is readily possible if the state of balance that is the goal has been defined during the planning phase before the implementation.

Assessment

In the assessment phase of the nursing process, questions related to specific subsystems are developed. Holaday (1980), Damus (1980), and Small (1980) propose that the assessment focus on the subsystem related to the presenting health problem. An assessment based on the behavioral subsystems does not easily permit the nurse to gather detailed information about the biological system. Assessment questions related to the affiliative subsystem might focus on the presence of a significant other or on the social system of which the individual is a member. In the assessment of the dependency subsystem, attention is placed on understanding how the individual makes needs known to significant others so that the significant others in the environment can assist the individual in meeting those needs. Assessment of the ingestive subsystem examines patterns of food and fluid intake, including the social environment in which the food and fluid are ingested. The eliminative subsystem generates questions related to patterns of defecation and urination and the social context in which the patterns occur. The sexual subsystem assessment includes information about sexual patterns and behaviors. The aggressive subsystem generates questions about how individuals protect themselves from perceived threats to safety. Finally, the achievement subsystem allows for assessment of how the individual changes the environment to facilitate the accomplishment of goals.

There are many gaps in information about the whole individual if only Johnson's Behavioral System Model is used to guide the assessment. There are few physiological data on the individual's present or past health status. The exception might be when an impaired health state is demonstrated in the ingestive or eliminative subsystems. Family interaction and patterns are touched on only in the affiliative and dependency subsystems. Basic information relating to education, socioeconomic status, and type of dwelling is tangentially related to most of the subsystems. However, these factors are not clearly identified as an important aspect of any of the subsystems.

Diagnosis

Diagnosis using Johnson's Behavioral System Model becomes cumbersome. Diagnosis tends to be general to a subsystem rather than specific to a problem. Grubbs (1980) has proposed four categories of nursing diagnoses derived from Johnson's Behavioral System Model, as follows:

1. *Insufficiency*—a state "which exists when a particular subsystem is not functioning or developed to its fullest capacity due to inadequacy of functional requirements . . .
2. *Discrepancy*—a behavior that does not meet the intended goal. The incongruity usually lies between the action and the goal of the subsystem, although the set and choice may be strongly influencing the ineffective action . . .
3. *Incompatibility*—the goals or behaviors of two subsystems in the same situation conflict with each other to the detriment of the individual . . .
4. *Dominance*—the behavior in one subsystem is used more than any other subsystem regardless of the situation or to the detriment of the other subsystems" (pp. 240–241).

Since Johnson has never written about the use of nursing diagnosis with her model, it is difficult to know whether these diagnostic classifications are Johnson's or if they are an extension of Johnson's work by Grubbs.

Planning and Implementation

Planning for implementation of the nursing care related to the diagnosis may be difficult because of the lack of client input into the plan. The plan focuses on the nurse's action to modify client behavior. These plans, then, have a goal: to bring about homeostasis in a subsystem that is based on the nurse's assessment of the individual's drive, set, behavioral repertoire, and observable behavior. The plan may include protection, nurturance, or stimulation of the identified subsystem.

Planning and implementation for clients that are based on Johnson's Behavioral System Model focus on maintaining or returning an individual's subsystem to a state of equilibrium. Implementation focuses on achieving the goals of nursing as identified by Johnson (1980). Although Johnson refers to the biological system in her goals of nursing, it is not included in her Behavioral System Model and can and does produce incongruities for the planning and implementation of nursing care in relation to a specific diagnosis.

Evaluation

Evaluation is based on the attainment of a goal of balance in the identified subsystems. If base-line data are available for the individual, the nurse may have a goal for the individual to return to the baseline behavior. If the alterations in behavior that are planned do occur, the nurse should be able to observe the return to previous behavior patterns.

There is little or no recognition by either Johnson (1980) or Grubbs (1980) of the client's input into plans for nursing implementation. They use the term *nursing intervention.* Holaday's (1980) example of implementation also does not contain strong client input. Using Johnson's Behavioral System Model with the nursing process is a nurse-centered activity, with the nurse determining the client's needs and the state of behavior appropriate to those needs.

Holaday (1980) demonstrates the flexibility available in the use of the Johnson Behavioral System Model with the nursing process by using a very specific assessment tool to determine appropriate interventions. Holaday uses tests of cognitive development developed by Piaget to determine the level of information to present to a child during a preoperative teaching session.

Situation. An example of the use of the nursing process with Johnson's Behavioral System Model is demonstrated with Johnny Smith, age 6 weeks, brought into the clinic for a routine checkup. He presents with no weight gain since his checkup at age 2 weeks. His mother states that she feeds him but that he does not seem to eat much. He sleeps 4 to 5 hours between feedings. His mother holds him in her arms without making trunk-to-trunk contact. As the assessment is made, the nurse notes that Mrs. Smith never looks at Johnny and never speaks to him. She states that he was a planned baby but that she never "realized how much work an infant could be." She says her mother has told her she was not a good mother because Johnny is not gaining weight as he should. She states that she has not called the nurse when she knew Johnny was not gaining weight because she thought the nurse would think she was a "bad mother" just as her own mother thought she was a "bad mother."

Based on the information available and using the Johnson Behavioral System Model, assessment focuses on the affiliative and dependency subsystems between mother and Johnny. Further assessment of Mrs. Smith's relationship with her own mother needs to be done. The critical need is for

Johnny to begin gaining weight. The secondary need is for Mrs. Smith to resolve her conflict with her own mother. The assessment of the affiliative subsystem focuses on the specific behaviors manifested by Johnny to indicate attachment to his mother. The assessment of the dependency subsystem focuses on the specific behaviors manifested by Johnny to cue his mother to his needs. Because of the nature of his problem, a decision is made to use a tool that specifically focuses on parent–infant interaction during a feeding situation. Thus, the Nursing Child Assessment Feeding Scale (Barnard, 1978) is used during a feeding that takes place at a normal feeding time for Johnny. Johnny cries at the beginning of the feeding and turns toward his mother's hand when she touches his cheek. Mrs. Smith does not speak to Johnny or in any verbal way acknowledge his hunger. When Johnny slightly chokes on some formula, she does not remove the bottle from his mouth. Mrs. Smith does not describe any of the environment to Johnny, nor does she stroke his body or make eye contact with him. Johnny does not reach out to touch his mother nor does he make any vocalizations. The assessment scale indicates that both mother and baby are not cueing each other at a level at which they can respond appropriately.

The diagnoses based on this assessment, using Johnson's Behavioral System Model, are, "insufficient development of the affiliative subsystem" and "insufficient development of the dependency subsystem." Based on these diagnoses, nursing implementation focuses on increasing Mrs. Smith's awareness of the meaning of Johnny's infrequent cues. By increasing her awareness of the meaning of his cues, she can begin to reinforce them so that he begins to know there is someone in the environment who cares about him, thus fostering his attachment to her. Further assistance needs to be given in helping Mrs. Smith in communicating with her infant. If further assessment indicates Mrs. Smith is uncomfortable talking with an infant who does not respond with words, it may be suggested that she read to Johnny from a book, thus providing him with needed verbal stimulation. Another implementation may include the nurse placing herself in Johnny's role and "talking" for him to his mother. The nurse may sit, watching Mrs. Smith hold Johnny, and say such things as "I like it when you pat me," "It feels good when you cuddle me," "When I turn my head like this, I'm hungry."

Evaluation of these implementations are based on two criteria. First, Johnny's weight gains or losses are carefully assessed. Not gaining weight places him in a life-threatening situation; therefore, it is critical that a pattern of weight gain be initiated. Second, the mother–infant interaction can be reassessed, again using the Nursing Child Assessment Feeding Scale (Barnard, 1978), which allows for comparison of the first observation with a series of subsequent observations.

JOHNSON'S WORK AND THE CHARACTERISTICS OF A THEORY

Johnson states that she is presenting a model related to subsystems of the human being that have observable behaviors leading to specific outcomes, although the method of attaining the specific outcomes may vary according to the culture of the individual. Using the characteristics of a theory discussed in Chapter 1 as a guide, it is clear that Johnson has indeed developed a model. Johnson's Behavioral System Model is based on general system concepts. However, the definitions related to the terms used to label her concepts have not been made explicit by Johnson. Grubbs (1980) has presented her definitions of Johnson's terms, and those are the definitions most often reflected in the literature of other investigators claiming to use Johnson's model.

1. Theories can interrelate concepts in such a way as to create a different way of looking at a particular phenomenon. Johnson does not clearly interrelate her concepts of subsystems that comprise the Behavioral System Model.

2. Theories must be logical in nature. The lack of clear interrelationships among the concepts creates difficulty in following the logic of Johnson's work. The definitions of the concepts are so abstract that they are difficult to use. For example, intimacy is identified as an aspect of the affiliative subsystem, but the concept is not defined or described. An advantage of the abstract definition is that individuals using the model may identify an assessment tool that most specifically fits a problem and use it in their work. There are two major disadvantages. First, the abstract level and multiplicity of definitions make it difficult to compare the same subsystem across studies. Second, the lack of clear definitions for the interrelationships among and between the subsystems makes it difficult to view the entire behavioral system as an entity.

3. Theories should be relatively simple yet generalizable. Johnson's behavioral model can be generalized across the lifespan and across cultures. However, the focus on the behavioral system may make it difficult for nurses working with physically impaired individuals to use the model. Johnson's model is also very individual oriented, so that nurses working with groups of individuals with similar problems would have difficulty using the model. The subsystems in Johnson's Behavioral System Model are individual oriented to such an extent that the family can be considered only as the environment in which the individual presents behaviors and not as the focus of care.

4. Theories are the bases for hypotheses that can be tested or for theory to be expanded, and

5. Theories contribute to and assist in increasing the general body of knowledge within the discipline through the research implemented to validate them. It is difficult to test Johnson's model by the development of hypotheses. Subsystems of the model can be examined because relationships within the subsystems can be identified. The lack of definitions and connections between the subsystems creates a barrier for stating relationships in the form of hypotheses to be tested. Although such relationships may be predicted, the lack of definitions in the original work makes impossible to identify whether it is Johnson's work or someone's interpretation of her work that is being tested.

6. Theories can be used by practitioners to guide and improve practice. Johnson does not clearly define the expected outcomes when one of the subsystems is being affected by nursing implementation. An implicit expectation is made that all humans in all cultures will attain the same outcome—homeostasis. Because of the lack of definitions, the model does not allow for control of the areas of interest, so it is difficult to use the model to guide practice. The authors reportedly using the model to guide practice have not integrated the subsystems to the degree necessary to label this model a theory.

7. Theories must be consistent with other validated theories, laws, and principles but will leave open unanswered questions that need to be investigated. Johnson's Behavioral System Model provides a framework for organizing human behavior. However, it is a different framework from that provided by other nursing theorists, such as Roy (1989) or Rogers (1970). Johnson believes that she is the first person to view "man as a behavioral system." Others have viewed the behavioral subsystem as just one piece of the biopsychosocial human being. Johnson's framework does contribute to the general body of nursing knowledge but needs further development. Johnson's Behavioral System Model is based on principles of general system theory. Her statements on the multiple modes of attaining the same subsystem goal, regardless of culture, are an example of the principle of "equifinality." As with Rogers (1970), this allows individuals to develop and change through time at unique rates but with the same outcomes at the end of the process: mature, adult behaviors that are culturally acceptable.

Johnson's Behavioral System Model is not as flexible as Rogers's (1970) concept of homeodynamics or Roy's (1989) adaptation model. Rogers' concepts are so broadly applicable that nursing care can take place at any level: individual, family, or community. All systems within the human being can be considered for the focus of nursing implementations. With Roy's model, the focus is still at the individual level, but the total human being can be considered. Roy's assumptions include that the human being is a biopsychosocial being, which allows for all the subsystems of a human being to be included for nursing assessment and implementation.

Johnson's Behavioral System Model is congruent with many of the nursing models in the belief that the individual is influenced by the environment. Since Nightingale (1859) first presented her beliefs about nursing, nurses have been concerned with the individual's relationship with the environment. In practice, nurses often have the necessary control over the environment to promote a healthier state for the individual.

In general, the Johnson Behavioral System Model does not meet the criteria for a theory. However, it must be stressed that Johnson does not suggest that she has developed a theory, although other nurse scholars have identified and used Johnson as a theorist.

SUMMARY

Although Johnson's Behavioral System Model has many limitations, she does provide a frame of reference for nurses concerned with specific client behaviors. It must also be noted that Johnson, through her work at the University of California, Los Angeles, has had a profound influence on the development of nursing models and nursing theories. Through her position as a faculty member she influenced Roy, Grubbs, Holaday, and others. As a peer, she influenced Riehl, Neuman, Wu, and others, scholars who have generated many ideas about nursing concepts and theories.

Johnson's Behavioral System Model is a model of nursing care that advocates the fostering of efficient and effective behavioral functioning in the patient to prevent illness. The patient is identified as a behavioral system composed of seven behavioral subsystems: affiliative, dependency, ingestive, eliminative, sexual, aggressive, and achievement. Each subsystem is composed of four structural characteristics: drive, set, choices, and observable behaviors. The three functional requirements for each subsystem include protection from noxious influences, provision for a nurturing environment, and stimulation for growth. An imbalance in any of the behavioral subsystems results in disequilibrium. It is nursing's role to assist the client to return to a state of equilibrium.

REFERENCES

Auger, J. R. (1976). *Behavioral systems and nursing.* Englewood Cliffs, NJ: Prentice-Hall.

Barnard, K. E. (1978). *Nursing Child Assessment Feeding Scale.* Seattle: University of Washington.

Chin, R. (1961). The utility of system models and developmental models for practitioners. In K. Benne, W. Bennis, & R. Chin (Eds.), *The planning of change.* New York: Holt.

Conner, S. S., Harbour, L. S., Magers, J. A., & Watt, J. K. (1994). Dorothy E. Johnson: Behavioral System Model. In A. Marriner-Tomey (Ed.), *Nursing theorists and their work* (3rd ed.) (pp. 231–245). St Louis: Mosby.

Damus, K. (1980). An application of the Johnson Behavioral System Model for Nursing Practice. In J. P. Riehl, & C. Roy (Eds.), *Conceptual models for nursing practice* (2nd ed.) (pp. 274–289). New York: Appleton-Century-Crofts.

Grubbs, J. (1980). An interpretation of the Johnson Behavioral System Model for nursing practice. In J. P. Riehl, & C. Roy (Eds.), *Conceptual models for nursing practice* (2nd ed.) (pp. 217–254). New York: Appleton-Century-Crofts.

Holaday, B. (1980). Implementing the Johnson Model for Nursing Practice. In J. P. Riehl, & C. Roy (Eds.), *Conceptual models for nursing practice* (2nd ed.) (pp. 255–263). New York: Appleton-Century-Crofts.

Johnson, D. E. (1959). The nature of a science of nursing. *Nursing Outlook, 7,* 291–294.

Johnson, D. E. (1961). The significance of nursing care. *American Journal of Nursing, 61,* 63–66.

Johnson, D. E. (1968, April). *One conceptual model of nursing.* Paper presented at Vanderbilt University, Nashville, Tennessee.

Johnson, D. E. (1968). Theory in nursing: Borrowed and unique. *Nursing Research, 17,* 206–209.

Johnson, D. E. (1974). Development of theory: A requisite for nursing as a profession. *Nursing Research, 23*, 372–377.

Johnson, D. E. (1978). State of the art of theory development in nursing. In *Theory development: What, why, how?* (pp. 1–10). New York: National League for Nursing.

Johnson, D. E. (1980). The Behavioral System Model for Nursing. In J. P. Riehl, & C. Roy (Eds.), *Conceptual models for nursing practice* (2nd ed.) (pp. 207–216). New York: Appleton-Century-Crofts.

Johnson, D. E. (1992). The origins of the Behavioral Systems Model. In F. Nightingale, *Notes on nursing: What it is and what it is not* (Com. ed.). Philadelphia: Lippincott. (Originally published, 1859).

Loveland-Cherry, C., & Wilkerson, S. A. (1989). Dorothy Johnson's Behavioral System Model. In J. Fitzpatrick, & A. Whall (Eds.), *Conceptual models of nursing: Analysis and application* (2nd ed.) (pp. 147–164). Norwalk, CT: Appleton & Lange.

Nightingale, F. (1992). *Notes on nursing: What it is, and what it is not* (Com. ed.). Philadelphia: Lippincott. (Originally published, 1859).

Rogers, M. (1970). *The theoretical basis for nursing.* Philadelphia: Davis.

Roy, C. (1989). The Roy Adaptation Model. In J. Riehl-Sisca (Ed.), *Conceptual models for nursing practice* (3rd ed.) (pp. 105–114). Norwalk, CT: Appleton & Lange.

Skolny, M. A., & Riehl, J. P. (1974). Hope: Solving patient and family problems by using a theoretical framework. In J. P. Riehl, & C. Roy (Eds.), *Conceptual models for nursing practice* (pp. 206–217). New York: Appleton-Century-Crofts.

Small, B. (1980). Nursing visually impaired children with Johnson's Model as a conceptual framework. In J. P. Riehl, & C. Roy (Eds.), *Conceptual models for nursing practice* (2nd ed.) (pp. 264–273). New York: Appleton-Century-Crofts.

Torres, G. (1986). *Theoretical foundations of nursing.* Norwalk, CT: Appleton-Century-Crofts.

Wu, R. (1973). *Behavior and illness.* Englewood Cliffs, NJ: Prentice-Hall.

BIBLIOGRAPHY

Hardy, M. E. (1974). Theories: Components, development, evaluation. *Nursing Research, 23*, 100-107.

Johnson, D. E. (1978). *Behavioral System Model for Nursing.* Supplemental materials for Nursing Theorists General Session, the Second Annual Nurse Education Conference.

Neuman, B. (1995). *The Neuman Systems Model* (3rd ed.). Norwalk, CT: Appleton & Lange.

BETTY JO HADLEY'S
JOHNSON–HADLEY CONNECTION

Julia B. George

Betty Jo Hadley earned a BA in general studies from the University of California, Berkeley; a diploma in nursing from the California Hospital School of Nursing; a masters in counseling and guidance from the University of Southern California; and a PhD in sociology from the University of California, Los Angeles. She entitled her theory the Johnson–Hadley Connection, because she built her conceptions upon those of Dorothy Johnson (Hadley, 1986). These conceptions were first published in 1969. Hadley has conducted research using her theory as a framework and has guided graduate students in similar research.

Hadley believes the focus of nursing is to prevent or reduce the tensions associated with entrance into the health care system. She defines entrance into the health care system as any contact with a health care provider from a question over the back fence to a neighbor who is a nurse to a hospital admission through the emergency room. She views man as a bio-psycho-social being who functions in a physical and a psycho-social environment. Man has patterned ways of achieving goals within these environments, as well as patterned ways of coping with the stresses of everyday life. Disruptions of these patterned behaviors lead to the primary stress of illness, whereas the stresses of everyday life offer the threat of illness. Either illness or the threat of illness may lead to entrance into the health care system (see Fig. 8–2). Such entrance leads to changes in structure, function, the psycho-social environment, and/or the physical environment, which are the secondary stresses.

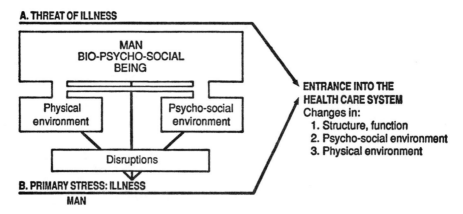

Figure 8–2. Entrance into health care system. *(From Hadley. B. J. (1969). Evolution of a conception of nursing. Nursing Research, 18, 400–405. Used with permission.)*

Entrance into the health care system and the consequent secondary stresses lead to patient situations that comprise the stress syndrome of entrance. Hadley identifies patient situations as the internal and/or external environmental consequences of the secondary stresses (see Fig. 8–3). She also suggests that these are situations equivalent to Johnson's Behavioral System Disturbances (personal communication, April, 1984). These patient situations may include such examples as body image distortions, sensory overload, affectional deprivation, immobility, inability to meet own needs, perceptual incongruence, and biochemical imbalance. The assumption that connects the patient situation with nursing problems is that stress results in tension. The nursing problems are the tensions that include bio-physical tensions such as pain, dyspnea, tightness of skin, anorexia, nausea, bladder distention, bowel distention, heat, cold, dizziness, sleepiness, wakefulness, hunger, itchiness, weakness, thirst, and fatigue. Psycho-social tensions include anxiety, fear, loneliness, emptiness, powerlessness, frustration, grief, depression, anger, irritableness, helplessness, self-consciousness, boredom, embarrassment, confusion, uncertainty, guilt, and disgust. These tensions are nursing's objects of analysis and are manifested by behavioral instability.

Nursing needs to use systematic ways of ordering knowledge about man's behaviors in order to interpret what tensions the patient is experiencing as a consequence of entrance into the health care system. Nursing action represents the manipulation of man, his environments, or both to maintain or restore behavioral stability. Maintaining and restoring behavioral stability focuses on real or anticipated nursing problems. Nursing's goal is achieved when the tensions are prevented or reduced.

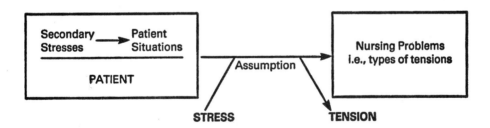

Patient Situations: Consequence of Secondary Stresses
Example: Body image distortions; sensory overload or deprivation; affectional deprivation; immobility; inability to meet needs; perceptual incongruities; biochemical imbalance; etc.
Nursing Problems: Bio–Psycho–Social Tensions
Example: Bio–physical pain; dyspnea; tightness of skin; anorexia; thirst; fatigue; etc. Psycho–social anxiety; fear; loneliness; frustration; grief; depression; anger; etc.

Figure 8–3. Consequence of entrance. *(From Hadley. B. J. (1969). Evolution of a conception of nursing,* Nursing Research, 18, 400–405. *Used with permission.)*

REFERENCES

Hadley, B. J. (1969). Evolution of a conception of nursing. *Nursing Research, 18,* 400–405.

Hadley, B. J. (1986). The author comments. In L. H. Nicoll (Ed.), *Perspectives on nursing theory* (p. 214). Boston: Little, Brown.

FAYE GLENN ABDELLAH

Suzanne M. Falco

■ ■ ■

Faye Glenn Abdellah was born in New York City. She graduated magna cum laude from Fitkin Memorial Hospital School of Nursing in Neptune, New Jersey, in 1942 and received her BS (1945), MA (1947), and EdD (1955) from Teachers College, Columbia University. She has been granted honorary doctorates by a number of institutions, including Case Western Reserve, Rutgers, University of Akron, Catholic University of America, Eastern University, and Monmouth College.

Dr. Abdellah served as Deputy Surgeon General and as Chief Nurse Officer for the U.S. Public Health Service, Department of Health and Human Services, Washington, DC. She is the recipient of both national and international awards and is a Fellow in the American Academy of Nursing. Now retired, she has more than one hundred publications related to nursing care, education for advanced practice in nursing, and nursing research, and she continues to provide leadership in nursing.

In 1960, influenced by the desire to promote client-centered comprehensive nursing care, Abdellah described nursing as a service to individuals, to families, and, therefore, to society. According to Abdellah, nursing is based on an art and science that mold the attitudes, intellectual competencies, and technical skills of the individual nurse into the desire and ability to help people, sick or well, cope with their health needs. Nursing may be carried out under general or specific medical direction. As a comprehensive service, nursing includes the following:

1. Recognizing the nursing problems of the patient [client]
2. Deciding the appropriate courses of action to take in terms of relevant nursing principles
3. Providing continuous care of the individual's total health needs
4. Providing continuous care to relieve pain and discomfort and provide immediate security for the individual
5. Adjusting the total nursing care plan to meet the patient's [client's] individual needs
6. Helping the individual to become more self-directing in attaining or maintaining a healthy state of mind and body

7. Instructing nursing personnel and family to help the individual do for himself that which he can within his limitations
8. Helping the individual to adjust to his limitations and emotional problems
9. Working with allied health professions in planning for optimum health on local, state, national, and international levels
10. Carrying out continuous evaluation and research to improve nursing techniques and to develop new techniques to meet the health needs of people (Abdellah, Beland, Martin, & Matheney, 1960, pp. 24–25).

These original premises have undergone an evolutionary process. As a result, in 1973, Item 3—"providing continuous care of the individual's total health needs"—was eliminated (Abdellah, Beland, Martin, & Matheney, 1973). Although no reason was given, it can be hypothesized that the words *continuous* and *total* render that service virtually impossible to provide. From these premises, Abdellah's theory was derived.

ABDELLAH'S THEORY

Although Abdellah's writings are not specific as to a theoretical statement, such a statement can be derived by using her three major concepts of health, nursing problems, and problem solving. Abdellah's theory would state that nursing is the use of the problem-solving approach with key nursing problems related to the health needs of people. Such a theoretical statement maintains problem solving as the vehicle for the nursing problems as the client is moved toward health—the outcome. It is also a relatively simple statement and can be used as a basis for nursing practice, education, and research.

Health

Although Abdellah never defined it per se, her concept of health may be defined as the dynamic pattern of functioning whereby there is a continued interaction with internal and external forces that results in the optimal use of necessary resources that serve to minimize vulnerabilities (Abdellah & Levine, 1986; Torres & Stanton, 1982). Emphasis should be placed upon prevention and rehabilitation with wellness as a lifetime goal. By performing nursing services through a holistic approach to the client, the nurse helps the client achieve a state of health. However, to effectively perform these services, the nurse must accurately identify the lacks or deficits regarding health that the client is experiencing. These lacks or deficits are the client's health needs.

Nursing Problems

The client's health needs can be viewed as problems, which may be *overt* as an apparent condition, or *covert* as a hidden or concealed one. Because covert problems can be emotional, sociological, and interpersonal in nature, they are often missed or perceived incorrectly. Yet, in many instances, solving the covert problems may solve the overt problems as well (Abdellah, et al., 1960).

Such a view of problems implies a client-centered orientation. Abdellah, however, seems to imply a different viewpoint (Abdellah et al., 1960). She says a nursing problem presented by a client is a condition faced by the client or client's family that the nurse, through the performance of professional functions, can assist them to meet. Abdellah's use of the term *nursing problems* is more consistent with "nursing functions" or "nursing goals" than with client-centered problems. This viewpoint leads to an orientation that is more nursing-centered than client-centered (Nicholls & Wessells, 1977).

This nursing-centered orientation to client care seems contrary to the client-centered approach that Abdellah professes to uphold (Abdellah et al., 1960). The apparent contradiction can be explained by her desire to move away from a disease-centered orientation. In her attempt to bring nursing practice into its proper relationship with restorative and preventive measures for meeting total client needs, she seems to swing the pendulum to the opposite pole, from the disease orientation to nursing orientation, while leaving the client somewhere in the middle (see Fig. 9–1).

It is noted that Abdellah recognized the need to shift from nursing problems to patient/client outcomes (Abdellah & Levine, 1986). However, there has been no further development of the framework to accomplish this.

Problem Solving

Quality professional nursing care requires that nurses be able to identify and solve overt and covert nursing problems. These requirements can be met by the problem-solving approach. The problem-solving process involves identifying the problem, selecting pertinent data, formulating hypotheses, testing

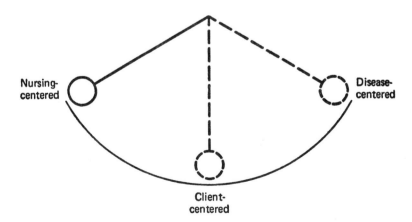

Figure 9–1. The focus of care pendulum.

hypotheses through the collection of data, and revising hypotheses when necessary on the basis of conclusions obtained from the data (Abdellah & Levine, 1986).

Many of these steps parallel the steps of the nursing process of assessment, diagnosis, planning, implementation, and evaluation. The problem-solving approach was selected because of the assumption that the correct identification of nursing problems influences the nurse's judgment in selecting the next steps in solving the client's nursing problems (Abdellah & Levine, 1986). The problem-solving approach is also consistent with such basic elements of nursing practice espoused by Abdellah as observing, reporting, and interpreting the signs and symptoms that comprise the deviations from health and constitute nursing problems, and with analyzing the nursing problems and selecting the necessary course of action (Abdellah et al., 1960).

THE TWENTY-ONE NURSING PROBLEMS

The crucial element within Abdellah's theory is the correct identification of nursing problems. To assist in identification, the need was defined for a systematic classification of nursing problems presented by the client. It was believed that such problems could be classified into the following three major categories.

1. Physical, sociological, and emotional needs of the patient [clients].
2. Types of interpersonal relationships between the nurse and the patient [client].
3. Common elements of patient [client] care (Abdellah, et al, 1960, p. 11).

Over a five-year period, several studies were carried out to establish the classification. As the result of this research, 21 groups of common nursing problems were identified (see Table 9–1). It is these 21 common nursing problems of Abdellah's that are most widely known, and they are the focus of the rest of the chapter.

These twenty-one nursing problems focus on the physical, biological, and socio-psychological needs of the client and attempt to provide a more meaningful basis for organization than the categories of systems of the body. The most difficult problems were thought to be Numbers 12, 14, 15, 17, 18, and 19 (Abdellah et al., 1973). Although a rationale is not provided for this conclusion, it is interesting that all these problems fall into the realm of sociopsychological needs and tend to be covert in nature.

Within the practice of nursing, it was anticipated that these 21 problems as broad groupings would encourage the generalization of principles and would thereby guide care and promote the development of the nurse's judgmental ability. In each of the broad nursing problems are numerous specific overt

TABLE 9–1. ABDELLAH'S TWENTY-ONE NURSING PROBLEMS

1. To maintain good hygiene and physical comfort.
2. To promote optimal activity: exercise, rest, and sleep.
3. To promote safety through the prevention of accidents, injury, or other trauma and through the prevention of the spread of infection.
4. To maintain good body mechanics and prevent and correct deformities.
5. To facilitate the maintenance of a supply of oxygen to all body cells.
6. To facilitate the maintenance of nutrition of all body cells.
7. To facilitate the maintenance of elimination.
8. To facilitate the maintenance of fluid and electrolyte balance.
9. To recognize the physiological responses of the body to disease conditions—pathological, physiological, and compensatory.
10. To facilitate the maintenance of regulatory mechanisms and functions.
11. To facilitate the maintenance of sensory function.
12. To identify and accept positive and negative expressions, feelings, and reactions.
13. To identify and accept the interrelatedness of emotions and organic illness.
14. To facilitate the maintenance of effective verbal and nonverbal communication.
15. To promote the development of productive interpersonal relationships.
16. To facilitate progress toward achievement of personal spiritual goals.
17. To create and/or maintain a therapeutic environment.
18. To facilitate awareness of self as an individual with varying physical, emotional, and developmental needs.
19. To accept the optimum possible goals in the light of limitations, physical and emotional.
20. To use community resources as an aid in resolving problems arising from illness.
21. To understand the role of social problems as influencing factors in the case of illness.

From Abdellah, F.G., and others. (1960). *Patient-centered approaches to nursing,* New York: Macmillan pp. 16–17. Used with permission.

and covert problems. It was also anticipated that the constant relating of the broad basic nursing problems to the specific problems of the individual client and vice versa would encourage the development of increased ability to use theory in clinical practice. Thus, a greater understanding of the relationship between theory and practice would strengthen the usefulness of the nursing problems (Abdellah et al., 1960).

COMPARISON WITH OTHER THEORIES

An examination of the 21 problems yields similarities to other theories. Most notable is their similarity to Henderson's (1991) 14 components of basic nursing care (see Table 9–2). As can be seen in this table, Abdellah has consolidated some components (such as Number 7—Select suitable clothing, and Number 8—Keep body clean and well groomed;) and has expanded others (most notably Number 14—Learn, discover, and satisfy curiosity). The

TABLE 9–2. COMPARISON OF MASLOW'S, HENDERSON'S, AND ABDELLAH'S FRAMEWORKS

Maslow	Henderson	Abdellah[a]
1. Physiological needs	1. Breathe normally 2. Eat and drink adequately	5. To facilitate the maintenance of a supply of oxygen to all body cells 6. To facilitate the maintenance of nutrition of all body cells 8. To facilitate the maintenance of fluid and electrolyte balance
	3. Eliminate body waste	7. To facilitate the maintenance of elimination
	4. Move and maintain desirable posture	4. To maintain good body mechanics and prevent and correct deformities
	5. Sleep and rest	2. To promote optimal activity: exercise, rest, and sleep
	6. Select suitable clothing	10. To facilitate the maintenance of regulatory mechanisms and functions
	7. Maintain body temperature 8. Keep body clean and well groomed & protect the integument	1. To maintain good hygiene and physical comfort
2. Safety needs	9. Avoid environmental dangers and avoid injuring others	3. To promote safety through the prevention of accidents, injury, or other trauma and through the prevention of the spread of infection 11. To facilitate the maintenance of sensory function
3. Belonging and love needs	10. Communicate with others	14. To facilitate the maintenance of effective verbal and nonverbal communication 15. To promote the development of productive interpersonal relationships
	11. Worship according to faith	16. To facilitate progress toward achievement of personal spiritual goals
4. Esteem needs	12. Work at something providing a sense of accomplishment 13. Play or participate in various forms of recreation 14. Learn, discover, or satisfy curiosity	19. To accept the optimum possible goals in the light of limitations, physical and emotional 9. To recognize the physiological responses of the body to disease conditions—pathological, physiological, and compensatory

(Continued)

TABLE 9–2. (CONTINUED)

Maslow	Henderson	Abdellah[a]
		12. To identify and accept positive and negative expressions, feelings, and reactions
		13. To identify and accept the interrelatedness of emotions and organic illness
		17. To create and/or maintain a therapeutic environment
		18. To facilitate awareness of self as an individual with varying physical, emotional, and developmental needs
		20. To use community resources as an aid in resolving problems arising from illness
		21. To understand the role of social problems as influencing factors in the case of illness
5. Self-actualization needs		

[a]Numbers in column 3 refer to the twenty-one problems as listed in Table 9–1.

strong similarity may be the result of both Henderson's and Abdellah's exposure to the same environment—Teachers College, Columbia University, New York. It might be hypothesized that Abdellah moved from the rather simplistic form of Henderson's theory to a more complex structure.

Despite the noted similarity, a major difference is evident. Henderson's components are written in terms of client behaviors, whereas Abdellah's problems are formulated in terms of the nursing services that should be incorporated into the determination of the client's needs (DeYoung, 1976). This emphasis on nursing services is consistent with Abdellah's apparent nurse-centered orientation mentioned earlier. Henderson seems to have maintained the client orientation, whereas Abdellah seems to have moved beyond it (see Table 9–2).

Abdellah's nursing problems are also comparable to Maslow's (1954) hierarchy of needs. In contrast to Henderson's components, which have a strong physiological orientation, Abdellah's expansion in the area of *esteem needs* provides a more balanced set of nursing problems between the physical and nonphysical areas (Table 9–2). As with Henderson's components, Abdellah's problems do not meet the self-actualization needs of Maslow. This is not surprising, for self-actualization is not a goal to be accomplished but a process that is ongoing—the dynamic process of becoming. To place elements in this area would negate the dynamism of self-actualization. From a different viewpoint, if Henderson's components and Abdellah's problems are fulfilled, then the client will move toward becoming and self-actualization.

ABDELLAH'S THEORY AND NURSING'S METAPARADIGM

Abdellah does not clearly specify each of the four major concepts—the individual or human, health, environment/society, and nursing. She does describe the recipients of nursing as *individuals* (and families), although she does not delineate her beliefs or assumptions about the nature of human beings. Her 21 nursing problems deal with biological, psychological, and social areas of individuals and can be considered to represent areas of importance to them.

Health, or the achieving of it, is the purpose of nursing services. Although Abdellah does not give a definition of health, she speaks to "total health needs" and "a healthy state of mind and body" in her description of nursing as a comprehensive service (Abdellah et al., 1960).

Society is included in "planning for optimum health on local, state, national, and international levels" (Abdellah et al., 1960). However, as Abdellah further delineates her ideas, the focus of nursing service is clearly the individual. Society is negated when she discusses implementation.

Nursing is broadly grouped into the 21 problem areas to guide care and promote the use of nursing judgment. Abdellah considers nursing to be a comprehensive service that is based on an art and science and aims to help people, sick or well, cope with their health needs.

USE OF THE TWENTY-ONE PROBLEMS IN THE NURSING PROCESS

Because of the strong nurse-centered orientation in the 21 nursing problems, their use in the nursing process is primarily to direct the nurse. Indirectly, the client benefits. If the nurse helps the client reach all the goals stated in the nursing problems, then the client will be moved toward health.

Within the *assessment* phase, the nursing problems provide guidelines for the collection of data. A principle underlying the problem-solving approach is that for each identified problem, pertinent data are collected. Thus, for each of the identified 21 nursing problems, relevant data are collected. The overt or covert nature of the problems necessitates a direct or indirect approach, respectively. For example, the overt problem of nutritional status can be assessed by direct measures of weight, food intake, and body size, whereas the covert problem of maintaining a therapeutic environment requires more indirect approaches to data collection.

The nursing problems can be divided into those that are basic to all clients and those that reflect sustenal, remedial, or restorative care needs, as seen in

Table 9–3. By facilitating data collection, such a classification promotes investigating those problems consistent with the client's stage of illness. However, such a classification promotes the thinking that the client's stage of illness determines appropriate or acceptable problems. Such thinking is contrary to the philosophy of holism. If clients are holistic, then they can have needs in any and all areas regardless of the stage of illness. A varied multitude of nursing problems could then exist.

The results of the data collection would determine the client's specific overt and/or covert problems. These specific problems would be grouped under one or more of the broader nursing problems. This step is consistent with that involved in *nursing diagnosis*. Within this framework, the nursing diagnoses are derived from the exhibited nursing problems.

The 21 nursing problems can have a great impact on the *planning* phase of the nursing process. The statements of the nursing problems most closely resemble goal statements. Therefore, once the problem has been diagnosed, the goals have been established. Many of the nursing problem statements can be considered goals for either the nurse or the client. Given that these problems are called *nursing problems,* then it becomes reasonable to conclude that these goals are basically nursing goals.

Using the goals as the framework, a plan is developed and appropriate nursing interventions are determined. Table 9–3 summarizes the kinds of interventions that would be appropriate for the categories of nursing problems. Again, holism tends to be negated in *implementation* because of the isolated, particulate nature of the nursing problems.

Following implementation of the plan, *evaluation* takes place. According to the American Nurses' Association's *Standards of nursing practice,* the plan is evaluated in terms of the client's progress or lack of progress toward the achievement of the stated goals (Congress for Nursing Practice, 1973). This would be extremely difficult if not impossible to do for Abdellah's nursing problem approach because it has been determined that the goals are *nursing* goals, not *client* goals. Thus, the most appropriate evaluation would be the *nurse's* progress or lack of progress toward the achievement of the stated goals.

Abdellah postulates that criterion measures can be determined from the groupings of the nursing problems, as shown in Table 9–3. A criterion is a value-free name of a measurable variable believed or known to be a relevant indicator of the quality of client care (Bloch, 1977). Criteria can be used to measure client care. Although it is not clear in her writings, the measurement of criteria seems to have been substituted for evaluating a client's progress toward goal achievement.

The use of Abdellah's 21 nursing problems in an example might be beneficial. Consider the case of Ron, who experienced severe crushing chest pain following a board meeting at his place of business. In addition to the pain, he experienced shortness of breath, tachycardia, and profuse diaphoresis. Upon admission to the hospital, assessment indicated that Ron might have sustained some cardiac damage. Investigation into his history revealed that he had been having episodes of chest pain for the past two months. With this as

TABLE 9–3. THE RELATIONSHIPS AMONG THE CLASSIFICATION AND APPROACH OF THE TWENTY-ONE NURSING PROBLEMS AND STAGES OF ILLNESS, NURSING INTERVENTIONS, AND CRITERION MEASURES

Stages of Illness[a]	Nursing Problems	Classification and Approach[b]	Nursing Interventions[c]	Criterion Measures[a]
Basic to all patients	1. To maintain good hygiene and physical comfort 2. To promote optimal activity: exercise, rest, and sleep 3. To promote safety through prevention of accident, injury, or other trauma and through the prevention of the spread of infection 4. To maintain good body mechanics and prevent and correct deformities	Overt problems, covert problems, or both Direct methods, indirect methods, or both	Measures necessary to maintain hygiene, physical comfort, activity, rest and sleep, safety, and body mechanics	Related to preventive care needs
Sustenal care needs	5. To facilitate the maintenance of a supply of oxygen to all body cells 6. To facilitate the maintenance of nutrition of all body cells 7. To facilitate the maintenance of elimination 8. To facilitate the maintenance of fluid and electrolyte balance	Usually overt problems Direct methods	Measures necessary to maintain oxygen supply, nutrition, elimination, fluid and electrolyte balance, regulatory mechanisms, and sensory functions. Interventions imply recognition of body's response to disease	Related to sustenal and restorative care needs—the normal and disturbed physiological body processes that are vital to sustaining life

	9. To recognize the physiological responses of the body to disease conditions—pathological, physiological, and compensatory		
	10. To facilitate the maintenance of regulatory mechanisms and functions		
	11. To facilitate the maintenance of sensory function		
Remedial care needs	12. To identify and accept positive and negative expressions, feelings, and reactions	Usually covert problems Indirect methods	Measures that are helpful to the client and his or her family during their emotional reactions to client's illness
	13. To identify and accept the interrelatedness of emotions and organic illness		
	14. To facilitate the maintenance of effective verbal and nonverbal communication		
	15. To promote the development of productive interpersonal relationships		
	16. To facilitate progress toward achievement of personal spiritual goals		Related to rehabilitation needs, particularly those involving emotional and interpersonal difficulties

(Continued)

TABLE 9–3. (CONTINUED)

Stages of Illness[a]	Nursing Problems	Classification and Approach[b]	Nursing Interventions[c]	Criterion Measures[a]
	17. To create and maintain a therapeutic environment			
	18. To facilitate awareness of self as an individual with varying physical, emotional, and developmental needs			
Restorative care needs	19. To accept the optimum possible goals in the light of limitations, physical and emotional	Overt problems, covert problems, or both Direct methods, indirect methods, or both	Measures that will assist the client and his or her family to cope with the illness and necessary life adjustment	Related to sociological and community problems affecting client care
	20. To use community resources as an aid in resolving problems arising from illness			
	21. To understand the role of social problems as influencing factors in the cause of illness			

[a]From Abdellah, F.G., Levine, E. (1965). *Better patient care through nursing research*, New York: Macmillan, pp. 78–79, 280–281.
[b]From Abdellah, F.G., et al. (1960). *Patient-centered approaches to nursing*, New York: Macmillan, pp. 81–82.
[c]From Carter, J.H., et al. (1976). *Standards of nursing care*, New York: Springer, pp. 8–9.

the data base, the specific problems of pain, impaired cardiac functioning, work-related stress, and failure to seek medical assistance can be identified. These specific problems can be related to selected nursing problems defined by Abdellah, and the nursing problems can be related to the stage of Ron's illness. Nursing strategies and criterion measures can then be determined. Table 9–4 illustrates the implementation of Abdellah's framework. The results of fractionalizing care can be readily seen by the repetition of intervention strategies for the two problems of pain and impaired cardiac functioning. (This table is in no way designed to be inclusive. Rather, it is offered as an attempt to make the theory operational.)

ABDELLAH'S WORK AND THE CHARACTERISTICS OF A THEORY

1. Theories can interrelate concepts in such a way as to create a different way of looking at a particular phenomenon. Abdellah's theory has interrelated the concepts of health, nursing problems, and problem solving as she attempts to create a different way of viewing nursing phenomena. The result is the statement that nursing is the use of the problem-solving approach with key nursing problems related to the health needs of people.

2. Theories must be logical in nature. The theoretical statement places heavy emphasis on problem solving, an activity that is inherently logical in nature.

3. Theories should be relatively simple yet generalizable. Because of the failure of the framework to provide a perspective on humans and society in general, the theory appears to be limited to use which seems to focus quite heavily on nursing practice with individuals. This somewhat limits the ability to generalize, although the problem-solving approach is readily generalizable to clients with specific health needs and specific nursing problems.

4. Theories can be the bases for hypotheses that can be tested or for theory to be generated, and

5. Theories contribute to and assist in increasing the general body of knowledge within the discipline through the research implemented to validate them. One of the most important questions that arises when considering Abdellah's work is the role of the client within the framework, a question that could generate hypotheses for testing. The results of testing such hypotheses would contribute to the general body of nursing knowledge.

6. Theories can be used by practitioners to guide and improve their practice. As a logical and simple statement, Abdellah's problem-solving approach can easily be used by practitioners to guide various activities within their nursing practice. This is especially true when considering nursing practice that deals with clients who have specific needs and specific nursing problems.

7. Theories must be consistent with other validated theories, laws, and principles but will leave open unanswered questions that need to be investigated. Abdellah's theory is consistent with other theories, such as those of Maslow and Henderson. Although this consistency exists, many questions remained unanswered.

TABLE 9–4. AN ILLUSTRATION OF THE IMPLEMENTATION OF ABDELLAH'S FRAMEWORK IN RON'S CARE

Stages of Illness	Selected Abdellah Nursing Problems	Classification and Approach	Selected Nursing Interventions	Criterion Measures
Basic care	1. To maintain good hygiene and physical comfort	Overt problem of pain Direct and indirect methods	1. Administer oxygen 2. Elevate headrest 3. Reposition client 4. Administer prescribed analgesic 5. Remain with client	Amount of pain
Sustenal care needs	5. To facilitate the maintenance of a supply of oxygen to all body cells	Overt problem of impaired cardiac functioning Direct methods	1. Promote rest 2. Place in sitting position 3. Promote deep breathing and coughing 4. Implement exercise program as tolerated	Vital signs
Remedial care needs	13. To identify and accept the interrelatedness of emotional and organic illness	Covert problem of effects of work-related stress on cardiac functioning Indirect methods	1. Investigate the nature of his job and activities involved 2. Explore his work-related goals 3. Explore the kinds of stress associated with his job	Knowledge of relationship between stress and his illness
Restorative care needs	20. To use community resources as an aid in resolving problems arising from illness	Overt problem of failure to seek medical assistance when needed Direct methods	1. Teach early warning signs and symptoms of cardiac distress 2. Teach course of action should specific symptoms occur	Knowledge of appropriate use of certain community resources

LIMITATIONS

The major limitation to Abdellah's theory and the 21 nursing problems is their very strong nurse-centered orientation. With this orientation, appropriate uses might be the organization of teaching content for nursing students, the evaluation of a student's performance in the clinical area, or both. But in terms of client care, there is little emphasis on what the client is to achieve.

Abdellah's framework is inconsistent with the concept of holism. The classification of the 21 nursing problems according to stages of illness and the particulate nature of the problems attests to this inconsistency. As a result, the client may be diagnosed as having numerous problems that would lead to fractionalized care efforts, and potential problems might be overlooked because the client is not deemed to be in a particular stage of illness.

CONCLUSIONS

Abdellah's theory and framework provide a basis for determining and organizing nursing care. If all the problems are investigated, the client would be likely to be thoroughly assessed. The problems also provide a basis for organizing appropriate nursing strategies. It is anticipated that by solving the nursing problems, the client would be moved toward health. The nurse's philosophical frame of reference would determine whether this theory and the 21 nursing problems could be implemented in practice.

SUMMARY

Using Abdellah's concepts of health, nursing problems, and problem solving, the theoretical statement of nursing that can be derived is the use of the problem-solving approach with key nursing problems related to the health needs of people. From this framework, 21 nursing problems were developed. These problems are compared to Henderson's 14 components of nursing and Maslow's hierarchy of needs. Ways to use the nursing problems in the nursing process are explored. The major limitation of Abdellah's theory is its strong nursing-centered orientation. Some modification of the nursing problems to promote a more client-centered orientation would encourage effective use of the theory in professional nursing practice.

REFERENCES

Abdellah, F. G., Beland, I. L., Martin, A., & Matheney, R. V. (1960). *Patient-centered approaches to nursing*. New York: Macmillan. [out of print]

Abdellah, F. G., Beland, I. L., Martin, A., & Matheney, R. V. (1973). *New directions in patient-centered nursing*. New York: Macmillan.

Abdellah, F. G., & Levine, E. (1986). *Better patient care through nursing research* (3rd ed.). New York: Macmillan.

Bloch, D. (1977). Criteria, standards, norms—Crucial terms in quality assurance. *Journal of Nursing Administration, 7,* 22.

Carter, J. H., Hilliard, M., Castles, M. R., Stoll, L. D., & Cowan, A. (1976) *Standards of nursing care.* NY: Springer.

Congress for Nursing Practice. (1973). *Standards of nursing practice.* Kansas City: American Nurses' Association.

DeYoung, L. (1976). *The foundations of nursing.* St. Louis: Mosby.

Henderson, V. (1991). *The nature of nursing: Reflections after 25 years.* New York: National League for Nursing.

Maslow, A. (1954). *Motivation and personality.* New York: Harper & Row.

Nicholls, M. E., & Wessells, V. G. (Eds.). (1977). *Nursing standards and nursing process.* Wakefield, Mass.: Contemporary Publishing.

Torres, G., & Stanton, M. (1982). *Curriculum process in nursing: A guide to curriculum development.* Englewood Cliffs, NJ: Prentice-Hall.

BIBLIOGRAPHY

Dycus, D. K., McClure, E. A., Schmeiser, D. N., Taggart, F. M., & Yancey, R. (1994). Faye Glenn Abdellah: Twenty-one Nursing Problems. In A. Marriner-Tomey (Ed.), *Nursing theorists and their work* (3rd ed.) (pp. 116–137). St. Louis: Mosby.

See, E. M. (1989). Abdellah's model for nursing: Twenty-one Nursing Problems. In J. J. Fitzpatrick, & A. L. Whall (Eds.), *Conceptual models of nursing: Analysis and application* (2nd ed.) (pp. 123–136). Norwalk, CT: Appleton & Lange.

IDA JEAN ORLANDO

Mary Kathryn Leonard
Julia B. George*

■ ■ ■

*Ida Jean Orlando Pelletier (b. 1926) has had a varied career as a practitioner,
educator, researcher, and consultant in nursing. During the early part of her
career, she worked as a staff nurse in such areas as obstetrics, medicine, and
surgery, and the emergency room. She also held supervisory positions and the title
of Second Assistant Director of Nurses. She received a diploma in nursing from
New York Medical College, Flower Fifth Avenue Hospital School of Nursing in
1947, and a BS in Public Health Nursing from St. John's University in Brooklyn,
New York, in 1951. In 1954, she received her MA in mental health consultation
from Columbia University, New York. She then went to Yale University as a
research associate and principal investigator on a project studying the integration
of mental health concepts into the basic nursing curriculum. This led to the
publication of her first book,* The dynamic nurse–patient relationship: Function,
process, and principles, *in 1961 (reprinted 1990). She also served as director of the
graduate program in mental health and psychiatric nursing at Yale.*

*In 1962, Orlando married Robert Pelletier and moved to Massachusetts. She
became a clinical nursing consultant to a psychiatric hospital, McLean Hospital,
and at a veterans' hospital. At McLean Hospital, she carried out the research that
led to the publication in 1972 of her second book,* The discipline and teaching of
nursing process.

*Since 1972, Orlando has been associated intermittently with Boston University
School of Nursing, teaching nursing theory and supervising graduate students in
the clinical area. She also served as a project consultant for The New England
Board of Higher Education in their Mental Health Project for Associate Degree
Faculties. Her most recent position is as a nurse educator at Metropolitan State
Hospital in Waltham, Massachusetts.*

*Throughout her career, Orlando has been active in a variety of organizations,
including the Massachusetts Nurses' Association and the Harvard Community
Health Plan. She has also lectured and offered workshops and consultation to a
wide variety of agencies.*

---

*Gratitude is expressed to Mary D. Crane for her contributions to this chapter in earlier editions.

Ida Jean Orlando Pelletier describes a nursing process based on the interaction between a patient and a nurse. Her nursing process discipline was developed through research and presented in two books. Her initial work, *The dynamic nurse–patient relationship: Function, process and principles,* was originally published in 1961 and reprinted in 1990. *The discipline and teaching of nursing process,* showing further testing and refinement of her work, appeared in 1972.

Orlando's educational background and the work that led to her publications provide insight into the content of her theory. Her advanced nursing preparation and area of teaching responsibility and practice were in mental health and psychiatric nursing. Although she applied her ideas to many nursing specialty areas, the focus of her work is interaction.

The dynamic nurse–patient relationship was written to report the results of a five-year project at Yale University in the mid-1950s. The purpose of this project, supported by a grant from the National Institute of Mental Health, was "to identify the factors which enhanced or impeded the integration of mental health principles in the basic nursing curriculum" (Orlando, 1961/1990, p. vii). This research resulted in identification that a nurse's statement of her perception, thought, or feeling about the patient's behavior differentiated between effective and ineffective communication. The book describes the curriculum content developed from the study. Its stated purpose is "to offer the professional nursing student a theory of effective nursing practice" (p. viii). This book was completed in 1958 and was initially rejected for publication as not being marketable in nursing. Finally, in 1961, it was recognized as having an important contribution to make to the practice of nursing.

Orlando refined her ideas and put them into practice at a private psychiatric facility, McLean Hospital in Belmont, Massachusetts. Again with a National Institute of Mental Health grant, she studied an objective means to evaluate her process and training in its discipline. The discipline variable was found to make a statistically significant difference in patient outcomes. This work, done during the 1960s, led to *The discipline and teaching of nursing process* (1972), in which she was concerned with the specific definition of nursing function and with incorporating nursing activities beyond the nurse–patient relationship into a total nursing system. She also developed more readily measured criteria to guide the nurse in her reaction to patient behavior.*

Orlando's work spans a fertile period of nursing thinking. She was probably influenced by, as well as an influence upon, other nursing theorists. For example, Orlando sounds similar to Nightingale when she states, "It is important for the nurse to concern herself with the patient's distress because the treatment and prevention of disease proceed best when conditions extraneous to the disease itself and its management do not cause the

---

*In this chapter, the feminine pronoun is used when referring to the nurse and the masculine pronoun when referring to the patient. This is consistent with Orlando's use of these pronouns and terms.

patient additional suffering" (Orlando, 1961/1990, pp. 22–23). Another nursing theorist, Peplau (1952/1988), published her highly interpersonal theory two years before Orlando began her first study. Henderson also was redefining her definition of nursing during Orlando's first study. Henderson's 1955 definition is consistent with Orlando when she states, "Nursing is primarily assisting the individual . . . in the performance of those activities . . . that he would perform unaided if he had the necessary strength, will, or knowledge" (Harmer & Henderson, 1955, p. 4). Ernestine Wiedenbach's interest in the initial study led to an increased concentration of data collection about nursing practice in the maternal/newborn area (Trench, Wallace, & Coberg, 1987).

ORLANDO'S KEY CONCEPTS

Certain major concepts are evident in Orlando's theory of nursing. She believes that nursing is *unique* and *independent* because it concerns itself with an *individual's need for help,* real or potential, in an *immediate* situation. The process by which nursing resolves this helplessness is *interactive* and is pursued in a *disciplined* manner that requires *training.* She believes one's actions should be based on rationale, not protocols.

Throughout her career, Orlando has been concerned with identifying that which is *uniquely* nursing. In her first book, she presents principles to guide nursing practice (Orlando, 1961/1990). She believes that the use of general principles from other fields is not sufficient to help the nurse in her interaction with patients. In this book, she identifies nursing's role as follows, "It is the nurse's direct responsibility to see to it that the patient's needs for help are met either by her own activity or by calling in the help of others" (p. 22).

Orlando (1972) also suggests that nursing's failure to establish its uniqueness is a result of the lack of a clearly identifiable function, which leads to inadequate care and insufficient attention to the patient's reactions to his immediate experiences. Thus, she identifies nursing's function as being "concerned with providing direct assistance to individuals in whatever setting they are found for the purpose of avoiding, relieving, diminishing, or curing the individual's sense of helplessness" (p. 12).

It is this unique function that gives nurses the authority to work *independently.* Orlando recommends that "nurses . . . must radically shift their focus from assistance to physicians and institutions to assisting patients with what they cannot do alone" (Pelletier, 1967, p. 28). Physicians' orders are directed to patients, not to nurses. Moreover, at times nurses may even assist patients in *not* complying with medical orders when such orders are in conflict with the patient's need for help. Nurses must also resolve conflicts between the patient's need for help and institutional policies. Nursing's unique function allows nurses to work in any setting where persons experience a need for help that they cannot resolve themselves. Thus, nurses may practice with well or ill persons in an independent practice or in an institutional setting.

Orlando's theory focuses on the patient as an *individual*. Each person, in each situation, is different. To be appropriate, nursing actions for two patients with the same presenting behavior, or the same patient at different times, are to be individualized. Nurses cannot automatically act only on the basis of principles, past experience, or physicians' orders. They must first ascertain that their actions will meet the patient's specific need for help.

Nursing is concerned with "individuals who suffer or anticipate a sense of helplessness" (Orlando, 1961/1990, p. 12). Orlando (1972) defines need as "a requirement of the patient which, if supplied, relieves or diminishes his immediate distress or improves his immediate sense of adequacy or well-being" (p. 5). In many instances, people can meet their own needs, do so, and do not require the help of professional nurses. When they cannot do so, or do not clearly understand these needs, a *need for help* is present. The nurse's function is to correctly identify and relieve this need.

The *immediacy* of the nursing situation is a vital concept in Orlando's theory. Each patient's behavior must be assessed to determine whether it expresses a need for help. Furthermore, identical behaviors by the same patient may indicate different needs at different times. The nursing action must also be specifically designed for the immediate encounter. Long-term planning has no part in Orlando's theory except as it pertains to providing adequate staff coverage for a job setting.

Orlando describes a nursing process discipline that is totally *interactive*. It describes, step by step, what goes on between a nurse and a patient in a specific encounter. A patient behavior causes the process discipline to begin. The process discipline involves the nurse's reaction to this behavior and the nurse's consequent action. The nurse shares her reaction with the patient to identify the need for help and the appropriate action. The nurse also verifies that the action met the need for help. Orlando's principles are meant to guide the nurse at various stages of the interaction. She emphasizes the importance of interaction when she writes, "Learning how to understand what is happening between herself and the patient is the central core of the nurse's practice and comprises the basic framework for the help she gives to patients" (Orlando, 1961/1990, p. 4).

The actual *process* of a nurse–patient interaction may be the same as that of any interaction between two persons. When nurses use this process to communicate their reactions in caring for patients, Orlando calls it the "nursing process discipline." It is the tool that nurses use to fulfill their function to patients. In an attempt to extend her theory to encompass all nursing activities, Orlando (1972) broadens the use of the process discipline beyond the individual nurse–patient relationship in her book, *The discipline and teaching of nursing process*. She applies the process discipline to contacts between a nurse leader and those she supervises or directs. When it is used in this manner, she refers to the process discipline as the "directive or supervisory job process in nursing" (p. 29).

If the nursing process is the same as the interactive process between any two individuals, how can nursing call itself a profession? The key is *discipline* in use of the process. Orlando (1972) provides three criteria to evaluate this discipline. These criteria differentiate an "automatic personal response" from a "disciplined professional response" (p. 31). Only the latter leads to effective nursing care, that is, relief of the patient's sense of helplessness. Learning to employ the process discipline requires *training*. This justifies the need for specific education in nursing. Orlando's nursing process discipline and the criteria for its use are discussed in more detail.

ORLANDO'S NURSING PROCESS DISCIPLINE

Orlando's (1972) nursing process discipline is based on the "process by which any individual acts" (p. 24). The purpose of the process discipline, when it is used between a nurse and a patient, is to meet the patient's immediate need for help. Improvement in the patient's behavior that indicates resolution of the need is the desired result. The process discipline is also used with other persons working in a job setting. The purpose here is to understand how the professional and job responsibilities of each affect the other. This understanding allows each nurse to effectively fulfill her professional function for the patient within the organizational setting.

Patient Behavior

The nursing process discipline is set in motion by *patient behavior*. All patient behavior, no matter how insignificant, must be considered an expression of need for help until its meaning to a particular patient in the immediate situation is understood. Orlando (1961/1990) stresses this in her first principle: "The presenting behavior of the patient, regardless of the form in which it appears, may represent a plea for help" (p. 40).

Patient behavior may be verbal or nonverbal. Inconsistency between these two types of behavior may be the factor that alerts the nurse that the patient needs help. Verbal behavior encompasses all the patient's use of language. It may take the form of "complaints . . . , requests . . . , questions . . . , refusals . . . , demands . . . , and . . . comments or statements" (Orlando, 1961/1990, p. 11). Nonverbal behavior includes physiological manifestations such as heart rate, perspiration, edema, and urination, and motor activity such as smiling, walking, and avoiding eye contact. Nonverbal patient behavior may also be vocal, including such actions as sobbing, laughing, shouting, and sighing.

When the patient experiences a need that he cannot resolve, a sense of helplessness occurs. The patient's behavior reflects this distress. In *The dynamic nurse–patient relationship*, Orlando (1961/1990) describes some categories of patient distress: "physical limitations, . . . adverse reactions to the setting and . . . experiences which prevent the patient from communicating his needs" (p. 11). Feelings of helplessness caused by physical limitations may result from incomplete development, temporary or permanent disability, or restrictions of the environment, real or imagined. Adverse reactions to the setting, on the other hand, usually result from incorrect or inadequate understanding of an experience there. Patients may become distressed by a negative reaction to any aspect of the setting, despite its helpful or therapeutic intent. A need for help may also arise from the patient's inability to communicate effectively. This inability may be due to such factors as ambivalence concerning dependency brought on by illness, embarrassment related to the need, lack of trust in the nurse, and inability to state the need precisely.

Although all patient behavior may indicate a need for help, the behavior may not effectively communicate that need. When the behavior does not communicate the need, problems in the nurse–patient relationship can arise. Ineffective patient behavior "prevents the nurse from carrying out her concerns for the patient's care or from maintaining a satisfactory relationship to the patient" (Orlando, 1961/1990, p. 78). Ineffective patient behavior may also indicate difficulties in the initial establishment of the nurse–patient relationship, inaccurate identification of the patient's need by the nurse, or negative patient reaction to automatic nursing action. Resolution of ineffective patient behavior deserves high priority, for the behavior usually becomes worse over time if the need for help that it expresses remains unresolved. The nurse's reaction and action are designed to resolve ineffective patient behaviors as well as to meet the immediate need.

Nurse Reaction

The patient behavior stimulates a *nurse reaction*, which marks the beginning of the nursing process discipline. This reaction is comprised of three sequential parts (Orlando, 1972). First, the nurse perceives the behavior through any of her senses. Second, the perception leads to automatic thought. Finally, the thought produces an automatic feeling. For example, the nurse sees a patient grimace, thinks he is in pain, and feels concern. The nurse then shares her reaction with the patient to ascertain that she has correctly identified the need for help and to identify the nursing action appropriate to resolve it. Orlando (1961/1990) offers a principle to guide the nurse in her reaction to patient behavior. "The nurse does not assume that any aspect of her reaction to the patient is correct, helpful, or appropriate until she checks the validity of it in exploration with the patient" (p. 56).

Perception, thought, and feeling occur automatically and almost simultaneously. Therefore the nurse must learn to identify each part of her reaction. This helps her to analyze the reaction to determine why she responded as she did. The process becomes logical rather than intuitive and, thus, disciplined rather than automatic. The nurse is able to use her reaction for the purpose of helping the patient.

The discipline in the nursing process prescribes how the nurse shares her reaction with the patient. Orlando (1961/1990) offers a principle to explain the usefulness of this sharing: "Any observation shared and explored with the patient is immediately useful in ascertaining and meeting his need or finding out that he is not in need at that time" (pp. 35–36).

Orlando (1972) also provides three criteria to ensure that the nurse's exploration of her reaction with the patient is successful:

1. What the nurse says to the individual in the contact must match (*be consistent with*) any or all of the items contained in the immediate reaction, and what the nurse does nonverbally must be verbally expressed and the expression must match one or all of the items contained in the immediate reaction; 2. The nurse must clearly communicate to the individual that the item being expressed belongs to herself; 3. The nurse must ask the individual about the item expressed in order to obtain correction or verification from that same individual (pp. 29–30).

Which aspect of her reaction the nurse shares with the patient is not as important as that it be shared in the manner described in the criteria. From a practical standpoint, it may be more expeditious to share a perception than a thought or feeling. "You are grimacing" contains less assumption than "Are you in pain?" In this way the patient can more easily express his need for help without having to correct the nurse's misconception.

Feelings can and should be shared even when they are negative. The nonverbal action of the nurse will usually show her feelings even if they are not verbally expressed. Thus, the nurse's verbal and nonverbal behavior may be inconsistent. Proper sharing of feelings can effectively help the patient to express his need for help. For example, a nurse may react to a patient's refusal of a medication with anger. If she says, "I am angry with your refusal of your medication. Could you explain to me why you have refused?" she invites the patient to explain the need for help that his refusal expressed. Her expression meets the three criteria, and the patient's need for help can be identified and resolved.

This example shows the importance of the nurse sharing her reaction as a fact about herself. She states, "I am angry," rather than, "You make me angry." This clear identification of the reaction as her own reduces the chance of misinterpretation by the patient. The sharing of the nurse's immediate reaction creates a climate in which the patient is more able to share his own reaction.

Adequate identification of the three aspects of the nurse's reaction helps to resolve extraneous feelings that may interfere with the patient's care. The nurse may find that her feelings come from her personal belief of how people should act or from stresses in the organizational setting or in her personal life. These feelings or stresses are unrelated to meeting the patient's need. If they are not resolved, the nurse's verbal and nonverbal behavior will again be inconsistent. This same process should be employed with nurses or other professionals in the job setting to resolve any conflicts that interfere with the nurse's fulfilling her professional function for the patient.

Orlando (1972) used her three criteria in the study described in *The discipline and teaching of nursing process* and found that use of the process discipline is positively related to improvement in patient behavior. The study also showed a positive relationship between the nurse's use of the process discipline and its use by the patient. Thus, use of the process discipline alone can help the patient communicate his need more effectively.

Orlando (1972) offers a diagram depicting open sharing of the nurse's reaction versus keeping the reaction secret (see Figs. 10–1 and 10–2). The nurse action that results from the reaction becomes a behavior which stimulates a reaction by the patient. Only openness in sharing of the nurse's reaction assures that the patient's need will be effectively resolved. This sharing, in the manner prescribed, differentiates professional nursing practice from automatic personal response.

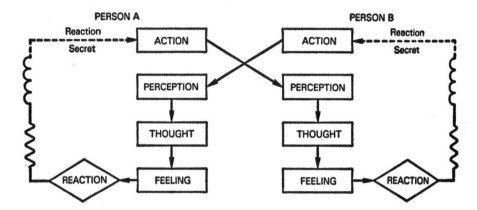

Figure 10–1. The action process in a person-to-person contact functioning in secret. The perceptions, thoughts, and feelings of each individual are not directly available to the perception of the other individual through the observable action. *(From Orlando, I.J. (1972).* The discipline and teaching of nursing process, *New York: G. P. Putnam's Sons, p. 26. Used with permission.)*

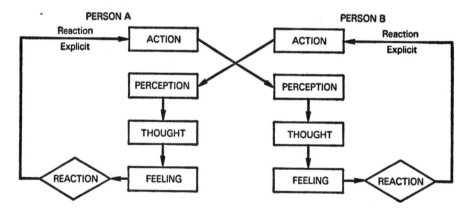

Figure 10–2. The action process in a person-to-person contact functioning by open disclosure. The perceptions, thoughts, and feelings of each individual are directly available to the perception of the other individual through the observable action. *(From Orlando, I.J. (1972). The discipline and teaching of nursing process, New York: G. P. Putnam's Sons, p. 26. Used with permission.)*

Nurse's Action

Once the nurse has validated or corrected her reaction to the patient's behavior through exploration with him, she can complete the nursing process discipline with the *nurse's action*. Orlando (1961/1990) includes "only what she [the nurse] says or does with or for the benefit of the patient" as professional nursing action (p. 60). The nurse must be certain that her action is appropriate to meet the patient's need for help. Orlando's principle for guiding nursing action states, "The nurse initiates a process of exploration to ascertain how the patient is affected by what she says or does" (p. 67).

The nurse can act in two ways: automatic or deliberative. Only the second manner fulfills her professional function. Automatic actions are "those decided upon for reasons other than the patient's immediate need," whereas deliberative actions ascertain and meet this need (Orlando, 1961/1990, p. 60). There is a distinction between the purpose an action actually serves and its intention to help the patient. For example, a nurse administers a sleeping pill because the physician orders it. Carrying out the physician's order is the purpose of the action. However, the nurse has not determined that the patient is having trouble sleeping or that a pill is the most appropriate way to help him sleep. Thus, the action is automatic, not deliberative, and the patient's need for help is unlikely to be met. The following list identifies the criteria for deliberative actions:

1. Deliberative actions result from the correct identification of patient needs by validation of the nurse's reaction to patient behavior.
2. The nurse explores the meaning of the action with the patient and its relevance to meeting his need.
3. The nurse validates the action's effectiveness immediately after completing it.
4. The nurse is free of stimuli unrelated to the patient's need when she acts.

Automatic actions fail to meet one or more of these criteria. Automatic actions are most likely to be done by nurses primarily concerned with carrying out physicians' orders, routines of patient care, or general principles for protecting health or by nurses who do not validate their reactions to patient behaviors. Although any nursing action may be purported to have occurred with the intention of helping the patient, deliberation is needed to determine if the action achieved its purpose and to identify if the patient was helped.

Professional Function

Nurses often work within organizations with other professionals and are subject to the authority of the organization that employs them. It is inevitable, therefore, that at times conflicts will arise between the actions appropriate to the nurse's profession and those required by the job. Nonprofessional actions can prevent the nurse from carrying out her professional function, and this can lead to inadequate patient care. A well-defined function of the profession can help to prevent and resolve this conflict.

Nurses should not accept positions that do not allow them to meet their patients' needs for help. If a conflict does arise, the nurse must present data to show that nursing is unable to fulfill its professional function. Orlando (1972) believes that an employer is unlikely to continue to require job activities that interfere with a well-defined function of a profession. For an agency to do so "would be to completely abandon the whole point of having enlisted the services of that profession in the agency or institution" (p. 16).

Nurses must be constantly aware that their "activity is professional only when it deliberately achieves the purpose of helping the patient" (Orlando, 1961/1990, p. 70). Some automatic activities may be necessary to the running of an institution. These should, however, be kept to a minimum and should be carried out as much as possible by support personnel. The nurse must attend to helping the patients resolve any conflict between these routines and their needs for help.

In most acute care institutions today, the potential demand for nursing skill and judgment exceeds the availability of such qualities. As a result, nursing care delivery systems are being evaluated and revised to enable the nurse to practice in those situations or areas where she is most needed. Some of these situations have been specifically identified by the Professional Nursing Accreditation Committee and, through their input, reflected in the accreditation standards of the Joint Commission on Accreditation for Health Care Organizations. These are: (1) when the patient is admitted, a professional nursing assessment is needed to identify the patient's need for help; (2) when the patient has a need for education commonly called patient education; and (3) when the patient is being prepared for discharge. In each of these situations, the use of Orlando's theory would guide the nurse in expeditiously meeting the patient's need. At this time, nurses in acute care facilities are being looked to to use their professional skills and knowledge to recognize and resolve the patient's need for help. Some of this recognition of the nursing contribution may be related to the situational pressures arising out of the prospective payment reimbursement system affecting health care institutions today. Under this system, emphasis is placed on the patient being treated and discharged within a predetermined number of days. Nursing can capitalize on this situation and use it to the patient's and profession's best interests. Orlando's theory, although simple in nature, provides direction and focus for identifying and understanding the patient's need.

Thus, the nursing process discipline is set in motion by a patient behavior that may indicate a need for help. The nurse reacts to this behavior with perceptions, thoughts, and feelings. She shares an aspect of her reaction with the patient, making sure that her verbal and nonverbal actions are consistent with her reaction, that she identifies the reaction as her own, and that she invites the patient to comment on the validity of her reaction. A properly shared reaction by the nurse helps the patient to use the same process to more effectively communicate his need. Next, an appropriate action to resolve the need is mutually decided upon by the patient and nurse. After the nurse acts, she immediately asks the patient if the action has been effective. Throughout the interaction, the nurse makes sure that she is free of any extraneous stimuli that interfere with her reaction to the patient.

ORLANDO'S THEORY AND NURSING'S METAPARADIGM

Orlando includes material specific to three of the four major concepts: the human, health, and nursing. The fourth concept, society, is not included in her theory.

She uses the concept of *human* as she emphasizes individuality and the dynamic nature of the nurse–patient relationship. For Orlando, humans in need are the focus of nursing practice.

Although *health* is not specified by Orlando, it is implied. In her initial work, Orlando focused on illness. Later, she indicated that nursing deals with the individual whenever there is a need for help. Thus, a sense of helplessness replaces the concept of health or illness as the initiator of a need for nursing.

Orlando largely ignores *society*. She deals only with the interaction between a nurse and a patient in an immediate situation and speaks to the importance of individuality. She does make some attempt to discuss the overall nursing system in an institutional setting. However, she does not discuss how the patient is affected by the society in which he lives nor does she use society as a focus of nursing action. It is possible the immediate need could involve persons other than the patient. However, Orlando does not discuss nursing action with families or groups.

Nursing is, of course, the focus of Orlando's work. She speaks of nursing as unique and independent in its concerns for an individual's need for help in an immediate situation. The efforts to meet the individual's need for help are carried out in an interactive situation and in a disciplined manner that requires proper training.

COMPARISON OF ORLANDO'S PROCESS DISCIPLINE AND THE NURSING PROCESS

Orlando's nursing process discipline may be compared with the nursing process described in Chapter 2. Figure 10–3 helps to guide this comparison.

Certain overall characteristics are similar in both processes. For example, both are interpersonal in nature and require interaction between patient and nurse. The patient is asked for input throughout the process. Both processes also view the patient as a total person. He is not merely a disease process or body part. Orlando does not use the term *holistic,* but she effectively describes a holistic approach. Both processes are also used as a method to provide nursing care and as a means to evaluate that care. Finally, both are deliberate intellectual processes.

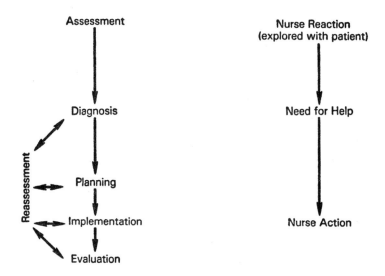

Figure 10–3. Comparison of Orlando's process with the nursing process.

The *assessment* phase of the nursing process corresponds to the sharing of the nurse reaction to the patient behavior in Orlando's process discipline. Patient behavior initiates the assessment. The collection of data includes only information relevant to identifying the patient's need for help. An ongoing data base is not useful to the immediate situation of the patient. The nurse's reaction, however, is probably influenced by her past experiences with the patient and other patients.

Orlando (1961/1990) discusses data collection in her first book, *The dynamic nurse–patient relationship*. She defines observation as "any information pertaining to a patient which the nurse acquires while she is on duty" (p. 31). Direct data are comprised of "any perception, thought, or feeling the nurse has from her own experience of the patient's behavior at any or several moments in time" (p. 32). Indirect data come from sources other than the patient, such as records, other health team members, or the patient's significant others. Both types of data require exploration with the patient to determine their relevance to the specific situation. Both verbal and nonverbal patient behaviors are important. Their consistency or inconsistency is a data piece in itself. This corresponds somewhat with subjective and objective data in the nursing process.

The sharing of the nurse's reaction in Orlando's process discipline has components similar to the analysis in the nursing process. Although the nurse's reaction is automatic, her awareness of it and the way she shares it is a deliberate intellectual activity. Orlando's sharing of the reaction, however, is a process of exploration with the patient. The nursing process, on the other hand, makes use of nursing's theoretical base and principles from the physical and behavioral sciences.

The product of the analysis in the nursing process is the *nursing diagnosis.* Exploration of the nurse's reaction with the patient in Orlando's process discipline leads to identification of his need for help. The statement of the nursing diagnosis is a more formal process than that of need. Many nursing diagnoses may be made, given priority ratings, and resolved over time. Orlando deals with immediate nurse–patient interaction; only one need is dealt with at a time. Current efforts to develop a taxonomy of nursing diagnosis would be inappropriate in Orlando's theory because each patient encounter is different. Using Orlando's theory, nursing might develop categories of such areas as causes of patient's needs for help. These categories would, of course, have to be modified to fit the particular patient situation.

The *planning* phase of the nursing process involves writing goals and objectives and deciding upon appropriate nursing action. This corresponds to the nurse's action phase of Orlando's process discipline. Any type of goal beyond the immediate situation is not possible in Orlando's process discipline. Her goal is always relief of the patient's need for help; the objective relates to improvement in the patient's behavior. The nursing process mandates a more formal action of writing and giving priority to goals and objectives.

Both processes require patient participation in determining the appropriate action. In the nursing process this participation occurs mostly in goal setting. Orlando's process discipline sees the patient as an active participant in determining the actual nurse action. The nursing process, on the other hand, relies more heavily on scientific principles and nursing theories in deciding how the nurse will act.

Implementation involves the final selection and carrying out of the planned action and is also part of the nurse's action phase of Orlando's process discipline. Both processes mandate that the action be appropriate for the patient as a unique individual. The nursing process expects the nurse to consider all possible effects of the action upon the patient. Orlando's process discipline is concerned only with the effectiveness of the action in resolving the immediate need for help.

Evaluation is inherent in Orlando's action phase of her process discipline. For an action to be deliberative, the nurse must evaluate its effectiveness when it is completed. Failure to evaluate can result in a series of ineffective actions including failure to meet the patient's need and an increase in the cost of nursing care and materials.

Evaluation in both processes is based on objective criteria. In the nursing process, evaluation asks whether the behaviorally stated objectives were met. In Orlando's process discipline, the nurse observes patient behavior to see whether the patient has been helped. Thus, both processes evaluate in terms of outcomes of care.

Both the nursing process and Orlando's process discipline are described as a series of sequential steps. The steps do not actually occur discretely and in order in either process. As new information becomes available, earlier steps may be repeated. Thus, new assessment data may alter the nursing diagnosis or the plan. Orlando's process discipline is almost a continuous interchange in which patient behavior leads to nurse reaction, which leads to nurse behavior, which leads to patient reaction (see Figs. 10–2 and 10–3). Thus, both processes are dynamic and responsive to changes in the patient's situation.

The nursing process used today and Orlando's process discipline have many similarities. They do, however, have important differences. The nursing process is far more formal and has more detailed phases than does Orlando's process discipline. It requires the nurse to use her knowledge of scientific principles and nursing theory to guide her behavior. Orlando demands only that the nurse follow the principles she lays down to guide nursing care. Long-term planning is part of the nursing process but is not relevant to Orlando's process discipline. Although both processes call for patient involvement in his care, Orlando's demands this participation more comprehensively.

ORLANDO'S WORK AND THE CHARACTERISTICS OF A THEORY

Can Orlando's work be called a theory of nursing, as described in Chapter 1? In the sense of a "vision" of what nursing is, her work certainly qualifies. Does she combine concepts for the purpose of deriving hypotheses about practice? An exploration to see whether Orlando's work meets all the basic characteristics of a theory helps to answer this question.

Before this exploration, a comment on Orlando's use of the term *principle* is appropriate. Principles, as are laws, are truly predictable. They are most useful in the pure sciences. Human beings are too individualistic to be predictable, especially in relation to their behavior. Orlando's principles tell the nurse how to act. They predict only in the general sense that if the nurse uses the principles, the patient's behavior will improve. Thus, *guides for practice* would be a more appropriate term for them than principles.

1. **Theories can interrelate concepts in such a way as to create a different way of looking at a particular phenomenon.** Nursing is the focus of Orlando's work. Her theory views nursing as a unique discipline that interacts with an individual in an immediate situation to relieve a sense of helplessness. She does relate concepts into a new and meaningful whole.

2. **Theories must be logical in nature.** Orlando's work does provide a reasonable and sequential process for nursing. Patient behavior initiates the nurse reaction. Exploration of this reaction with the patient leads to identification of a need and of an action to resolve that need. The nurse must react in a carefully prescribed manner to be certain she meets her goal of helping the patient. She must evaluate her action to be certain of its effectiveness. Thus, Orlando provides a logical rather than an intuitive approach to practice.

3. **Theories should be relatively simple yet generalizable.** Although Orlando's theory is simple in nature, it does generalize well to all nursing practice. The theory remains simple by revolving around the nurse–patient interaction, the basic unit of nursing. This simplicity also makes the theory generalizable. This basic unit is applicable regardless of the setting of nursing care or the type of patient receiving care.

4. Theories can be the bases for hypotheses that can be tested or for therapy to be expanded. Orlando did derive hypotheses from her theory and tested them. Although her initial study was observational, she tested her ideas in a variety of nursing situations. In her second study, she developed criteria for the nurse's reaction that were specific enough for the development of hypotheses and statistical testing.

5. Theories contribute to and assist in increasing the general body of knowledge within the discipline through the research implemented to validate them. In testing her theory, Orlando (1972) added to the general body of nursing knowledge. She was able to test the effectiveness of her process discipline in a nurse's contacts with the patients, staff, and workers the nurse supervises. Her findings showed a positive relationship between use of the process discipline and helpful outcomes of contacts. She also provided support for the idea that the process can be taught in a specified period. Although her hypotheses need retesting, they provide a basis for other nurses to develop new theories. Other nursing theorists, such as Orem and Rogers, show consistency with, if not the influence of, aspects of Orlando's work.

6. Theories can be used by practitioners to guide and improve their practice. Orlando has been quite successful in developing a theory useful to practice. Nurses can easily use her principles and process discipline in their interactions with patients and fellow workers. By using her theory, nurses are assured that they will not provide care in a way that is inappropriate for an individual patient. If Orlando's theory were more consciously applied by nurses at all levels, collegiality within the profession would develop at a faster pace. Professional differences and alternative approaches could be shared and resolved in a constructive manner. Some institutions are changing their nursing delivery systems to a more professional model—for example, the case management system or a shared governance system. When such a delivery system is used, there is less need to invoke hierarchial authority to resolve differences and enforce compliance with institutional policies and practices. Currently, within health care much energy, time, and financial resources are being spent on teaching hospital personnel, including nurses, to communicate with patients, visitors, and each other. The goals of many of these programs are to teach people to listen to the needs expressed and to meet these needs. These programs encompass the essence of Orlando's theory. However, Orlando's theory does not guide all aspects of nursing practice. Areas for further study include long-term planning, dealing with family and community, and caring for patients who do not recognize that their health is endangered.

7. Theories must be consistent with other validated theories, laws, and principles but will leave open unanswered questions that need to be investigated. Orlando's theory does not conflict with other validated theories if it is viewed in the somewhat limited sense of a nurse–patient interaction. It is most consistent with interaction theory, but general system theory relates to it with difficulty. Orlando (1972) does discuss a "system of nursing practice" (p. 18), which encompasses both the nurse–patient interaction and the relationship of nurses among themselves and with others in an organized work setting. She does not, however, view the patient in relation to his subsystems and suprasystems. For this reason, Orlando's theory does not relate well to family theory. The family is mentioned only as a source of indirect data.

Thus, Orlando's work contains many of the characteristics of a theory. Despite her intent, however, it does not provide a comprehensive theory to guide nursing practice. Nonetheless, this deficit does not negate its usefulness in guiding nurse–patient interaction. Nor does it deny its value as a stimulus to other nurses to carry theory development further.

STRENGTHS AND LIMITATIONS

Orlando's theory has much to offer to nursing. The predominant strength of her work is its usefulness in nursing practice. It guides nurses through their interactions with patients. Use of her theory virtually assures that patients will be treated as individuals and that they will have an active and constant input into their own care. The nurse's focus must remain on the patient rather than on the demands of the work setting. Use of the process discipline helps the nurse deal with her personal reactions and leads her to value her own individuality as a thinking person.

The nurse can keep Orlando in mind while applying the nursing process of today. Use of her theory prevents inaccurate diagnosis or ineffective plans because the nurse has to constantly explore her reactions with the patient. No nurse, following Orlando's principles, could fail to evaluate the care she has given.

Another of Orlando's strengths is her assertion of nursing's independence as a profession and her belief that this independence must be based on a sound theoretical framework. She bases this belief on her definition of nursing function. She believes that this clearly defined function will assist nursing in establishing its independence and in structuring the work setting so that nurses can effectively meet their patients' needs for help. The function of finding and meeting the patient's immediate needs for help is broad enough to encompass nurses practicing in all settings and in all specialty areas. It allows nursing to evolve over time by avoiding a rigid list of nursing activities.

Orlando guides the nurse to evaluate her care in terms of objectively observable patient outcomes. It is not the structure of the setting or the number of nurses on duty that determines effective care. Orlando has found a positive relationship between the use of her process and favorable outcomes of patient behavior. In planning to implement standards for nursing practice, the American Nurses' Association has described patient outcomes as "the ultimate indicators of quality patient care" (Congress of Nursing Practice, 1975, p. 16). The immediate and interactive nature of her process does, however, make evaluation a time-consuming process.

As previously alluded to, the nursing profession's input into accreditation standards for health care organizations has placed great emphasis on the evaluation of interventions in terms of patient outcomes. Consistent use of Orlando's theory by nurses could make evaluation a less time-consuming and more deliberate function, the results of which would be documented in patient charts. Such documentation of patient needs, planned interventions, and evaluation of interventions would provide data for analysis that would contribute to the general body of knowledge within the field of nursing.

Orlando's testing of her theory in the practice setting lends further support to its usefulness. Her first study, published in *The dynamic nurse–patient relationship,* provided a basis for future work. For a second study, described in *The discipline and teaching of the nursing process,* she developed specific criteria amenable to statistical testing. Nursing can pursue Orlando's work by retesting and further developing her work.

Although Orlando's ideas contain many of the characteristics of a theory, there are limitations. Her mental health background is probably responsible for the highly interactive nature of her theory. Although this interactive nature is one of the theory's strengths, it also provides limitation in her ideas. Nurses deal extensively with monitoring and controlling the physiological processes of patients to prevent illness and restore health. Orlando scarcely mentions this aspect of the nurse's role other than to question if monitoring machines is practicing nursing. The highly interactive nature of Orlando's theory makes it hard to include the highly technical and physical care that nurses give in certain settings, such as intensive care units. Her theory does, however, prevent the nurse from forgetting the patient in her efforts to fulfill the technical aspects of her job.

Orlando's theory is also limited by its focus on interaction with an individual, whereas the patient should be viewed as a member of a family and within a community. Often it is vital to deal with the family as a whole to help the patient. Orlando does not deal with these areas.

Long-term care and planning are not applicable to Orlando's focus on the immediate situation. She views long-term planning only as it is related to adequate staffing within an institution. Orlando herself recognizes this problem. In *The dynamic nurse–patient relationship* she speculated that "repeated experiences of having been helped undoubtedly culminate over periods of time in greater degrees of improvement" (p. 90). She also identified the cumulative effect of nursing as an area for further study.

In *The discipline and teaching of nursing process,* Orlando tried to define the entire nursing system. She described the system as the "regularly, interacting parts of a nursing service" (p. 18). This part of her theory attempts to incorporate nurses' relationships with other nurses and with members of different professions in the job setting. Her theory struggles with the authority derived from the function of the profession and that of the employing institution's commitment to the public. The same process is offered for dealing with others as for working with an individual patient. This part of her process is somewhat confusing. It appears to be more of a description of the administration of nursing services than a theory of nursing practice.

When a nurse–manager deals with staff, Orlando's theory provides a framework for an interaction that leads to a positive result. As the nurse executive listens to the needs of the staff, she must decide if deliberate action is needed; such action may take the form of a policy or procedure change, staffing variation, or institutional policy change. The nurse executive may need to influence another department, group, or level within the organization to effect a positive intervention with staff. On the administrative level, Orlando's theory is used, but the time span needed to complete all components varies depending on the situations. An organization that consistently and methodically uses Orlando's theory can positively respond to all issues that need to be confronted. In such an environment, needs can be met and emphasis placed on the present rather than the past or the way it has always been done. Thus, the organization is able to maintain its competitive edge.

Orlando can be considered a nursing theorist who made a significant contribution to the advancement of nursing practice. She helped nurses to focus on the patient rather than on the disease or institutional demands. The nurse is firmly viewed as the handmaiden of the patient, not of the physician. Nurses must base their practice on logical thinking rather than on intuition. Orlando's nursing process disciplines continues to be useful to nurses in their interactions with patients.

SUMMARY

Orlando's nursing process discipline is rooted in the interaction between a nurse and a patient at a specific time and place. A sequence of interchanges involving patient behavior and nurse reaction takes place until the patient's need for help, as he perceives it, is clarified. The nurse then decides on an appropriate action to resolve the need in cooperation with the patient. This action is evaluated after it is carried out. If the patient behavior improves, the action was successful and the process is completed. If there is no change or the behavior gets worse, the process recycles with new efforts to clarify the patient's behavior or the appropriate nursing action. Orlando (1961/1990) summarizes her process as follows:

> A deliberative nursing process has elements of continuous reflection as the nurse tries to understand the meaning to the patient of the behavior she observes and what he needs from her in order to be helped. Responses comprising this process are stimulated by the nurse's unfolding awareness of the particulars of the individual situation (p. 67).

REFERENCES

Congress of Nursing Practice. (1975). *A plan for implementation of the standards of nursing practice.* Kansas City, MO: American Nurses' Association.

Harmer, B., & Henderson, V. (1955). *Textbook of the principles and practice of nursing* (5th ed.). New York: Macmillan.

Orlando, I. J. (1990). *The dynamic nurse–patient relationship: Function, process and principles*. New York: National League for Nursing. (reprinted from 1961, New York: G. P. Putnam's Sons.)

Orlando, I. J. (1972). *The discipline and teaching of nursing process*. New York: G. P. Putnam's Sons. [out of print]

Pelletier, I. O. (1967). The patient's predicament and nursing function. *Psychiatric Opinion, 4,* 25–30.

Peplau, H. E. (1988). *Interpersonal relations in nursing*. London: Macmillan Education. (Original work published 1952, New York: G. P. Putnam's Sons).

Trench, A. S. (Executive producer), Wallace, D. (Producer), & Coberg, T. (Director). (1987). *Ida Jean Orlando—The nurse theorists: Portraits of excellence* [Videotape]. Oakland, CA: Studio Three Production, Samuel Merritt College of Nursing.

ERNESTINE WIEDENBACH*

Agnes M. Bennett
Peggy Coldwell Foster

■ ■ ■

Ernestine Wiedenbach (b. 1900) graduated from Wellesley College, Wellesley, Massachusetts, in 1922 with a liberal arts degree. She received her nursing diploma from the Johns Hopkins School of Nursing, Baltimore, Maryland, in 1925. Her master's degree in public health nursing is from Teachers College, Columbia University, New York, in 1934. Wiedenbach also obtained a certificate in nurse midwifery from the Maternity Center Association in New York in 1946. She practiced as a nurse midwife and a public health nurse, and taught in a number of schools of nursing. She is an Associate Professor Emeritus from Yale University School of Nursing. She served as a visiting professor at California State University, Los Angeles, and at the College of Nursing, University of Florida, Gainesville. In 1978, she received the Hattie Hemschemeyer award from the American College of Nurse Midwives for exceptional achievements in her professional life. Wiedenbach is retired and lives in Miami, Florida. She relates that she is well but is not publishing additional nursing material (personal communication, March, 1993).

Ernestine Wiedenbach, a progressive nursing leader, began her nursing career in the 1920s. Wiedenbach first published *Family-centered maternity nursing* in 1958. It is of interest that in that book she recommended that babies be in hospital rooms with their mothers rather than in a central nursery. This innovative concept was not widely implemented until 20 years later. In 1964 she wrote *Clinical nursing—A helping art,* in which she described her ideas about nursing as a "concept and philosophy" derived from 40 years of nursing experience. She credits Patricia James, James Dickoff, and Ida Orlando Pelletier as great influences in her nursing writing and theory development. In collaboration with Dickoff and James, Wiedenbach presented the symposium and co-authored, "Theory in a Practice Discipline" (1968a, 1968b). In 1970 Wiedenbach defined the essentials of her prescriptive theory in "Nurses' wisdom in nursing theory."

---

* Wiedenbach consistently uses the term *patient* and refers to the nurse as *her* in all her writings. This approach will be used in this chapter.

According to Ernestine Wiedenbach (1964), nursing is nurturing and caring for someone in a motherly fashion. That care is given in the immediate present and can be given by any caring person. Nursing is a helping service that is rendered with compassion, skill, and understanding to those in need of care, counsel, and confidence in the area of health (Wiedenbach, 1977).

Nursing wisdom is acquired through meaningful experience (Wiedenbach, 1964). Sensitivity alerts the nurse to an awareness of inconsistencies in a situation that might signify a problem. It is a key factor in assisting the nurse to identify the patient's need for help (Wiedenbach, 1977).

The nurse's beliefs and values regarding reverence for the gift of life, the worth of the individual, and the aspirations of each human being determine the quality of the nursing care. The nurse's purpose in nursing represents a professional commitment (Wiedenbach, 1970).

Wiedenbach (1964) states that the characteristics of a professional person that are essential for the professional nurse include the following [italics added]:

1. *Clarity* of purpose.
2. *Mastery* of skills and knowledge essential for fulfilling the purpose.
3. *Ability* to establish and sustain purposeful working relationships with others, both professional and nonprofessional individuals.
4. *Interest* in advancing knowledge in the area of interest and in creating new knowledge.
5. *Dedication* to furthering the good of mankind rather than to self-aggrandizement (p. 2).

The practice of nursing comprises a wide variety of services, each directed toward the attainment of one of its three components: (1) *identification* of the patient's need for help, (2) *ministration* of the help needed, and (3) *validation* that the help provided was indeed helpful to the patient (Wiedenbach, 1977). Within Wiedenbach's (1964) "identification of the patient's need for help," she presents three principles of helping: (1) the principle of inconsistency/consistency, (2) the principle of purposeful perseverance, and (3) the principle of self-extension. The *principle of inconsistency/consistency* refers to the assessment of the patient to determine some action, word, or appearance that is different from that expected—that is, something out of the ordinary for this patient. It is important for the nurse to observe the patient astutely and then critically analyze her observations. The *principle of purposeful perseverance* is based on the nurse's sincere desire to help the patient. The nurse needs to strive to continue her helping efforts in spite of difficulties she encounters while seeking to use her resources and capabilities effectively. The *principle of self-extension* recognizes that each nurse has limitations that are both personal and situational. It is important that she recognize when these limitations are reached and that she seek help from others.

WIEDENBACH'S PRESCRIPTIVE THEORY

Theory may be described as a system of conceptualizations invented to some purpose. Prescriptive theory (a situation-producing theory) may be described as one that conceptualizes both a desired situation and the prescription by which it is to be brought about. Thus, a prescriptive theory directs action toward an explicit goal. Wiedenbach's (1969) prescriptive theory is made up of three factors, or concepts, (see Fig. 11–1) [italics added]:

1. The *central purpose* which the practitioner recognizes as essential to the particular discipline.
2. The *prescription* for the fulfillment of the central purpose.
3. The *realities in the immediate situation* that influence the fulfillment of the central purpose (p. 2).

The Central Purpose

The nurse's central purpose defines the quality of health she desires to effect or sustain in her patient and specifies what she recognizes to be her special responsibility in caring for the patient (Wiedenbach, 1970). This central purpose (or commitment) is based on the individual nurse's philosophy. Wiedenbach (1964) states:

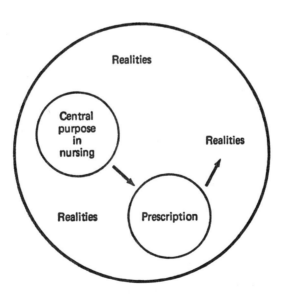

Figure 11–1. Wiedenbach's prescriptive theory. *(Adapted from Wiedenbach, E. (1969). Meeting the realities in clinical teaching, New York: Springer, p. x. Used with permission.)*

Purpose and philosophy are, respectively, goal and guide of clinical nursing. . . . Purpose—that which the nurse wants to accomplish through what she does—is the overall goal toward which she is striving, and so is constant. It is her reason for being and doing . . . Philosophy, an attitude toward life and reality that evolves from each nurse's beliefs and code of conduct, motivates the nurse to act, guides her thinking about what she is to do and influences her decisions. It stems from both her culture and subculture, and is an integral part of her. It is personal in character, unique to each nurse, and expressed in her *way* of nursing. Philosophy underlies purpose, and purpose reflects philosophy (p. 13).

Wiedenbach (1970) identifies three essential components for a nursing philosophy: (1) a reverence for the gift of life, (2) a respect for the dignity, worth, autonomy, and individuality of each human being, and (3) a resolution to act dynamically in relation to one's beliefs. Any of these concepts might be further developed. However, Wiedenbach (1964, 1970) emphasizes the second in her work, formulating the following beliefs about the individual:

1. Human beings are endowed with unique potential to develop within themselves the resources that enable them to maintain and sustain themselves.
2. Human beings basically strive toward self-direction and relative independence, and desire not only to make the best use of their capabilities and potentialities but also to fulfill their responsibilities.
3. Human beings need stimulation in order to make the best use of their capabilities and realize their self-worth.
4. Whatever individuals do represents their best judgment at the moment of doing it.
5. Self-awareness and self-acceptance are essential to the individual's sense of integrity and self-worth.

Thus, the central purpose is a concept the nurse has thought through—one she has put into words, believes in, and accepts as a standard against which to measure the value of her action to the patient. It is based on her philosophy and suggests the nurse's reason for being, the mission she believes is hers to accomplish (Wiedenbach, 1970).

The Prescription

Once the nurse has identified her own philosophy and recognizes that the patient has autonomy and individuality, she can work *with* the individual to develop a *prescription* or plan for his or her care.

A *prescription* is a directive to activity (Wiedenbach, 1969). It "specifies both the *nature of the action* that will most likely lead to fulfillment of the nurse's central purpose and the *thinking process* that determines it" (Wiedenbach, 1970, p. 1059). A prescription may indicate the broad general action appropriate to implementation of the basic concepts as well as suggest the kind of behavior needed to carry out these actions in accordance with the central purpose. These actions may be voluntary or involuntary. Voluntary action is an intended response, whereas involuntary action is an unintended response.

A prescription is a directive to at least three kinds of voluntary action: (1) *mutually understood and agreed upon* action ("the practitioner has . . . evidence that the recipient understands the implications of the intended action and is psychologically and physiologically receptive to it . . ."); (2) *recipient-directed* action ("the recipient of the action essentially directs the way it is to be carried out"); and (3) *practitioner-directed* action ("the practitioner carries out the action") (Wiedenbach, 1969, p. 3). Once the nurse has formulated a central purpose and has accepted it as a personal commitment, she not only has established the prescription for her nursing but also is ready to implement it (Wiedenbach, 1970).

The Realities

When the nurse has determined her central purpose and has developed the prescription, she must then consider the *realities* of the situation in which she is to provide nursing care. Realities consist of all factors—physical, physiological, psychological, emotional, and spiritual—that are at play in a situation in which nursing actions occur at any given moment. Wiedenbach (1970) defines the five realities as: (1) the agent, (2) the recipient, (3) the goal, (4) the means, and (5) the framework.

The *agent* who is the practicing nurse or her delegate is characterized by personal attributes, capacities, capabilities, and most importantly, commitment and competence in nursing. As the agent, the nurse is the propelling force that moves her practice toward its goal. In the course of this goal-directed movement, she may engage in innumerable acts called forth by her encounter with actual or discrepant factors and situations within the realities of which she herself is a part (Wiedenbach, 1967). The agent or nurse has the following four basic responsibilities:

1. To reconcile her assumptions about the realities . . . with her central purpose.
2. To specify the objectives of her practice in terms of behavioral outcomes that are realistically attainable.
3. To practice nursing in accordance with her objectives.
4. To engage in related activities which contribute to her self-realization and to the improvement of nursing practice (Wiedenbach, 1970, p. 1060).

The *recipient,* the patient, is characterized by personal attributes, problems, capacities, aspirations, and most important, the ability to cope with the concerns or problems being experienced (Wiedenbach, 1967). The patient is the recipient of the nurse's actions or the one on whose behalf the action is taken. The patient is vulnerable, depending on others for help and risking losing individuality, dignity, worth, and autonomy (Wiedenbach, 1970).

The *goal* is the desired outcome the nurse wishes to achieve. The goal is the end result to be attained by nursing action. The stipulation of an activity's goal gives focus to the nurse's action and implies her reason for taking it (Wiedenbach, 1970).

The *means* comprise the activities and devices through which the practitioner is enabled to attain her goal. The means include skills, techniques, procedures, and devices that may be used to facilitate nursing practice. The nurse's way of giving treatments, of expressing concern, of using the means available is individual and is determined by her central purpose and the prescription (Wiedenbach, 1970).

The *framework* consists of the human, environmental, professional, and organizational facilities that not only make up the context within which nursing is practiced but also constitute its currently existing limits (Wiedenbach, 1967). The framework is composed of all the extraneous factors and facilities in the situation that affect the nurse's ability to obtain the desired results. It is a conglomerate of "objects, existing or missing, such as policies, setting, atmosphere, time of day, humans, and happenings that may be current, past, or anticipated" (Wiedenbach, 1970, p. 1061).

The realities offer uniqueness to every situation. The success of professional nursing practice is dependent on them. Unless the realities are recognized and dealt with, they may prevent the achievement of the goal.

The concepts of central purpose, prescription, and realities are interdependent in Wiedenbach's theory of nursing. The nurse develops a prescription for care that is based on her central purpose, which is implemented in the realities of the situation.

WIEDENBACH'S CONCEPTUALIZATION OF NURSING PRACTICE AND PROCESS

According to Wiedenbach (1967), nursing practice is an art in which the nursing action is based on the principles of helping. Nursing action may be thought of as consisting of the following four distinct kinds of actions:

- Reflex   (spontaneous)
- Conditioned   (automatic)
- Impulsive   (impulsive)
- Deliberate   (responsible)

Nursing as a practice discipline is goal-directed. The nature of the nursing act is based on thought. The nurse thinks through the kind of results she wants, gears her actions to obtain those results, then accepts responsibility for the acts and the outcome of those acts (Wiedenbach, 1970). Since nursing requires thought, it can be considered a deliberate responsible action.

Nursing practice has three components: (1) identification of the patient's need for help; (2) ministration of the help needed, and (3) validation that the action taken was helpful to the patient (Wiedenbach, 1977). Within the identification component, there are four distinct steps. First, the nurse observes the patient, looking for an inconsistency between the expected behavior of the patient and the apparent behavior. Second, she attempts to clarify what the inconsistency means. Third, she determines the cause of the inconsistency. Finally, she validates with the patient that her help is needed.

The second component is the ministration of the help needed. In ministering to her patient, the nurse may give advice or information, make a referral, apply a comfort measure, or carry out a therapeutic procedure. Should the patient become uncomfortable with what is being done, the nurse will need to identify the cause and if necessary make an adjustment in the plan of action.

The third component is validation. After help has been ministered, the nurse validates that the actions were indeed helpful. Evidence must come from the patient that the purpose of the nursing actions has been fulfilled (Wiedenbach, 1964).

Wiedenbach (1977) views the nursing process essentially as an internal personalized mechanism. As such, it is influenced by the nurse's culture, purpose in nursing, knowledge, wisdom, sensitivity, and concern.

In Wiedenbach's (1977) nursing process (see Fig. 11–2), she identifies seven levels of awareness: sensation, perception, assumption, realization, insight, design, and decision. Wiedenbach's nursing process begins with an activating situation. This situation exists among the realities and serves as a stimulus to arouse the nurse's consciousness. This consciousness arousal leads to a subjective interpretation of the first three levels, which are defined as: *sensation* (experienced sensory impression), *perception* (the interpretation of a sensory impression), and *assumption* (the meaning the nurse attaches to the perception). These three levels of awareness are obtained through the focus of the nurse's attention on the stimulus; they are intuitive rather than cognitive and may initiate an involuntary response. For example, a nurse enters a patient's room and states, "My, it's hot in here!" She immediately goes to the window and opens it. The *sensation* is the room temperature. The *perception* is "It feels hot." The *assumption* is "If I am hot, then the patient must be hot." The involuntary response is to open the window.

Progressing from intuition to cognition, the nurse's actions become voluntary rather than involuntary. The next four levels of awareness occur in the voluntary phase: *realization* (in which the nurse begins to validate the assumption previously made about the patient's behavior); *insight* (which includes joint planning and additional knowledge about the cause of the problem); *design* (the plan of action decided upon by the nurse and confirmed by the patient); and *decision* (the nurse's performance of a responsible action) (Wiedenbach, 1977).

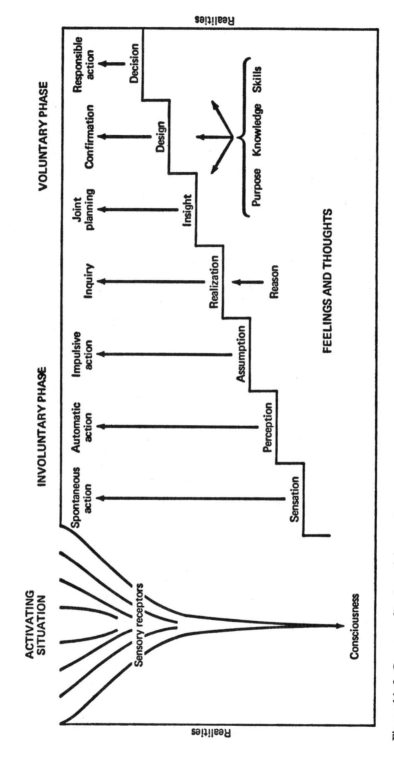

Figure 11–2. Conceptualization of the nursing process. *(Reproduced from Clausen, J. P. and others (1977). Maternity nursing today, New York: McGraw-Hill, p. 43. Used with permission.)*

To continue with the previous example: The nurse asks, "Are you too warm?" and the patient replies, "No, I'm not. I have felt cold since I washed my hair." The nurse responds, "I will close the window and get you a blanket." The patient agrees, "That would be fine." The nurse shuts the window and gets a blanket for the patient.

The *realization* is the validation of the patient's perception of temperature comfort. The *insight* is the additional information that the patient had washed his or her hair. The *design* is the plan to close the window and get a blanket as confirmed by the patient. The *decision* is the nurse shuts the window and gets a blanket for the patient.

In summary, the comparison of Wiedenbach's prescriptive theory, the practice of nursing, and the nursing process as outlined in Chapter 2 of this book is as follows: In the practice of nursing, a nurse with her unique personality, philosophy, education, and life experiences (her central purpose), assesses the individual's health status and potential for development. She identifies the patient's need for help (makes a *nursing diagnosis*). She formulates a *plan* with the patient, setting goals that they will act upon (implement). This plan or prescription and its implementation are affected by the realities, or the strengths and limitations of the situation (the *environment*). Their plan is implemented or the nurse provides the help needed. Validation is then obtained that the help provided was indeed helpful to the patient (*evaluation*).

WIEDENBACH'S THEORY AND NURSING'S METAPARADIGM

Wiedenbach (1964) emphasizes that the human or *individual* possesses unique potential, strives toward self-direction, and needs stimulation. Whatever the individual does represents his or her best judgment at the moment. Self-awareness and self-acceptance are essential to the individual's sense of integrity and self-worth. Wiedenbach believes these characteristics require respect from the nurse.

Wiedenbach (1977) does not define the concept of *health*. However, she supports the World Health Organization's definition of health as a state of complete physical, mental, and social well-being, and not merely the absence of disease and infirmity.

In Wiedenbach's work, she incorporates the *environment* within the realities—a major component of her theory. One element of the realities is the framework. According to Wiedenbach (1970), the framework is a complex of extraneous factors and circumstances that are present in every nursing situation. The framework may include objects "such as policies, setting, atmosphere, time of day, humans, and happenings" (p. 1061).

According to Wiedenbach (1969), *nursing,* a clinical discipline, is a practice discipline designed to produce explicit desired results. The art of nursing is a goal-directed activity requiring the application of knowledge and skill toward meeting a need for help experienced by a patient. Nursing is a helping process that extends or restores the patient's ability to cope with demands implicit in the situation.

COMPARISON OF THE NURSING PROCESS WITH WIEDENBACH'S WORK

The comparison of the nursing process described in Chapter 2 and Wiedenbach's conceptualization of the nursing process and nursing practice yields some similarities and several significant differences (see Table 11–1). In Wiedenbach's nursing practice, the steps of (1) observation, (2) ministration of help, and (3) validation are comparable with the nursing process's phases of *assessment, implementation, and evaluation.*

Assessment, the first phase of the nursing process, considers the person holistically and requires extensive data collection. In Wiedenbach's (1977) model (see Fig. 11–3), there is a stimulus to which the nurse reacts. This

TABLE 11–1. COMPARISON OF THE NURSING PROCESS WITH WIEDENBACH'S NURSING PROCESS AND NURSING PRACTICE

Nursing Process	Weidenbach's Nursing Process		Weidenbach's Nursing Practice
1. Nursing assessment	Stimulus		1. Observation
	Involuntary 1. Sensation 2. Perception 3. Assumption	Voluntary	
1. (a) Analysis and synthesis 2. Nursing Diagnosis		4. Realization with reason—Inquiry	
3. (a) Goals and objectives 3. (b) Plans		5. Insight— Joint planning 6. Design— Confirmation	
	1. (a) Spontaneous action 2. (a) Automatic action 3. (a) Impulsive action		2. Ministration of help
4. Implementation with scientific rationale		7. Decision with responsible action	
5. Nursing evaluation			3. Validation

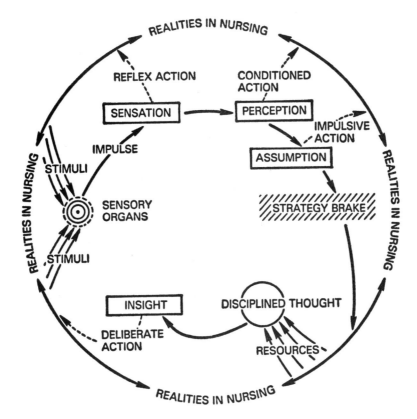

Figure 11–3. Genesis of nursing action. Diagrammatic presentation of how an impulse to act originates and how it is converted into action. Broken lines represent overt processes; solid lines represent covert processes. *(Reprinted by permission of G. P. Putnam's Sons from Family-Centered Maternity Nursing (2nd ed.) by Wiedenbach, E., 1967, G. P. Putnam's Sons.)*

stimulus produces a reaction at the level of sensation or perception. These levels are involuntary and intuitive. The nurse then makes an assumption about the situation and may act involuntarily. Such acts are spontaneous, automatic, or impulsive. They occur on the spur of the moment and are precipitated by unchecked, rampant thoughts and feelings. Occasionally in an emergency they may be lifesaving. However, these involuntary acts can frequently do more harm than good.

If the nurse makes an assumption, she might act impulsively. However, Wiedenbach (1964) points out that the nurse needs to willfully apply a strategy brake (see Fig. 11–3). This provides time for her to assemble the resources necessary for disciplined thought to control her action. This strategy brake then is applied just before Wiedenbach's realization level. At the realization level the process becomes voluntary, for the nurse uses reason and inquiry.

Within the *assessment* phase of the nursing process (as presented in Chapter 2), the components of *analysis* and *synthesis* require much conscious thought and deliberation about the corrected data before the nurse can make a *nursing diagnosis*. Once the nursing diagnosis has been determined, the nurse sets goals and objectives and *plans* the nursing care. This planning phase can be compared to Wiedenbach's levels of insight and design, which are part of her voluntary phase. The insight level of her nursing process model includes joint planning. This joint planning is between the nurse and the patient and does not involve other health care professionals.

Wiedenbach (1964) does not directly incorporate the concept of goal as part of the nursing process. However, the nurse's central purpose could be considered a goal. On the design level the nurse plans a course of action. After the plan is decided on, the nurse confirms it with the patient. Once the plan has been decided on and confirmed, the nurse performs the responsible, deliberate nursing action. This level is comparable to the *implementation* phase of the nursing process.

In Wiedenbach's (1977) model of the nursing process, she does not identify *evaluation*. However, she does refer to evaluation in her discussion of nursing practice, emphasizing that the nurse needs "validation that the help provided was indeed helpful to the patient" (p. 39).

WIEDENBACH'S WORK AND THE CHARACTERISTICS OF A THEORY

1. Theories can interrelate concepts in such a way as to create a different way of looking at a particular phenomenon. Wiedenbach's work does interrelate concepts in such a way as to create a different way of looking at a particular phenomenon. She defines and interrelates the concepts of realities and central purpose to devise a prescription for nursing care.

2. Theories must be logical in nature. When using Wiedenbach's theory, it is difficult, if not impossible, to follow a logical thought process and predict the outcome of nursing care because the prescription and desired outcome will vary from one nurse to another depending on each nurse's central purpose. However, Wiedenbach (1970) stated that she was presenting a prescriptive rather than a predictive theory.

3. Theories should be relatively simple yet generalizable. Wiedenbach's theory is simple yet generalizable to all of nursing. Although the theory is situation producing, it is not situation specific. The situation is produced by the nurse's central purpose and prescription within the existing realities. The situation is not site oriented and thus could be a hospital, a community setting, a school, or in the home.

4. Theories can be the bases for hypotheses that can be tested or for theory to be expanded, and

5. Theories contribute to and assist in increasing the general body of knowledge within the discipline through the research implemented to validate them. Although Wiedenbach's theory presents a philosophical approach that has not been tested, hypotheses can be formed. For example, how does the central purpose affect care when the realities and prescription remain fairly constant? That is, according to a patient or family survey, is there a perceived difference in the quality of nursing care between a group of nurses who work in a nursing care facility because it is close to their home and a group of nurses who chose to work in this setting because it has a specialized unit for patients with Alzheimer's disease?

6. Theories can be used by practitioners to guide and improve their practice. Wiedenbach's theory can be used to support, guide, and assist the nurse to fulfill her commitment to nursing. The nurse's commitment to nursing is her central purpose that will influence prescriptions within the situational realities. Thus, the nurse whose central purpose is the holistic support of the optimal development of the individual will develop prescriptions that deal with a multitude of aspects of the individual rather than focusing solely on the problem that led to initial contact.

7. Theories must be consistent with other validated theories, laws, and principles but should leave open unanswered questions that need to be investigated. Wiedenbach does not use other theories or support her theory from other disciplines. However, her work is consistent with interaction and communication theories and principles.

SUMMARY

Nursing is a helping art. The nurse renders compassionate care to those in need of help. Nursing requires a professional commitment and is based on the individual nurse's philosophy. For Wiedenbach (1970) the concepts that epitomize the nurse's philosophy are the "reverence for the gift of life"; "respect for the dignity, worth, autonomy, and individuality of each human being"; and the "resolution to act dynamically in relation to one's beliefs" (p. 1058). The components of nursing practice are identification of the patient's need for help, ministration of help, and validation that the help given is beneficial.

Wiedenbach's theory for nursing, a prescriptive theory, contains three concepts: *central purpose, prescription,* and *realities.* The interrelationship of these three concepts is as follows: Within the realities, the nurse develops a prescription for nursing care based on her central purpose. The central purpose is the nurse's philosophy for care; the prescription is the directive to activity; the realities are the matrix in which the action occurs. These concepts are all interdependent.

Wiedenbach identifies seven levels within her nursing process: sensation, perception, assumption, realization, insight, design, and decision. Sensation through realization involves involuntary action, insight through design involves voluntary action. With increased purpose, knowledge, experience, and skill, the nurse moves from an involuntary response to voluntary action.

Wiedenbach's theory presents a philosophical, altruistic approach to nursing. The nurse is viewed as a loving, caring individual. The nurse's philosophy about the value and worth of the individual directs her care. Wiedenbach (1967) states: "Nursing [is] a service which ideally exemplifies man's humanity to man" (p. 5).

The reader perceives that the nurse acts with a self-sacrificing commitment to nursing. If a nurse values the life and dignity of human beings, then she will provide quality nursing care. Wiedenbach (1964) states that "although recognized as a humanitarian service, nursing in its entirety is hard to describe, and the nurse's responsibilities are hard to delineate" (p. 1).

Wiedenbach's nursing process is different from the nursing process outlined in Chapter 2 in this text. She identifies the nursing process as being activated by a stimulus that may result in an involuntary response unless this reflexive action is halted by a strategy brake. This brake, or pause, allows the nurse to think, gather more data, analyze, and then plan before a voluntary deliberate action is taken. The nursing process in Chapter 2 more closely parallels Wiedenbach's definition of nursing practice, that is, observation, ministration of help, and validation.

This theory is useful with an individual patient but not with groups. With this theory, Wiedenbach recognizes that the "need for help" must be verified with the patient. This factor would require the patient to be coherent and responsive.

Wiedenbach's work occurred early in the development of the theoretical nursing models. Her prescriptive theory defines her concepts of central purpose, prescription, and realities. However, these concepts are broad, vary with each nurse, each patient, each situation, and are difficult to use in research.

Although Wiedenbach's work does not fulfill all the characteristics of a theory, it is innovative within the nursing profession. Her classic writings, including those written with Dickoff and James, serve as a basis for the development of nursing theory. Wiedenbach is a "mother" of nursing theory development.

REFERENCES

Dickoff, J., James, P., & Wiedenbach, E. (1968a). Theory in a practice discipline I: Practice-orientated research. *Nursing Research, 17,* 415–435.

Dickoff, J., James, P., & Wiedenbach, E. (1968b). Theory in a practice discipline II: Practice-orientated research. *Nursing Research, 17,* 545–554.

Wiedenbach, E. (1958). *Family-centered maternity nursing.* New York: G. P. Putnam's.

Wiedenbach, E. (1964). *Clinical nursing—A helping art.* New York: Springer.

Wiedenbach, E. (1967). *Family-centered maternity nursing* (2nd ed.). New York: G. P. Putnam's.

Wiedenbach, E. (1969). *Meeting the realities in clinical teaching.* New York: Springer.

Wiedenbach, E. (1970). Nurse's wisdom in nursing theory. *American Journal of Nursing, 70,* 1057–1062.

Wiedenbach, E. (1977). The nursing process in maternity nursing. In J. P. Clausen, M. H. Flook, & B. Ford. *Maternity nursing today* (2nd ed.) (pp. 39–51). New York: McGraw-Hill.

BIBLIOGRAPHY

Burst, H. V. (1979). Presentation of the Hattie Hemschemeyer Award. *Journal of Nurse-Midwifery, 24, 35–36.*

Dickoff, J. J. (1968). Symposium in theory development in nursing: Researching research's role in theory development. *Nursing Research, 17, 204–206.*

Dickoff, J. J., & James, P. A. (1968). Symposium of theory development in nursing: A theory of theories: A position paper. *Nursing Research, 17, 197–203.*

Dunlop, M. J. (1986). Is a science of caring possible? *Journal of Advanced Nursing, 11, 661–670.*

Flaskerud, J. H. (1986). On toward a theory of nursing action: Skills and competency in nurse-patient interaction. *Nursing Research, 35, 250–252.*

Holland, M. A. (1989). *An examination of the propositions of James Dickoff, Patricia James: Implications for nursing research.* Unpublished doctoral dissertation, Temple University.

Wiedenbach, E. (1949). Childbirth as mothers say they like it. *Public Health Nursing, 51, 417–421.*

Wiedenbach, E. (1960). Nurse-midwifery, purpose, practice and opportunity. *Nursing Outlook, 8, 256.*

Wiedenbach, E. (1963). The helping art of nursing. *American Journal of Nursing, 63, 54–57.*

Wiedenbach, E. (1965). Family nurse practitioner for maternal and child care. *Nursing Outlook, 13, 50.*

Wiedenbach, E. (1968a). Genetics and the nurse. *Bulletin of the American College of Nurse Midwifery, 13, 8–13.*

Wiedenbach, E. (1968b). The nurse's role in family planning–A conceptual base for practice. *Nursing Clinics of North America, 3, 355–365.*

Wiedenbach, E. (1970). Comment on beliefs and values: Basis for curriculum design. *Nursing Research, 19, 427.*

Wiedenbach, E., & Falls, C. (1978). *Communication: Key to effective nursing.* New York: Tiresias Press.

MYRA ESTRIN LEVINE

Julia B. George

■ ■ ■

Myra E. Levine was born in 1920 in Chicago, the first child in a family of three siblings. Her experiences during her father's frequent illnesses contributed to her interest in and dedication to nursing. She received a diploma from Cook County School of Nursing in 1944, an SB from the University of Chicago in 1949, and a Masters of Science in nursing from Wayne State University in 1962. Her career in nursing has been varied. Clinically, she held positions as a private duty nurse, a civilian nurse for the U. S. Army, surgical supervisor, and director of nursing. She held faculty positions at Cook County School of Nursing, Loyola University, Rush University, and the University of Illinois, Chicago. She is now Professor Emerita, Medical-Surgical Nursing, University of Illinois, Chicago. Levine filled visiting professorships at Tel-Aviv University and Recanati School of Nursing, Ben Gurion University of the Negev, both in Israel.

Levine is a charter fellow in the American Academy of Nursing and has been honored by the Illinois Nurses Association. She was the first recipient of Sigma Theta Tau's Elizabeth Russell Belford Award for teaching excellence. She was granted an honorary doctorate by Loyola University, Chicago, in 1992.

Myra Levine has said that she had no intention of developing a theory when she first began putting her ideas about nursing into writing (Trench, Wallace, & Coberg, 1987). In fact, more than two decades after the initial publication of *Introduction to clinical nursing* (Levine, 1969) she has referred to her work as a theory but prefers to identify it as a conceptual model. She states that she was looking for a way to teach all the major concepts in medical-surgical nursing in three quarters and for a way to generalize the content, to move away from a procedurally oriented educational process. She was interested in helping nurses realize that every nurse–patient contact leads to a puzzle in relation to nursing care that needs to be solved in an individualized manner. Her work has evolved over the years, with the most recent comprehensive update of the theory published in 1989 and additional discussions in 1990 and 1991.

Levine (1990) believes that entry into the health care system is associated with giving up some measure of personal independence. To designate the person who has entered the health care system a client reinforces the state of dependency, for a client is a follower. She supports the term patient because patient means sufferer, and dependency is associated with suffering.

> It is the condition of suffering that makes it possible to set independence aside and accept the services of another person. It is the challenge of the nurse to provide the individual with appropriate care without losing sight of the individual's integrity, to honor the trust that the patient has placed in the nurse, and to encourage the participation of the individual in his or her own welfare. The patient comes in trust and dependence only for as long as the services of the nurse are needed. The nurse's goal is always to impart knowledge and strength so that the individual can . . . walk away . . . as an independent individual (p. 199).

It is Levine's intent that such dependency be a very temporary state of affairs (Trench, Wallace, & Coberg, 1987). In accord with Levine's belief, the term patient is used throughout this chapter.

In her writings, Levine (1989, 1990, 1991) is careful to credit the scientists' works upon which she has built. She speaks to the importance of recognizing and building upon these vital adjuncts to knowledge. This knowledge is not borrowed but, rather, is shared. In discussing physiological mechanisms, she drew upon Cannon's (1963) description of the flight or fight response. Selye's (1956) stress theories provided further information about protection from the hazards of living. Gibson's (1966) perceptual systems about how people are actively involved in gathering information from their environments to aid them in moving safely through those environments were drawn upon. Erikson's (1969, 1975) discussions of the influence of environment on development further expanded Levine's information about the person–environment interaction. Bates' (1967) description of three types of environment was also important. The works of Dubos (1966), Cohen (1968), and Goldstein (1963) contributed to Levine's concept of adaptation.

LEVINE'S THEORY

Levine discusses adaptation, conservation, and integrity. *Adaptation* is the process by which *conservation* is achieved, and the purpose for conservation is *integrity*. The core of Levine's theory are her four principles of conservation.

Adaptation

Adaptation is the life process by which, over time, people maintain their wholeness or integrity as they respond to environmental challenges; it is the consequence of interaction between the person and the environment (Trench, Wallace, & Coberg, 1987; Levine, 1989). Successful engagement with the environment depends on an adequate store of adaptations (Levine, 1990).

Both physiological and behavioral responses are different under different conditions—for example, responses to very quiet or very noisy environments will vary. It is possible to anticipate certain kinds of reactions, but the individuality of responses prevents accurate prediction. Adaptation is explanatory rather than predictive.

Adaptation includes the concepts of *historicity, specificity,* and *redundancy.* Adaptation is a historical process, responses are based on past experiences, both personal and genetic.

Adaptation is also specific. Each system has very specific responses. The physiological responses that "defend oxygen supply to the brain are distinct from those that maintain the appropriate blood glucose levels" (Levine, 1989, p. 328). Particular responses are called into action by a particular challenge; responses are task-specific. They are also synchronized. Although the changes that occur are sequential, they should not be viewed as linear. Rather, Levine (1989) describes them as occurring in "cascades" in which there is an interacting and evolving effect in which one sequence is not yet completed when the next begins.

"One of the most remarkable things about living species is the number of levels of response which permit them to confront the reality of their environment in ways that somehow maintain their well being" (Trench, Wallace, & Coberg, 1987). These redundant systems are both protective and adaptive. If one system does not adapt, another can take over. Levine (1989) indicates that redundant systems may function in a time frame; some are corrective whereas others permit a previously failed response to be re-established.

Levine describes adaptation as the best "fit of the person with his or her predicament of time and space" (Trench, Wallace, & Coberg, 1987). She differentiates between fit and congruence by using an example of shoes. Most of us have many pairs of shoes that are congruent with our feet. We also have certain pairs that we prefer to wear because they are the most comfortable—they are the best fit.

Conservation

The product of adaptation is conservation. Conservation is a universal concept, a natural law, that deals with defense of wholeness and system integrity (Levine, 1990, 1991). "Conservation defends the wholeness of living systems by ensuring their ability to confront change appropriately and retain their unique identity" (Levine, 1990, p. 192). Conservation describes how complex systems continue to function in the face of severe challenges; it provides not only for current survival but also for future vitality through facing challenges in the most economical way possible. An example Levine uses to illustrate conservation is that of the thermostat. The thermostat is set at a selected temperature. As long as the temperature in the room is the same as the set temperature, nothing occurs. When the room temperature falls below the selected temperature, the thermostat activates the heating system—but only until the room temperature again reaches the thermostat setting. When the setting is reached, the thermostat turns the heating system off. Levine (1990) describes this as conserving energy—using it in "the most frugal, economic, and energy-sparing fashion" (p. 192). The essence of conservation is the successful use of responses that cost the least (Levine, 1989). "Conservation is clearly the consequence of the multiple, interacting, and synchronized negative feedback systems that provide for the stability of the living organism" (Levine, 1989, p. 329). As long as systems are physiologically stable, or in balance, negative feedback systems can function at minimal cost. Energy resources are conserved for use when needed to restore balance. Homeostasis is a state of conservation, a state of synchronized sparing of energy.

Levine (1989) states that physiological and behavioral responses are essential components of the same activity. They are not parallel or simultaneous but part of the same whole. She also recognizes that it is difficult to break down a body of knowledge and that often information must be gathered piece by piece (Trench, Wallace, & Coberg, 1987). Thus, physiological and behavioral responses are often identified and described as separate things. Since they represent the same whole it is important to put the pieces together to represent that whole.

Levine (1989) describes four levels of behavior. The first is Cannon's (1963) "fight or flight" response, the adrenocortical-sympathetic reactions that provide both physiological and behavioral readiness in the face of sudden and unexplained challenges in the environment. The second is the inflammatory-immune response, which we rely upon for restoration of physical wholeness and healing. The third is Selye's (1956) stress response, described as an integrated defense that occurs over time and is "influenced by the accumulated experience of the individual" (p. 330). The fourth is Gibson's (1966) perceptual systems, in which the senses not only provide access to environmental energy sources but also convert these sources into meaningful experiences; people not only see, they *look;* they not only hear, they *listen.* These levels of behavior support the individual as an active participant with the environment, not merely as a reactive being. The levels of responses are not sequential but rather redundant and integrated within the individual.

Nursing's role in conservation is to help the person with the process of "keeping together" the total person through the least expense of effort. Levine (1989) proposed the following four principles of conservation:

1. The conservation of energy of the individual.
2. The conservation of the structural integrity of the individual.
3. The conservation of the personal integrity of the individual.
4. The conservation of the social integrity of the individual (p. 331).

The conservation of *energy* is basic to the natural, universal law of conservation. Levine (1989) states that energy is not hidden; "it is eminently identifiable, measurable, and manageable" (p. 331). Within nursing practice, the measurement of vital signs is a daily measurement of energy parameters. For example, body temperature is an indication of the heat (energy) generated by living cells as they accomplish their work. Energy conservation is encouraged

through the limitation of activities for coronary patients or the planned gradual resumption of activities postoperatively. It is important that, even at rest,
energy costs are incurred through the activities necessary to support living.
Levine (1989) identifies these as those activities involved in growth, transport, and biochemical and bioelectrical change. She states, "The conservation
of energy is clearly evident in the very sick, whose lethargy, withdrawal, and
self-concern are manifested while, in its wisdom, the body is spending its
energy resources on the processes of healing" (p. 332).

The second, third, and fourth principles continue the theme of conservation and also include integrity—structural integrity, personal integrity, and
social integrity. Levine (1990) also describes the conservation of energy as
protecting functional integrity. Levine presents the idea that "health" and
"whole" are derived from the same root word and that another synonym for
"whole" is "integrity." "Integrity means being in control of one's life . . .
having the freedom to choose: to move without constraint . . . to exercise
decisions on all matters . . . without apology, indebtedness, or guilt" (Levine,
1990, p. 193). We are concerned with the integrity of the whole person; the
essence of wholeness is integrity.

Conservation of *structural integrity* focuses on the healing process (Levine,
1989). Through multiple experiences with scraped knees and such that heal
with no scarring, humans develop a mind-set that expects perfect restoration
of structural integrity throughout life. "Healing is the defense of wholeness"
(p. 333). Nurses support structural integrity through efforts to limit injury
and thus limit scarring, through proper positioning and range of motion to
prevent skeletal deformity, pressure areas or loss of muscle tone. To Levine
the phantom limb phenomenon (Sacks, 1985) supports the idea that a sense
of structural integrity is more than a physiological need.

Conservation of *personal integrity* focuses on a sense of self (Levine, 1989).
Levine describes Goldstein's (1963) identification of self-actualization as
observed in efforts of severely brain injured persons to retain their personal
identity. She points out that both Maslow (1968) and Rogers (1961) discussed
self-actualization as a reaching beyond. Goldstein's concept, the one supported
by Levine, is a reaching into the person rather than a reaching beyond.
Humans have both a public and a very private self. At least some portion of
the private self is not known even to those who are closest to the person. The
self "is defined, defended, and described only by the soul that owns it. That
private self is unique and whole. A person can share mere fragments of it with
others" (Levine, 1990, p. 194). In this way a separation between self and other
is maintained. Levine (1989) states that efforts at collecting a complete psychosocial data base may well violate this need to maintain separation, and therefore these efforts violate personal integrity. She states, "the most generous
psycho–social approach would be to limit the recording of confidences to only
those generalizations that actually make a difference in the choice of treatment
plans" (p. 334). She likens the awareness of self to independence.

Conservation of *social integrity* involves a definition of self that goes
beyond the individual (Levine, 1989). Individuals use their relationships to

define themselves. One's identity is connected to family, community, culture, ethnicity, religion, vocation, education, and socioeconomic status. To function successfully in this wide variety of social environments requires a broad behavioral repertoire. The ultimate direction for social integrity is derived from the ethical values of the social system. "The health care system is a vast social order with its own rules, but it is an instrument of society and must guarantee privacy, personhood, and respect as moral imperatives" (p. 336). Levine (1990) points out that disease prevention is an issue of social integrity and discusses the need both to discuss and to fund studies and programs to deal with overwhelming health problems such as smoking, drug abuse, HIV, and cancer.

> The conservation principles do not, of course, operate singly and in isolation from each other. They are joined within the individual as a cascade of life events, churning and changing as the environmental challenge is confronted and resolved in each individual's unique way. The nurse as caregiver becomes part of that environment, bringing to every nursing opportunity his or her own cascading repertoire of skill, knowledge, and compassion. It is a shared enterprise and each participant is rewarded. (Levine, 1989, p. 336).

LEVINE'S THEORY AND NURSING'S METAPARADIGM

Levine skillfully weaves her beliefs about human beings, environment, health, and nursing throughout her discussions of conservation and adaptation. They are fundamental to her work.

In relation to *human beings,* Levine (1990) states that when a person is being studied, the focus should be on wholeness. She also maintains that a person cannot be understood outside the context of the place and time in which he or she is functioning or separated from the influence of everything that is happening around him or her. Not only are human beings influenced by their current circumstances, they also are "burdened by a lifetime of experience" which has been recorded on the tissues of the body as well as on the mind and spirit (p. 197). Human beings are continually adapting in their interactions with their environment. The process of adaptation results in conservation. Human beings have need for nursing when they are suffering and can set aside independence and accept the services of another.

Levine (1984) indicates that *health* and disease are patterns of adaptive change. Some adaptations are more successful than others; all adaptations are seeking the best fit with the environment. The most successful adaptations are the ones that achieve the best fit in the most conserving manner. Health is the goal of conservation (Levine, 1990). She also discusses the words *health, whole,* and *integrity* as all being derived from the same root word and that, even with a multiplicity of definitions of health, each individual still defines health for him or her self (Levine, 1991).

In defining *environment* Levine (1990) draws upon Bates's (1967) classifications. There are three aspects of environment. The *operational environment* consists of those undetected natural forces that impinge on the individual. The *perceptual environment* consists of information that is recorded by the sensory organs. The *conceptual environment* is influenced by language, culture, ideas, and cognition. Levine also says that even with definition, the environment is difficult to measure. However, because adaptation and conservation are based upon the human being's interaction with the environment, efforts to understand the environment and the role it plays in an individual's predicament are vital. The s*ocial context* is also important to consideration of the wholeness of an individual. Levine (1991) includes the individual's "ethnic and cultural heritage, economic niche, the opportunities ignored or seized" in social context (p. 9). She states, "It is the social system that, in every place and in every generation, establishes the values that direct it and sets the rules by which its members are judged. The social integrity of the individual mirrors the community to which he or she belongs" (p. 9).

For Levine (1989) the purpose of *nursing* is to take care of others when they need to be taken care of. The dependency created by this need is a very temporary state. Nursing takes place wherever there is an individual who needs care to some degree. Levine discusses the fact that the person who provides nursing care has special burdens of concern since the "permission to enter into the life goals of another human being bears onerous debts of responsibility and choice" (p. 336). The nurse–patient relationship is based on the willful participation of both parties, and in such a relationship there cannot be "a substitute for honesty, fairness, and mutual respect" (p. 336). Nursing theory "is tested finally in the pragmatic, humble daily exchanges between nurse and patient . . . [its] success [is demonstrated in its ability to] equip individuals with renewed strength to pursue their lives in independence, fulfillment, hope, and promise" (pp. 336–337).

LEVINE'S THEORY AND THE NURSING PROCESS

Levine's concepts of adaptation, conservation, and integrity can be used to guide patient care within the nursing process.

In *assessment,* an understanding of the wholeness of the patient needs to be the end result. However, because we lack the mechanisms for assessing the whole as such, the principles of conservation can be used as a guide to structure the assessment. The assessment would not be initiated unless the person is suffering and willing to become to some degree dependent upon the nurse. The overarching question could be, "What adaptation is needed, or has not been successful?" The history, specificity, and potential for redundancy in this area of adaptation need to be investigated. For example, with the cardiac patient it is important to gather information about the signs and symptoms that brought the person into the health care system. Is there a family or personal history of cardiac problems or of being at risk for such problems? Can the incident that initiated this problem be identified (eg, response to sudden change in temperature would indicate a different specific response than to overexertion)? Have compensating efforts been made?

Under the first principle, conservation of energy, assessment data would relate to energy sources and expenditure. Data would include vital signs, laboratory values related to uptake and use of oxygen and nutrients, activities of daily living, nutrition, exercise, elimination, menstrual cycles . . . any aspect of living that requires energy. The primary focus would be on identifying the areas of energy expenditure that are related to the suffering that brought the patient into contact with the nurse. Information about the balance between energy input and output is also important.

Assessment data in relation to conservation of structural integrity would relate to information about injury and disease processes. Data would include laboratory values that reflect the immune/inflammatory response, direct observations of wounds, and any visible indications of disease (eg, the "pox" in chicken pox), and information from the patient about symptoms which are not observable (eg, nausea, pain).

Assessment data related to conservation of personal integrity need to be collected very carefully. Levine (1989) warns about the threat to the self of the patient that can be created if the nurse seeks a too thorough investigation of the self of that patient. Her guideline to use "only those generalizations that actually make a difference in the choice of treatment plans" is helpful (p. 334). For example, knowing that the person prefers to learn from reading material and receiving individual instruction rather than in a group setting would influence the choice of treatment plans. The patient will be comfortable in sharing his or her public self but reluctant to share the private self. To assist in maintaining independence, assessment needs to be limited to those portions of the self that the person is willing to, and capable of, sharing.

Assessment data related to the conservation of social integrity includes information about others who have influenced the person's identification of self. Again, the kind and amount of data collected in this area need to be constructed carefully, with due sensitivity to the needs of the person to maintain privacy. Information may be obtained about family, the community in which the person lives and works, religious preferences, cultural and ethnic influences, and any other social information that the person deems important to share and that could influence the plan of care.

Assessment of the patient's nursing requirements leads to the development of *trophicognosis*. Trophicognosis is a nursing care judgment that is arrived at through the use of the scientific method (Trench, Wallace, & Coberg, 1987). Levine proposed the use of the term trophicognosis as an alternative to nursing diagnosis in 1966. In her more recent writings (1989, 1990) she does not include trophicognosis. She does state, "No diagnosis should be made that does not include the other persons whose lives are entwined with that of the individual (1989, p. 336). The *nursing diagnosis* focuses on the cause of the patient's suffering—what has put him or her in the predicament of need—and on the areas in which adaptation needs to be supported in order to achieve conservation and integrity.

Planning focuses on what the nurse needs to do to aid the patient in again becoming independent. The goals that are set will reflect the patient's behavior and the planned activities will include both willing participants—the nurse and the patient. Levine has made no effort to be prescriptive about the kinds of actions that would be planned. She is very clear, however, that the intent is to return the patient to a state of independence as quickly and fully as possible.

Implementation is structured according to the four conservation principles. For conservation of energy, actions will seek to balance energy input with energy output. The actions may focus on increasing energy input through improved nutrition or in decreasing energy output through changes in activity. The classic example of decreasing energy output is full bed rest. However, it is important to remember, as Levine (1989) points out, even at purportedly complete rest, the body is still using energy. Levine reports that Winslow's research demonstrates that energy conservation can be *predicted* (personal communication, 1994). For structural integrity, nursing actions will be "based on limiting the amount of tissue involvement in infections and disease" (Trench, Wallace, & Coberg, 1987). Such actions could include appropriate positioning to prevent the formation of decubiti, dressing changes, and administration of antibiotics. For personal integrity, efforts will be "based on helping the person to preserve his or her identity and selfhood" (Trench, Wallace, & Coberg, 1987). These actions may begin in deciding to protect the private self by *not* collecting complete psycho-social data and continue through the design of treatment plans that take individual characteristics into account. Levine indicates it is important to observe a strict moral approach. For structural integrity, nursing actions are "based on helping the patient to preserve his or her place in a family, community, and society" (Trench, Wallace, & Coberg, 1987). Such nursing actions may include teaching the family about the patient's care needs or teaching persons with new colostomies how to handle food and fluid intake and how to change the ostomy bag in a manner that helps to minimize its being evident to those they meet.

Evaluation is not specifically discussed by Levine but outcomes were discussed by Taylor (1974) for neurological patients. However, Levine's emphasis on the importance of assisting the person to return to independence as soon as possible supports the need for evaluation. It is important to know that the person's suffering has been relieved and that he or she is willing and capable of being no longer dependent. The evaluation data focus on the effectiveness of adaptation in achieving conservation and integrity in the four areas of energy, structural integrity, personal integrity, and social integrity.

LEVINE'S THEORY AND THE CHARACTERISTICS OF A THEORY

1. Theories can interrelate concepts in such a way as to create a different way of looking at a particular phenomenon. Levine has interrelated the concepts of adaptation, conservation, and integrity in a way that provides a nursing view different from that of the adjunctive disciplines with which nursing shares these concepts. Adaptation is identified as a process the product of which is conservation. The purpose of conservation is integrity or wholeness. Levine's writings clearly discuss the interrelationships of these concepts and specify how they influence the practice of nursing.

2. Theories must be logical in nature. Levine's work is logical. One thought or idea flows from the previous one and into the next. She is attuned to the origin of words and takes care in her use of words and how they relate to one another.

3. Theories should be relatively simple yet generalizable. There are only three major concepts in Levine's theory. This is the essence of simplicity. Because these three concepts apply to all living human beings and, according to Levine, nursing is not setting specific, the theory is generalizable. It can be used in any setting with any human being who is suffering and willing to seek assistance from a nurse.

4. Theories can be the bases for hypotheses that can be tested or for theory to be generated, and

5. Theories contribute to and assist in increasing the general body of knowledge within the discipline through the research implemented to validate them. Hypotheses have been developed from Levine's theory, and research has been conducted to test these hypotheses. The results of these research studies have contributed to the general body of knowledge in nursing. Levine (1989) discusses the studies conducted by Wong (1968) and Winslow, Lane, and Gaffney (1985) that support the importance of energy conservation for patients with myocardial infarctions. Research has also been conducted in using Levine's theory with confused patients over age 60 and caring for neonates and for women in labor (Foreman, 1989; 1991; Newport, 1984; Yeates & Roberts, 1984). Other studies have also been conducted. A number of these are included in Schaefer and Pond (1991). Others are unpublished master's theses or doctoral dissertations, and thus are less accessible than published materials.

6. Theories can be used by practitioners to guide and improve their practice. Levine developed her work to teach nursing students the practice of medical-surgical nursing. She had a practice-oriented focus in doing so. The work certainly provides a guide to practice and if used consistently can improve practice. Areas of nursing practice that have been reported in the literature as using Levine's work include the homeless; patients with burns, congestive heart failure, chronic pain, and epilepsy; and clinical settings which include critical care, emergency room, long term care, pediatrics, and perioperative nursing (Bayley, 1991; Brunner, 1985; Cox, 1991; Crawford-Gamble, 1986; Dever, 1991; Fawcett, et al., 1987; McCall, 1991; Pasco & Halupa, 1991; Pond, 1991; Pond & Taney, 1991: Schaefer, 1991). Levine's work has also been used in both undergraduate and graduate education (Grindley & Paradowski, 1991; Schaefer, 1991).

7. Theories must be consistent with other validated theories, laws, and principles but will leave open unanswered questions that need to be investigated.

Levine has clearly identified those ideas from adjunctive disciplines that she has used in her work. These include Cannon's (1963) flight or fight response, Selye's (1956) stress theories, Gibson's (1966) perceptual systems, Erikson's (1969, 1975) discussions of the influence of environment on development, Bates's (1967) three types of environment, and the works of Dubos (1966), Cohen (1968), and Goldstein (1963) in relation to adaptation. Her work is consistent with these works but builds on them in a way that creates questions to be answered. Such questions could include: Does change in one type of environment have a greater effect on adaptation than changes in the other two types? Why are some people more (or less) effective than others in adapting, conserving, and thus maintaining integrity? What are the most effective ways of conserving social integrity through disease prevention activities?

SUMMARY

Myra Levine's theory has evolved from a publication whose initial intention was the organization of medical-surgical nursing content to facilitate student learning. Her theory interrelates the concepts of adaptation, conservation, and integrity. Adaptation is the process by which conservation occurs. Human beings are constantly in interaction with their environments. It is this interaction that creates the need for adaptation. As the environment changes, the human must adapt. Successful adaptation will achieve the best fit with the environment and will do so in a manner that conserves energy, structural integrity, personal integrity, and social integrity. The purpose of conservation is health, or integrity—the wholeness of the individual. This theory has been tested through research and its usefulness demonstrated in clinical practice and education.

REFERENCES

Bates, M. (1967). Naturalist at large. *Natural history, 76,* 10.

Bayley, E. W. (1991). Care of the burn patient. In K. M. Schaefer, & J. B. Pond (Eds.), *Levine's conservation model: A framework for nursing practice* (pp. 91–99). Philadelphia: Davis.

Brunner, M. (1985). A conceptual approach to critical care nursing using Levine's model. *Focus on Critical Care, 12*(2), 39–44.

Cannon, W. B. (1953). *Bodily changes in pain, hunger, fear and rage.* New York: Harper Torchbooks.

Cohen, Y. (1968). *Man in adaptation: The biosocial background.* Chicago: Aldine.

Cox, S. R. A. (1991). A tradition of caring: Use of Levine's model in long-term care. In K. M. Schaefer, & J. B. Pond (Eds.), *Levine's conservation model: A framework for nursing practice* (pp. 179–197). Philadelphia: Davis.

Crawford-Gamble, P. E. (1986). An application of Levine's conceptual model. *Perioperative Nursing Quarterly, 2*(1), 64–70.

Dever, M. (1991). Care of children. In K. M. Schaefer, & J. B. Pond (Eds.), *Levine's conservation model: A framework for nursing practice* (pp. 71–82). Philadelphia: Davis.

Dubos, R. (1966). *Man adapting.* New Haven, CT: Yale University Press.

Erikson, E. (1969). *Ghandi's truth.* New York: Norton.

Erikson, E. (1975). *Life history and the historical moment.* New York: Norton.

Fawcett, J., Cariello, F. P., Davis, D. A., Farley, J., Zimmaro, D. M., & Watts, R. J. (1987). Conceptual models of nursing: Application to critical care nursing practice. *Dimensions of Critical Care Nursing, 6,* 202–213.

Foreman, M. D. (1989). Confusion in the hospitalized elderly: Incidence, onset, and associated factors. *Research in Nursing and Health, 12,* 21–29.

Foreman, M. D. (1991). Conserving cognitive integrity of the hospitalized elderly. In K. M. Schaefer, & J. B. Pond (Eds.), *Levine's conservation model: A framework for nursing practice* (pp. 133–149). Philadelphia: Davis.

Gibson, J. E. (1966). *The senses considered as perceptual systems.* Boston: Houghton-Mifflin.

Goldstein, K. (1963). *Human nature.* New York: Schocken.

Levine, M. E. (1966). Trophicognosis: An alternative to nursing diagnosis. In *American Nurses' Association Regional Clinical Conference Vol. 23* (pp. 55–70). New York: American Nurses' Association.

Levine, M. E. (1969). *Introduction to clinical nursing.* Philadelphia: Davis. [out of print]

Levine, M. E. (1973). *Introduction to clinical nursing* (2nd ed.). Philadelphia: Davis. [out of print]

Levine, M. E. (1984, August). *Myra Levine.* Paper presented at the Nurse Theorist Conference, Edmonton, Alberta, Canada. (Cassette recording).

Levine, M. E. (1989). The conservation principles of nursing: Twenty years later. In J. Riehl-Sisca (Ed.), *Conceptual models for nursing practice* (3rd ed.) (pp. 325–337). Norwalk, CT: Appleton & Lange.

Levine, M. E. (1990). Conservation and integrity. In M. E. Parker (Ed.), *Nursing theories in practice* (pp. 189–201). New York: National League for Nursing.

Levine, M. E. (1991). The conservation principles: A model for health. In K. M. Schaefer, & J. B. Pond (Eds.), *Levine's conservation model: A framework for nursing practice* (pp. 1–11). Philadelphia: Davis.

McCall, B. H. (1991). Neurological intensive monitoring system: Unit assessment tool. In K. M. Schaefer, & J. B. Pond (Eds.), *Levine's conservation model: A framework for nursing practice* (pp. 83–90). Philadelphia: Davis.

Newport, M. A. (1984). Conserving thermal energy and social integrity in the newborn. *Western Journal of Nursing Research, 6,* 176–197.

Pasco, A., & Halupa, D. (1991). Chronic pain management. In K. M. Schaefer, & J. B. Pond (Eds.), *Levine's conservation model: A framework for nursing practice* (pp. 101–117). Philadelphia: Davis.

Pond, J. B. (1991). Ambulatory care of the homeless. In K. M. Schaefer, & J. B. Pond (Eds.), *Levine's conservation model: A framework for nursing practice* (pp. 167–178). Philadelphia: Davis.

Pond, J. B., & Taney, S. G. (1991). Emergency care in a large university emergency department. In K. M. Schaefer, & J. B. Pond (Eds.), *Levine's conservation model: A framework for nursing practice* (pp. 151–166). Philadelphia: Davis.

Rogers, C. R. (1961). *On becoming a person.* Boston: Houghton–Mifflin.

Sacks, O. (1985). *The man who mistook his wife for a hat.* New York: Summit.

Schaefer, K. M. (1991). Developing a graduate program in nursing: Integrating Levine's philosophy. In K. M. Schaefer, & J. B. Pond (Eds.), *Levine's conservation model: A framework for nursing practice* (pp. 209–217). Philadelphia: Davis.

Schaefer, K. M., & Pond, J. B. (Eds.). (1991). *Levine's conservation model: A framework for nursing practice.* Philadelphia: Davis.

Selye, H. (1956). *The stress of life.* New York: McGraw-Hill.

Taylor, J. W. (1974). Measuring the outcomes of nursing care. *Nursing Clinics of North America, 9,* 337–349.

Trench, A. S. (Executive producer), Wallace, D. (Producer), & Coberg, T. (Director). (1987). *Myra E. Levine—The nurse theorists: Portraits of excellence* [Videotape]. Oakland, CA: Studio Three Production, Samuel Merritt College of Nursing.

Winslow, E., Lane, L. D., & Gaffney, F. A. (1985). Oxygen consumption and cardiovascular response in control adults and acute myocardial infarction patients during bathing. *Nursing Research, 34,* 164–169.

Wong, S. (1968). *Rehabilitation of a patient following myocardial in/out.* Unpublished master's thesis, Loyola University of Chicago School of Nursing.

Yeates, D. A., & Roberts, J. E. (1984). A comparison of two bearing-down techniques during the second stage of labor. *Journal of Nurse-Midwifery, 29,* 3–11.

BIBLIOGRAPHY

Levine, M. E. (1967). The four conservation principles of nursing. *Nursing Forum, 6,* 45–59.

Levine, M. E. (1969). The pursuit of wholeness. *American Journal of Nursing, 69,* 93–98.

Levine, M. E. (1970). The intransgient patient. *American Journal of Nursing, 70,* 2106–2111.

Levine, M. E. (1971). Holistic nursing. *Nursing Clinics of North America, 6,* 253–264.

Levine, M. E. (1988). Antecedents from adjunctive disciplines: Creation of nursing theory. *Nursing Science Quarterly, 1,* 16–21.

C H A P T E R   1 3

IMOGENE M. KING
Julia B. George

■ ■ ■

Imogene M. King was born in 1923, the youngest of three children. She received her basic nursing education from St. John's Hospital School of Nursing in St. Louis, Missouri, graduating in 1946. Her BS in nursing education (1948) and MS in nursing (1957) are from St. Louis University and her EdD (1961) is from Teachers College, Columbia University, New York. She has done postdoctoral study in research design, statistics, and computers (King, 1986b).

King has had experience in nursing as an administrator, an educator, and a practitioner. Her area of clinical practice is adult medical-surgical nursing. She has been a faculty member at St. John's Hospital School of Nursing, St. Louis; Loyola University, Chicago; and the University of South Florida. She served as director of the School of Nursing at The Ohio State University, Columbus. She was an Assistant Chief of the Research Grants Branch, Division of Nursing, Department of Health, Education and Welfare in the mid-1960s and on the Defense Advisory Committee on Women in the Services for the Department of Defense in the early 1970s. She is retired from the University of South Florida and continues to consult and work on the further application of her theory.

From the early 1960s the rapidity of scientific and technologic advances has had as great an impact on the profession of nursing as on other components of society. In the 1960s, as emerging professionals, nurses were identifying the knowledge base specific to nursing practice and to an expanding role for nurses. In this environment, Imogene M. King (1971) sought to answer several questions:

1. What are some of the social and educational changes in the United States that have influenced changes in nursing?
2. What basic elements are continuous throughout these changes in nursing?
3. What is the scope of the practice of nursing, and in what kind of settings do nurses perform their functions?
4. Are the current goals of nursing similar to those of the past half century?
5. What are the dimensions of practice that have given the field of nursing unifying focus over time? (p. 19).

In exploring the literature on systems analysis and general system theory, King (1971) developed additional questions:

1. What kind of decisions are nurses required to make in the course of their roles and responsibilities?
2. What kind of information is essential for them to make decisions?
3. What are the alternatives in nursing situations?
4. What alternative courses of action do nurses have in making critical decisions about another individual's care, recovery, and health?
5. What skills do nurses now perform and what knowledge is essential for nurses to make decisions about alternatives? (pp. 19–20)

King's *Toward a theory for nursing: General concepts of human behavior* was published in 1971 and *A theory for nursing: Systems, concepts, process* in 1981 (reprinted in 1990). These publications grew from King's thoughts about the vast amount of knowledge available to nurses and the difficulty this presents to the individual nurse in choosing the facts and concepts relevant to a given situation.

In the preface to *Toward a theory for nursing* (1971), King clearly states she was proposing a conceptual framework for nursing and not a nursing theory. As she denoted in the title, her purpose was to help move *toward* a theory for nursing. In contrast, in the preface to *A theory for nursing* (1981/1990a), she indicates that she has expanded and built upon the original framework. In this second publication, she

presents a conceptual framework by linking concepts essential to understanding nursing as a major system within health care systems . . . offers one approach to developing concepts and applying knowledge in nursing . . . [and] demonstrates one strategy for theory construction by presenting a theory of goal attainment derived from the conceptual framework (p. vii).

King identifies the conceptual framework as an open systems framework and the theory as one of goal attainment. As her extensive documentation indicates, she has drawn from a wide variety of sources in developing the framework and deriving the theory from that framework.

Because the theory of goal attainment is derived from the open systems framework, the framework and its assumptions and concepts are presented first, and then the goal attainment theory is discussed.

KING'S OPEN SYSTEMS FRAMEWORK

The purposes of the conceptual framework are to organize concepts that represent essential knowledge that might be used by many disciplines and to construct theories from the framework and test them from the perspective of nursing as a discipline (King, 1990c). The concepts and knowledge may be similar across disciplines, but the way each profession uses them will differ (King, 1989). The framework represents knowledge essential for nursing and has an additional purpose of allowing the construction and testing of theories from the perspective of nursing. The conceptual framework includes goal, structure, function, resources, and decision making, which King says are essential elements. The framework has health as the *goal* for nursing. *Structure* is represented by the three open systems. *Function* is demonstrated in reciprocal relations of individuals in interaction. *Resources* include both people (health professionals and their clients) and money, goods, and services for items needed to carry out specific activities. *Decision making* occurs when choices are made in resource allocation to support attaining system goals.

King (1989) presents several assumptions that are basic to her conceptual framework. These include the assumptions that human beings are open systems in constant interaction with their environment, that nursing's focus is human beings interacting with their environment, and that nursing's goal is to help individuals and groups maintain health.

The conceptual framework is composed of three interacting systems: the personal systems, the interpersonal systems, and the social systems. Figure 13–1 presents a schematic diagram of these interacting systems. King (1989) summarizes the conceptual framework as follows:

> Nursing phenomena are organized within three dynamic interacting systems: (1) personal systems (individuals); (2) interpersonal systems (dyads, triads, and small and large groups); and (3) social systems (family, school, industry, social organizations, and health care delivery systems) (p. 151).

King identifies several concepts as relevant for each of these systems. However, she also states that the placement of concepts with each system is arbitrary because all the concepts are interrelated in the human–environment interaction. For each system a comprehensive or major concept with additional subconcepts is identified.

Personal Systems

Each individual is a personal system. For a personal system the relevant concepts are perception, self, growth and development, body image, space, learning, and time (King, 1986a). *Perception* is presented as the major concept of a personal system, the concept that influences all behaviors or to which all other concepts are related. The characteristics of perception are that it is universal, or experienced by all; subjective or personal; and selective for each person, meaning that any given situation will be experienced in a unique manner by each individual involved. Perception is action oriented in the present and based on the information that is available. Perception is transactions; that is, individuals are active participants in situations and their identities are

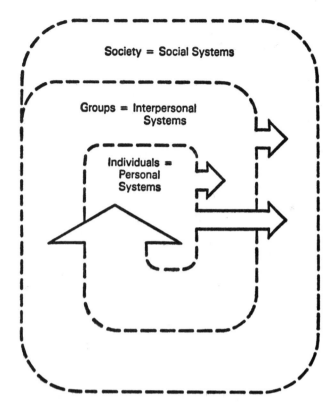

Figure 13–1. Dynamic interacting systems. *(Adapted from King, I. M. (1971).* Toward a theory for nursing, *New York: Wiley, p. 20. Copyright © 1971, by John Wiley & Sons, Inc. Used with permission.)*

affected by their participation (King, 1981/1990a). King further discusses perception as a process in which data obtained through the senses and from memory are organized, interpreted, and transformed. This process of human interaction with the environment influences behavior, provides meaning to experience, and represents the individual's image of reality.

The characteristics of *self* are a dynamic individual, an open system, and goal orientation. King (1981/1990a) accepts Jersild's (1952) definition of self:

> The self is a composite of thoughts and feelings which constitute a person's awareness of his individual existence, his conception of who and what he is. A person's self is the sum total of all he can call his. The self includes, among other things, a system of ideas, attitudes, values and commitments. The self is a person's total subjective environment. It is a distinctive center of experience and significance. The self constitutes a person's inner world as distinguished from the outer world consisting of all other people and

things. The self is the individual as known to the individual. It is that to which we refer when we say "I" (pp. 9–10).

The characteristics of *growth and development* include cellular, molecular, and behavioral changes in human beings. These changes usually occur in an orderly manner, one that is predictable but has individual variations and is a function of genetic endowment, of meaningful and satisfying experiences, and of an environment conducive to helping individuals move toward maturity (King, 1981/1990a). Growth and development can be defined as the processes in people's lives through which they move from a potential for achievement to actualization of self. Theorists mentioned are Freud (1966), Erikson (1950), Piaget (Inhelder & Piaget, 1964), Gesell (1952), and Havinghurst (1953), but no particular model, theory, or framework of growth and development is specifically selected.

Body image is characterized as very personal and subjective, acquired or learned, dynamic and changing as the person redefines self. Body image is part of each stage of growth and development. King (1981/1990a) defines body image as the way one perceives both one's body and others' reactions to one's appearance.

Space is characterized as universal because all people have some concept of it. It may be personal or subjective; individual; situational and dependent on the relationships in the situation; dimensional as a function of volume, area, distance, and time; and transactional or based on the individual's perception of the situation. King's (1981/1990a) operational definition of space includes that space exists in all directions, is the same everywhere, and is defined by the physical area known as "territory" and by the behaviors of those who occupy it.

Time is characterized as universal or inherent in life processes; relational or dependent on distance and the amount of information occurring; unidirectional or irreversible as it moves from past to future with a continuous flow of events; measurable; and subjective because it is based on perception. King (1981/1990a) defines time as "a duration between one event and another as uniquely experienced by each human being; it is the relation of one event to another event" (p. 45).

In 1986, King (1986a) added *learning* as a subconcept in the personal system. She did not further define learning as a concept.

Perception, self, growth and development, body image, space, and time are the concepts of the personal system. The focus of nursing in the personal system is the person (King, 1986a). When personal systems come in contact with one another, they form interpersonal systems.

Interpersonal Systems

Interpersonal systems are formed by human beings interacting. Two interacting individuals form a dyad, three form a triad, and four or more form small or large groups. As the number of interacting individuals increases, so does the complexity of the interactions. The relevant concepts for interpersonal systems are interaction, communication, transaction, role, and stress (King,

1981/1990a). The concepts from the personal system are also used in understanding interactions (King, 1989).

The comprehensive or major concept, *interaction*, is characterized by values; mechanisms for establishing human relationships; being universally experienced; being influenced by perceptions; reciprocity; being mutual or interdependent; containing verbal and nonverbal communication; learning occurring when communication is effective; unidirectionality; irreversibility; dynamism; and having a temporal-spatial dimension (King, 1981/1990a). Interactions are defined as the observable behaviors of two or more persons in mutual presence.

Characteristics of *communication* are that it is verbal; nonverbal; situational; perceptual; transactional; irreversible, or moving forward in time; personal; and dynamic (King, 1981/1990a). Symbols for verbal communications are provided by language, for such communication includes the spoken and written language that transmits ideas from one person to another. An important aspect of nonverbal behavior is touch. Other aspects of nonverbal behavior are distance, posture, facial expression, physical appearance, and body movements. King defines communication as "a process whereby information is given from one person to another either directly in face-to-face meeting or indirectly through telephone, television, or the written word" (p. 146). Communication as a fundamental social process develops and maintains human relations and facilitates the ordered functioning of human groups and societies. As the information component of human interactions, communication occurs in all behaviors.

Transactions, for this conceptual framework, are derived from cognition and perceptions and not from transactional analysis. The characteristics of transactions are that they are unique because each individual has a personal world of reality based on that individual's perceptions; they have temporal and spatial dimensions; and they are experience—a series of events in time. King (1981/1990a) defines transactions as "a process of interactions in which human beings communicate with the environment to achieve goals that are valued . . . goal-directed human behaviors (p. 82).

The characteristics of *role* include reciprocity in that a person may be a giver at one time and a taker at another time, with a relationship between two or more individuals who are functioning in two or more roles that are learned, social, complex, and situational (King, 1981/1990a). There are three major elements of role. The first is that role consists of a set of expected behaviors of those who occupy a position in a social system. The second is a set of procedures or rules that define the obligations and rights associated with a position in an organization. The third is a relationship of two or more persons who are interacting for a purpose in a particular situation. The nurse's role can be defined as interacting with one or more others in a nursing situation in which the nurse as a professional uses those skills, knowledge, and values identified as belonging to nursing to identify goals and help others achieve the goals.

The characteristics of *stress* are that it is dynamic as a result of open systems being in continuous exchange with the environment; the intensity varies;

there is a temporal-spatial dimension that is influenced by past experiences; it is individual, personal, and subjective—a response to life events that is uniquely personal. King (1981/1990a) derives a definition of stress to be "a dynamic state whereby a human being interacts with the environment to maintain balance for growth, development, and performance, which involves an exchange of energy and information between the person and the environment for regulation and control of stressors" (p. 96). In addition, stress involves objects, persons, and events as stressors that evoke an energy response from the person. Stress may be positive or negative, and may simultaneously help an individual to a peak of achievement and wear the individual down.

The concepts of interpersonal systems are interaction, communication, transaction, role, and stress. The focus of nursing in the interpersonal system is the environment (King, 1986a). Interpersonal systems join together to form larger systems known as social systems.

Social Systems

A social system is defined as an organized boundary system of social roles, behaviors, and practices developed to maintain values and the mechanisms to regulate the practices and rules (King, 1981/1990a, p. 115).

Examples of social systems include families, religious groups, educational systems, work systems, and peer groups. The concepts relevant to social systems are organization, authority, power, status, decision making, and control plus all the concepts from the personal and interpersonal systems (King, 1989).

King (1981/1990a) proposes four parameters for *organization:*

(1) human values, behavior patterns, needs, goals and expectations; (2) a natural environment in which material and human resources are essential for achieving goals; (3) employers and employees, or parents and children, who form the groups that collectively interact to achieve goals; (4) technology that facilitates goal attainment (p. 116).

The major concept, organization, is characterized by structure that orders positions and activities and relates formal and informal arrangements of individuals and groups to achieve personal and organizational goals; functions that describe the roles, positions, and activities to be performed; goals or outcomes to be achieved; and resources. King defines organization as being made up of human beings who have prescribed roles and positions and who make use of resources to meet both personal and organizational goals.

The characteristics of *authority* include that it is observable through provisions of order, guidance, and responsibility for actions; universal; essential in formal organizations; reciprocal because it requires cooperation; resides in a holder who must be perceived as legitimate; situational; essential to goal achievement; and associated with power (King, 1981/1990a). Assumptions about authority include that it can be perceived by individuals and be legitimate; it can be associated with a position in which the position holder distributes rewards and sanctions; it can be held by professionals through their competence in using special knowledge and skills; and it can be exercised through group leadership by those with human relations skills. King defines authority as an active, reciprocal process of transaction in which the actors' backgrounds, perceptions, and values influence the definition, validation, and acceptance of those in organizational positions associated with authority.

Power is characterized as universal, situational (ie, not a personal attribute), essential in the organization, limited by resources in a situation, dynamic, and goal directed (King, 1981/1990a). Premises about power are that it is potential energy, is essential for order in society, enhances group cohesiveness, resides in positions in an organization, is directly related to authority, is a function of human interactions, and is a function of decision making. King defines power in a variety of ways:

> Power is the capacity to use resources in organizations to achieve goals . . . is the process whereby one or more persons influence other persons in a situation . . . is the capacity or ability of a person or a group to achieve goals . . . occurs in all aspects of life and each person has potential power determined by individual resources and the environmental forces encountered. Power is social force that organizes and maintains society. Power is the ability to use and to mobilize resources to achieve goals (pp. 127–128).

Status is characterized as situational, position dependent, and reversible. King (1981/1990a) defines status as "the position of an individual in a group or a group in relation to other groups in an organization" and identifies that status is accompanied by "privileges, duties and obligations" (pp. 129–130).

Decision making is characterized as necessary to regulate each person's life and work, universal, individual, personal, subjective, situational, a continuous process, and goal directed. Decision making in organizations is defined as "a dynamic and systematic process by which goal-directed choice of perceived alternatives is made and acted upon by individuals or groups to answer a question and attain a goal" (King, 1981/1990a, p. 132).

In 1986, King (1986a) added *control* as a subconcept in the social system. She did not further define control as a concept.

As with the other two systems, King (1986a) has identified a focus for nursing in the social system. In this system, nursing's focus in health.

The major theses of King's (1981/1990a) conceptual framework are (1) that "each human being perceives the world as a total person in making transactions with individuals and things in the environment" (p. 141), and (2) that "transactions represent a life situation in which perceiver and thing perceived are encountered and in which each person enters the situation as an active participant and each is changed in the process of these experiences" (p. 142). Theories may be derived from conceptual frameworks. King has derived a theory of goal attainment from the concepts and systems of her conceptual framework.

KING'S THEORY OF GOAL ATTAINMENT

The major elements of the theory of goal attainment are seen "in the interpersonal systems in which two people, who are usually strangers, come together in a health care organization to help and be helped to maintain a state of health that permits functioning in roles" (King, 1981/1990a, p. 142). The theory's focus on interpersonal systems reflects King's belief that the practice of nursing is differentiated from that of other health professions by what nurses do with and for individuals. The concepts of the theory are interaction, perception, communication, transaction, self, role, stress, growth and development, time, and personal space (King, 1990c).

These concepts are interrelated in every nursing situation (King, 1989). Although these terms have already been defined as concepts in the conceptual framework, they are defined again here as part of the theory of goal attainment. King (1989) states that although all have been conceptually defined, only transaction has been operationally defined. However, the operational definition given for transaction is also used for interaction in another publication (King, 1990c).

Interaction is defined as "a process of perception and communication between person and environment and between person and person, represented by verbal and nonverbal behaviors that are goal directed" (King, 1981/1990a, pp. 141, 142). King diagrams interaction as seen in Figure 13–2. Each of the individuals involved in an interaction brings different ideas, attitudes, and perceptions to the exchange. The individuals come together for a purpose and perceive each other; each makes a judgment and takes mental action or decides to act. Then each reacts to the other and the situation (perception, judgment, action, reaction). King indicates that only the interaction and transaction are directly observable.

Perception is "each person's representation of reality" (King, 1981/1990a, p. 145). The elements of perception are the importing of energy from the environment and organizing it by information, transforming energy, processing information, storing information, and exporting information in the form of overt behaviors.

Communication is defined as "a process whereby information is given from one person to another either directly in face-to-face meetings or indirectly through telephone, television, or the written word" (King, 1981/1990a, p. 145). Communication represents, and is involved in, the information component of interaction.

Transaction is defined as "observable behaviors of human beings interacting with their environment" (King, 1981/1990a, pp. 145–146). Transactions

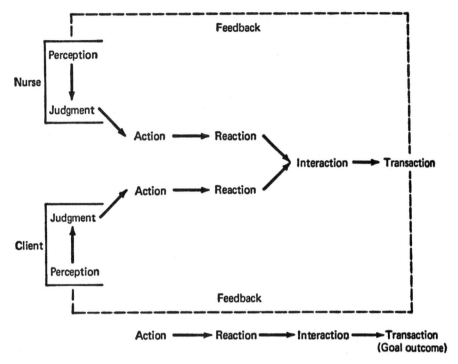

Figure 13–2. Interaction. *(Adapted from King, I. M. (1971). Toward a theory of nursing: General concepts of human behavior, New York: Wiley, pp. 26, 92. Copyright © 1971 by John Wiley & Sons, Inc. Used with permission.)*

represent the valuation component of human interactions and involve bargaining, negotiating, and social exchange. When transactions occur between nurses and clients, goals are attained.

Role is defined as "a set of behaviors expected of persons occupying a position in a social system; rules that define rights and obligations in a position; a relationship with one or more individuals interacting in specific situations for a purpose" (King, 1981/1990a, pp. 145–146). It is important that roles be understood and interpreted clearly to avoid conflict and confusion.

Stress is "a dynamic state whereby a human being interacts with the environment to maintain balance for growth, development, and performance . . . an energy response of an individual to persons, objects, and events called stressors" (King, 1981/1990a, p. 146). Although stress may be positive or negative, too high a level of stress may decrease an individual's ability to interact and to attain goals.

Growth and development can be defined as the "continuous changes in individuals at the cellular, molecular, and behavioral levels of activities . . . the processes that take place in the life of individuals that help them move from potential capacity for achievement to self-actualization" (King, 1981/1990a, p. 147).

Time is "a sequence of events moving onward to the future . . . a continuous flow of events in successive order that implies a change, a past and a future . . . a duration between one event and another as uniquely experienced by each human being . . . the relation of one event to another" (King, 1981/1990a, p. 147).

Space exists in every direction and is the same in all directions. Space includes that physical area named territory. Space is defined by the behaviors of those individuals who occupy it (King, 1981/1990a).

Health is not stated as a concept in the theory but is identified as an outcome variable. King (1986a) indicates the outcome is an individual's state of health or ability to function in social roles.

King's (1981/1990a, 1989, 1990c) operational definition of transaction has been used to identify the elements in interactions, at other times called a model of transactions. These elements are *action, reaction, disturbance (problem), mutual goal setting, exploration of means to achieve the goal, agreement on means to achieve the goal, transaction,* and *goal attainment.* The model essentially describes an interpersonal dyad (nurse and client) in interactions, using mutual goal setting or decision making as a process that leads to goal attainment.

From the theory of goal attainment, King (1990c) has developed predictive propositions:

- Perceptual accuracy, role congruence, and communication in a nurse–client interaction leads to transactions.
- Transactions lead to goal attainment and growth and development.
- Goal attainment leads to satisfaction and to effective nursing care (pp. 80–81).

She suggests that additional propositions may be generated.

In addition, King (1981/1990a) specifies internal and external boundary-determining criteria. Internal boundary criteria are derived from the characteristics of the concepts of the theory and speak to the theory itself. External boundary criteria speak to the area in which the theory is applicable. The internal boundary criteria for King's theory of goal attainment are the following:

1. Nurse and client do not know each other.
2. Nurse is licensed to practice professional nursing.
3. Client is in need of the services provided by the nurse.
4. Nurse and client are in a reciprocal relationship in that the nurse has special knowledge and skills to communicate appropriate information to help client set goals; client has information about self and perceptions of problems or concerns that when communicated to nurse will help in mutual goal setting.
5. Nurse and client are in mutual presence, purposefully interacting to achieve goals (p. 150).

The external boundary criteria for King's (1981/1990a) theory of goal attainment are the following:

1. Interactions in a two-person group
2. Interactions limited to licensed professional nurse and to client in need of nursing care
3. Interactions taking place in natural environments (p. 150).

In 1987, King added the boundary of client locus of control and states that it is difficult to achieve mutual goal setting with a client who has an external locus of control.

Thus, King is saying that a professional nurse, with special knowledge and skills, and a client in need of nursing, with knowledge of self and perceptions of personal problems, meet as strangers in a natural environment. They interact mutually to identify problems and to establish and achieve goals. The personal system of the nurse and the personal system of the client meet in interaction with the interpersonal system of their dyad. Their interpersonal system is influenced by the social systems that surround them as well as by each of their personal systems.

KING'S THEORY AND NURSING'S METAPARADIGM

In discussing her conceptual framework as an introduction to the presentation of her theory of goal attainment, King (1981/1990a) indicates that the abstract concepts of the framework are human beings, health, environment, and society. Because the theory is presented as a theory for nursing, King also defines nursing. Thus, the four major concepts of human beings, health, environment/society, and nursing are defined and discussed by King.

King (1981/1990a) identifies several assumptions about *human beings*. She describes human beings as social, sentient, rational, reacting, perceiving, controlling, purposeful, action-oriented, and time-oriented. From these beliefs about human beings, she has derived the following assumptions that are specific to nurse–client interaction:

- Perceptions of nurse and of client influence the interaction process.
- Goals, needs, and values of nurse and client influence the interaction process.
- Individuals have a right to knowledge about themselves.
- Individuals have a right to participate in decisions that influence their life, their health, and community services.
- Health professionals have a responsibility to share information that helps individuals make informed decisions about their health care.

- Individuals have a right to accept or to reject health care.
- Goals of health professionals and goals of recipients of health care may be incongruent (pp. 143–144).

King (1981/1990a) further states that "nurses are concerned with human beings interacting with their environment in ways that lead to self-fulfillment and to maintenance of health" (p. 3). Human beings have three fundamental health needs: (1) the need for health information that is usable at the time when it is needed and can be used, (2) the need for care that seeks to prevent illness, and (3) the need for care when human beings are unable to help themselves. She states, "nurses are in a position to assess what people know about their health, what they think about their health, how they feel about it, and how they act to maintain it" (p. 8).

King defines *health* as "dynamic life experiences of a human being, which implies continuous adjustment to stressors in the internal and external environment through optimum use of one's resources to achieve maximum potential for daily living" (King, 1989, p. 152) and as "a dynamic state of an individual in which change is constant and ongoing and may be viewed as the individual's ability to function in his or her usual roles (King, 1990b, p. 76). King (1990b) affirms that health is not a continuum but a holistic state. The characteristics of health are "genetic, subjective, relative, dynamic, environmental, functional, cultural, and perceptual" (p. 124). She discusses health as a functional state and illness as an interference with that functional state. She then defines illness as "a deviation from normal, that is, an imbalance in a person's biological structure or in his psychological make-up, or a conflict in a person's social relationships" (King, 1981/1990a, p. 5).

Environment and *society* are indicated as major concepts in King's framework but are not specifically defined in her work. Society may be viewed as the social systems portion of her open systems framework. In 1983, King extended the ability to interact in goal setting and selection of means to achieve the goal to include mutual goal setting with family members in relation to clients and families. Although her definition of health mentions both internal and external environment, and she has stated, "environment is a function of balance between internal and external interactions" (1990b, p. 127), the usual implication of the use of environment in *A theory for nursing* is that of external environment. Because she presents her material as based on open systems, it is assumed that a definition of external environment may be drawn from general system theory. Systems are considered to have boundaries that separate their internal components from the rest of the world. The external environment for a system is the portion of the world that exists outside of that boundary. Of particular interest as a system's external environment is the part of the world that is in direct exchange of energy and information with the system. King (1981/1990a) does say that the three systems form the environments that influence individuals.

Nursing is defined as "a process of action, reaction, and interaction whereby nurse and client share information about their perceptions in the nursing situation," and as "a process of human interactions between nurse and client whereby each perceives the other and the situation; and through communication, they set goals, explore means, and agree on means to achieve goals" (King, 1981/1990a, pp. 2, 144). *Action* is defined as a sequence of behaviors involving mental and physical action. The sequence is first mental action to recognize the presenting conditions; then physical action to begin activities related to those conditions; and finally, mental action in an effort to exert control over the situation, combined with physical action seeking to achieve goals. *Reaction* is not specifically defined but might be considered to be included in the sequence of behaviors described in action. *Interaction* has been discussed previously. Although King has altered her definition of nursing from that published in 1971, she has continued to refer to nursing as that which is done by nurses. "Lawyer" and "legal situation," "physical therapist," and "therapy situation," or any other practitioner who interacts with clientele could be substituted for "nurse" and "nursing situation" in her definitions of nursing. Such substitution would create definitions that could be applied to these other practices. This weakens her definition.

In addition to the foregoing definition of nursing, King (1981/1990a) discusses the goal, domain, and function of the professional nurse. The goal of the nurse is "to help individuals maintain their health so they can function in their roles" (pp. 3–4). Nursing's domain includes promoting, maintaining, and restoring health, and caring for the sick, injured, and dying. The function of the professional nurse is to interpret information in what is known as the nursing process to plan, implement, and evaluate nursing care.

THEORY OF GOAL ATTAINMENT AND THE NURSING PROCESS

The basic assumption of the theory of goal attainment—that nurses and clients communicate information, set goals mutually, and then act to attain those goals—is also the basic assumption of the nursing process. King (1990c) describes the steps of the nursing process as a system of interrelated actions and identifies concepts from her work that provide the theoretical basis for the nursing process as method.

According to King (1981/1990a), *assessment* occurs during the interaction of the nurse and client, who are likely to meet as strangers. Assessment may be viewed as paralleling action and reaction. The concepts King identifies are the perception, communication, and interaction of nurse and client. The nurse brings to this meeting special knowledge and skills, whereas the client brings knowledge of self and perceptions of the problems that are of concern. Assessment, interviewing, and communication skills are needed by the nurse as is the ability to integrate knowledge of natural and behavioral sciences for application to a concrete situation.

All concepts of the theory apply to assessment. Growth and development, knowledge of self and role, and the amount of stress influence perception and in turn influence communication, interaction, and transaction. In assessment, the nurse needs to collect data about the client's level of growth and development, view of self, perception of current health status, communication patterns, and role socialization, among other things. Factors influencing the client's perception include the functioning of the client's sensory system, age, development, sex, education, drug and diet history, and understanding of why contact with the health care system is occurring. The perceptions of the nurse are influenced by the cultural and socioeconomic background and age of the nurse and the diagnosis of the client (King, 1981/1990a). Perception is the basis for gathering and interpreting data, thus the basis for assessment. Communication is necessary to verify the accuracy of perceptions. Without communication, interaction and transaction cannot occur.

The information shared during assessment is used to derive a *nursing diagnosis,* defined by King (1981/1990a) as a statement that "identifies the disturbances, problems, or concerns about which patients seek help" (p. 177). The implication is that the nurse makes the nursing diagnosis as a result of the mutual sharing with the client during assessment. Stress may be a particularly important concept in relation to nursing diagnosis because stress, disturbance, and problem or concern may be closely connected.

After the nursing diagnosis is made, *planning* occurs. King (1981/1990a) says that the concepts involved are *decision making* about goals and *exploring means* and *identifying means* to attain goals. King describes planning as setting goals and making decisions about how to achieve these goals. This is part of transaction and again involves mutual exchange with the client. She specifies that clients are requested to participate in decision making about how the goals are to be met. Although King assumes that in nurse–client interactions clients have the right to participate in decisions about their care, she does not say they have the responsibility. Thus, clients are requested to participate, not expected to do so.

Implementation occurs in the activities that seek to meet the goals. Implementation is a continuation of transaction in King's theory. She states that the concept involved is the making of *transactions.*

Evaluation involves descriptions of how the outcomes identified as goals are attained. In King's (1981/1990a) description, evaluation not only speaks to the attainment of the client's goals but also to the effectiveness of nursing care. She also indicates that the involved concept is goal attainment or, if not, why not.

Although all the theory concepts apply throughout the nursing process, communication with perception, interaction, and transaction are vital for goal attainment and need to be apparent in each phase. King emphasizes the importance of mutual participation in interaction that focuses on the needs and welfare of the client and of verifying perceptions while planning and activities to achieve goals are carried out together. Although King emphasizes mutuality, she does not limit it to verbal communication, nor does she require the client's active physical participation in actions to achieve goal attainment.

In *A theory for nursing,* King presents an application of her theory of goal attainment that she identifies as the use of a goal-oriented nursing record.

Her description of this goal-oriented nursing record closely parallels the steps of the nursing process.

KING'S WORK AND THE CHARACTERISTICS OF A THEORY

King has stated that she has derived a theory of goal attainment from her open system framework of personal, interpersonal, and social systems. How her work compares with the characteristics of a theory presented in Chapter 1 is discussed below.

1. Theories can interrelate concepts in such a way as to create a different way of looking at a particular phenomenon. King has interrelated the concepts of interaction, perception, communication, transaction, self, role, stress, growth and development, time, and space into a theory of goal attainment. Her theory deals with a nurse–client dyad, a relationship to which each person brings personal perceptions of self, role, and personal levels of growth and development. The nurse and client communicate, first in interaction and then in transaction, to attain mutually set goals. The relationship takes place in space identified by their behaviors and occurs in forward-moving time. In particular, the specification of transaction as dealing with mutual goal attainment is a different way of looking at the phenomenon of nurse–client relationships.

2. Theories must be logical in nature. King's theory of goal attainment does describe a logical sequence of events. For the most part, concepts are clearly defined. However, a major inconsistency within her writing is the lack of a clear definition of environment, which is identified as a basic concept for the framework from which she derives her theory. In addition, she indicates that nurses are concerned about the health care of groups but concentrates her discussion on nursing as occurring in a dyadic relationship. Thus, the theory essentially draws on only two of the three systems described in the conceptual framework. The social systems portion of the framework is less clearly connected to the theory of goal attainment than are the personal and interpersonal systems. The definition of stress indicates that it is both negative and positive, but discussion of stress always implies that it is negative. Finally, King says that the nurse and client are strangers, yet she speaks of their working together for goal attainment and of the importance of health maintenance. Attainment of long-term goals, such as those concerning health maintenance, is not consistent with not knowing each other.

3. Theories should be relatively simple yet generalizable. Although the presentation appears to be complex, King's theory of goal attainment is relatively simple. Ten concepts are identified, defined, and their relationships considered; two concepts are identified only. Even though King indicates that many of the concepts are situation dependent, they are not situation specific; that is, they are influenced by the situation but may occur in many different situations. The theory of goal attainment is limited in setting only in regard to "natural environments" and, with growth and development as a major concept, is certainly not limited in age. The theory of goal attainment is generalizable to any dyadic nursing situation with a possible limitation relating to difficulties associated with seeking mutual goal setting with a client who has an external locus of control. The emphasis on mutuality would initially appear to limit the theory to dealing with those clients who can verbally interact with the nurse and physically participate in implementations to meet goals. However, King points to observable behaviors and to both verbal and nonverbal communication. Indeed, even the comatose individual has observable behaviors in the form of vital signs and does communicate nonverbally. The major limitation in relation to this characteristic is the effort required of the reader to sift through the presentation of a conceptual framework and a theory with repeated definitions to find the basic concepts. Another limitation relates to the lack of development of application of the theory in providing nursing care to groups, families, or communities.

   4. Theories can be the bases for hypotheses that can be tested or for theory to be expanded. King (1990c) presents the following hypotheses that she states are being tested:

- Mutual goal setting will increase ability to perform activities of daily living.
- Mutual goal setting by nurse and patient leads to goal attainment.
- Goal attainment will be greater in patients who participate in goal setting than those who do not participate in goal setting.
- Mutual goal setting will increase elderly patients' morale.
- Perceptual congruence in nurse–patient interactions increases mutual goal setting.
- Goal attainment decreases stress and anxiety in nursing situations.
- Congruence in role expectations and role performance increases transactions in nurse–patient interactions (pp. 81–82).

These and other hypotheses could be used to test the theory.

   5. Theories contribute to and assist in increasing the general body of knowledge within the discipline through the research implemented to validate them. King (1981/1990a) reports the results of a descriptive study conducted to test the theory of goal attainment. The study resulted in a classification system to analyze nurse–patient interactions and found that goal attainment is facilitated when the nurse and patient have accurate perceptions, adequate communication, and set goals mutually. She also states that data about interactions from two separate studies have confirmed the presence of transactions (King, 1990c). Studies reported in the literature include using King's conceptual framework and/or theory of goal attainment to investigate nurses' attitudes toward the elderly, attending behavior and mental status measurements, promoting postoperative participation in self-care (used in conjunction with Orem's theories), and parenting (Brower, 1981; Hanucharunkui & Vinya-nguag, 1991; Norris & Hayer, 1993; Rosendahl & Ross, 1982). These are examples of contributions to the general body of knowledge. The theory of goal attainment needs to be tested further. Such testing will expand the theory's contribution to the discipline.

6. Theories can be used by practitioners to guide and improve their practice. As demonstrated in the discussion of nursing process, King's theory of goal attainment can be used to guide and improve practice. Even though this theory in itself can be used as a guide to practice, King (1981/1990a) has also developed the goal-oriented nursing record in an effort to assist the practice of nursing. She presents the goal-oriented nursing record as an application of the theory of goal attainment in nursing. She has also developed a criterion-referenced tool for measuring attainment of health goals (King, 1988). Others have reported the use of King's work in nursing curricula (Daubenmire, 1989).

7. Theories must be consistent with other validated theories, laws, and principles but will leave open unanswered questions that need to be investigated. King's theory of goal attainment is not in apparent conflict with other validated theories, laws, and principles. She has clearly documented the sources on which she has based her characteristics and definitions of concepts, and she states that "the major technique used in developing concepts . . . has been a review of the literature in nursing and related fields to identify characteristics of the concept. From this information, an operational definition of the concept is formulated" (King, 1981/1990a, p. 22). Using the review of the literature as a base has helped to avoid being in conflict with others. King shares many similarities with other nursing theorists. As does Peplau (1952/1988), King indicates that the nurse and client usually enter the relationship as strangers when the client has a need. King's basic assumptions about human beings as thinking, sentient decision makers who have a right to information and to participation in decisions about themselves has a humanistic base similar to that of Paterson and Zderad (1976). The emphasis on the right to participate in decisions is similar to that of Orlando (1961/1990a, 1972), among others.

Throughout *A theory for nursing,* King identifies those theories from other fields that support what she is saying. Although there is no apparent conflict, many questions are open for exploration. A few of these are discussed in the hypotheses presented earlier in this chapter.

SUMMARY

Imogene King has presented an open systems framework from which she derived a theory of goal attainment. The framework consists of three systems—personal, interpersonal, and social—all of which are in continuous exchange with their environments. The concepts of the personal systems are perception, self, body image, growth and development, time, learning, and space. The concepts of the interpersonal systems are role, interaction, communication, transaction, and stress. Social systems concepts are organization, power, authority, status, decision making, control, and role.

From these systems and their abstract concepts of human beings, health, environment, and society, King derives a theory of goal attainment. The major concepts of the theory of goal attainment are interaction, perception, communication, transaction, role, stress, and growth and development. Each of these is defined, and overall propositions and criteria for determining internal and external boundaries of the theory are presented.

Imogene King has developed a theory of goal attainment that is based on a philosophy of human beings and an open systems framework. She presents the results of some of the research conducted to test the theory and proposes an application of the theory in the form of a goal-oriented nursing record.

The theory is useful, testable, and applicable to nursing practice. Although it is not the "perfect theory," it is widely generalizable and not situation specific. Dr. King's work is solidly based in the literature and provides the reader with a rich set of resources for further study.

REFERENCES

Brower, H. T. (1981). Social organization and nurses' attitudes toward older persons. *Journal of Gerontological Nursing, 7,* 293–298.

Daubenmire, M. J. (1989). A baccalaureate nursing curriculum based on King's conceptual framework. In J. Riehl-Sisca (Ed.), *Conceptual models for nursing practice* (3rd ed.). Norwalk, CT: Appleton & Lange.

Erikson, E. (1950). *Childhood and society.* New York: Norton. [out of print]

Freud, S. (1966). *Introductory lectures on psychoanalysis.* (J. Strachey, Trans.) New York: Norton. [out of print]

Gesell, A. (1952). *Infant development.* New York: Harper & Row. [out of print]

Hanucharunkui, S. & Vinya-nguag, P. (1991). Effects of promoting patient's participation in self-care on postoperative recovery and satisfaction with care *Nursing Science Quarterly, 4,* 14–20.

Havinghurst, R. (1953). *Human development and education.* New York: McKay. [out of print]

Inhelder, B. F. & Piaget, J. (1964). *The early growth of logic in the child.* New York: Norton. [out of print]

Jersild, A. T. (1952). *In search of self.* New York: Columbia University Teachers College Press. [out of print]

King, I. M. (1971). *Toward a theory for nursing: General concepts of human behavior.* New York: Wiley. [out of print]

King, I. M. (1983). King's theory of nursing. In I. W. Clements, & F. B. Roberts (Eds.), *Family health: A theoretical approach to nursing care.* New York: Wiley. [out of print]

King, I. M. (1986a). *Curriculum and instruction in nursing.* East Norwalk, CT: Appleton-Century-Crofts. [out of print]

King, I. M. (1986b). King's Theory of Goal Attainment. In P. Winstead-Fry (Ed.), *Case studies in nursing theory.* New York: National League for Nursing.

King, I. M. (1987). *King's theory.* Paper presented at Nurse Theorist Conference, Pittsburgh, PA. (cassette recording).

King, I. M. (1988). Measuring health goal attainment in patients. In C. Waltz, & O. Strickland (Eds.), *Measurement of nursing outcomes* (Vol I, pp. 109–117). New York: Springer.

King, I. M. (1989). King's general systems framework and theory. In J. Riehl-Sisca (Ed.), *Conceptual models for nursing practice* (3rd ed.) (pp. 149–158). Norwalk, CT: Appleton & Lange.

King, I. M. (1990a). *A theory for nursing: Systems, concepts, process.* Albany, NY: Delmar. (Originally published 1981, NY: Wiley.)

King, I. M. (1990b). Health as a goal for nursing. *Nursing Science Quarterly, 3,* 123–128.

King, I. M. (1990c). King's conceptual framework and Theory of Goal of Attainment. In M. E. Parker (Ed.), *Nursing theories in practice.* New York: National League for Nursing.

Norris, D. M., & Hayer, P. J. (1993). Dynamism in practice: Parenting within King's framework. *Nursing Science Quarterly, 6,* 79–85.

Orlando, I. J. (1990). *The dynamic nurse–patient relationship: Function, process and principles.* New York: National League for Nursing. (Originally published 1961, New York: Putnam's)

Orlando, I. J. (1972). *The discipline and teaching of nursing process.* New York: G. P. Putnam's. [out of print]

Peplau, H. E. (1988). *Interpersonal relations in nursing.* London: Macmillan Education. (Original work published 1952, New York: Putnam's)

Paterson, J., & Zderad, L. (1976). *Humanistic nursing.* New York: Wiley. [out of print]

Rosendahl, P. B., & Ross, V. (1982). Does your behavior affect your patient's response? *Journal of Gerontological Nursing, 8,* 572–575.

BIBLIOGRAPHY

Daubenmire, M. J., & King, I. M. (1973). Nursing process model: A systems approach. *Nursing Outlook, 21,* 512–517.

King, I. M. (1964, October). Nursing theory—Problems and prospects. *Nursing Science,* 394–403.

King, I. M. (1968). A conceptual frame of reference for nursing. *Nursing Research, 17,* 27–31.

King, I. M. (1970). Planning for change. *Ohio Nurses Review,* 4–7.

King, I. M. (1976). The health care system: Nursing intervention subsystem. In W. H. Werley, et al. (Eds.), *Health research: The systems approach.* New York: Springer. [out of print]

MARTHA E. ROGERS

Suzanne M. Falco
Marie L. Lobo

■ ■ ■

Martha E. Rogers was born in Dallas, Texas, May 12, 1914 and died in Phoenix, March 13, 1994. She was the eldest of four children. Her family heritage includes many active women suffragists and a strong belief in the necessity of a college education. Before entering the Knoxville General Hospital School of Nursing, she attended the University of Tennessee in Knoxville from 1931 to 1933. She received her diploma in 1936; a BS in public health nursing from George Peabody College, Nashville, Tennessee, in 1937; an MA in public health nursing supervision from Teachers College, Columbia University, New York, in 1945; and an MPH in 1952 and a ScD in 1954, both from Johns Hopkins University.

Following numerous leadership and staff positions in community health nursing, including establishing the first visiting nurse service in Arizona, she moved into higher education as a visiting lecturer and then as a research associate. For 21 years, Dr. Rogers was Professor and Head of the Division of Nurse Education at New York University. In 1975 she became Professor Emeritus at New York University.

Dr. Rogers was active in numerous professional organizations, received many awards and honors, and published extensively in numerous nursing journals. She wrote several books and contributed chapters to many others.

As "a humanistic science dedicated to compassionate concern for maintaining and promoting health, preventing illness, and caring for and rehabilitating the sick and disabled," nursing historically has meant service to humanity (Rogers, 1970, pp. vii, ix). Throughout nursing's evolution, from the earliest ages to the present, nurturance of the human race has been an ever-present and central concern. Over the years, the scientific extension of people's centuries-long interest in life and its many manifestations has become an integral component of nursing. Thus, the history of humanity is reflected in the evolutionary development of nursing. Consequently, Martha Rogers believed that knowledge of the past is a necessary foundation for the present understanding of nursing and for evolving the theories and principles that must guide nursing practice.

The concept that human life is valuable did not develop until people had begun to band together into tribes, villages, and towns (Rogers, 1970). Such communal living allowed for sharing work and responsibility and providing mutual support. This more settled life style made it possible for mothers to keep their newborns and care for more children. Thus, partly out of love and partly out of need, human beings began to develop strong feelings about and concern for fellow human beings.

As culture developed and more complex concepts in economic, political, and social structures increased, the value of human life increased (Rogers, 1970). Science, art, and religion brought a growing awareness of one's fellow human beings. The Hebrews developed a monotheistic faith, whereas the Greeks contributed philosophy, politics, and government. Humanism was becoming strongly entrenched in culture. Following the rise of Christianity, the medieval world was dominated by the Christian religions whose members assumed the responsibility for nursing. With the Dark Ages came a decline in religious, cultural, and political life. The end of this period led to the beginning of modern science.

As modern science evolved, new ideas mushroomed into new discoveries. The nature of the universe was explored. Descartes established the basis of modern philosophy. Einstein's theory of relativity brought a fourth dimension in the coordinate of space–time to man's previously three-dimensional world. Space research has multiplied scientific knowledge and has altered life styles. The reality of these evolutionary changes is reflected in man's growing complexity.

As a result of these factors, the rate at which society has been storing up useful knowledge about humanity and the universe has been spiraling upward for the past 10,000 years. This vast storehouse of knowledge coupled with a high degree of humanism and value of life has made advancement of nursing through scientific means and theoretical development a reality.

ROGERS'S DEFINITION OF NURSING

Capitalizing on the knowledge base gained from anthropology, sociology, astronomy, religion, philosophy, history, and mythology, Rogers in 1970 developed what she later called an abstract system for nursing. This abstract system has undergone changes over time as knowledge has expanded and new understandings have emerged. Through the years, terms and definitions have been refined, and as a work in progress, the abstract system continued to evolve. Consequently, what is reported here attempts to reflect the most current conceptualization, while preserving the richness of the preceding works. Throughout its development, some ideas have remained central to the abstract system. Since human beings are at the center of nursing's purpose, this abstract system looks at the total individual and is strongly based in general system theory. *Nursing,* then, is a humanistic and a humanitarian science directed toward describing and explaining the human being in synergistic wholeness and in developing the hypothetical generalizations and predictive principles basic to knowledgeable practice. The science of nursing is a science of humanity—the study of irreducible human beings and their environments (Rogers, 1971; 1990).

BASIC ASSUMPTIONS

Underlying Rogers's (1970) original work are five assumptions about human beings. First, the human being is a unified whole possessing an individual integrity and manifesting characteristics that are more than and different from the sum of the parts. The distinctive properties of the whole are also significantly different from those of its parts. Extensive knowledge of the subsystems is ineffective in enabling one to determine the properties of the living system—the human being. The human being is visible only when particulars disappear from view. Because of this wholeness, the individual's life process is a dynamic course that is continuous, creative, evolutionary, and uncertain, resulting in highly variable and constantly changing patterning.

Second, it is assumed that the individual and the environment are continuously exchanging matter and energy with each other. Environment for any individual is defined as "an irreducible, pandimensional energy field identified by pattern and integral with the human field" (Rogers, 1992, p. 29). This constant interchange of materials and energy between the individual and the environment characterizes each of them as open systems.

The third assumption holds that the life process of human beings evolves irreversibly and unidirectionally along a space–time continuum. Although Rogers's view of the continuum changed over time, the result continues to be the same. The individual can never go backward or be something he or she previously was. At any given point in time, then, the individual is the expression of the totality of events present at that given time and influenced by preceding events.

Identifying individuals and reflecting their wholeness are life's patterns. These patterns allow for self-regulation, rhythmicity, and dynamism. They give unity to diversity and reflect a dynamic and creative universe. Thus, the fourth assumption is that pattern identifies individuals and reflects their innovative wholeness.

Finally, the fifth assumption is that the human being is characterized by the capacity for abstraction and imagery, language and thought, sensation and emotion. Of all the earth's life forms, only the human is a sentient thinking being who perceives and ponders the vastness of the cosmos.

Based on these assumptions are the four building blocks identified by Rogers—energy fields, openness, pattern, and pandimensionality (Lutjens, 1991; Malinski, 1986; Rogers, 1992). A unifying concept for both animate and inanimate environments, *energy fields* have no boundaries; they are indivisible, extend to infinity, and are dynamic. Thus, these fields are *open,* allowing exchange with other fields. The interchange between and among energy fields has *pattern* that is perceived as a single wave; these patterns are not fixed but change as situations require. The interchanges occur in pandimensionality—a nonlinear domain that is not bounded by space or time. With these building blocks as the base, *unitary humans* are defined as irreducible, indivisible, pandimensional energy fields identified by pattern and manifesting characteristics that are different from those of the parts and cannot be predicted from knowledge of the parts, with the *environment* being an irreducible, indivisible, pandimensional energy field identified by pattern and manifesting characteristics different from, yet integral to, the person.

There is a strong parallel between Rogers's basic assumptions and general system theory. According to von Bertalanffy (1968), a system is a set of interrelated elements. The interrelated elements in this abstract system are human beings and their environments. As a living system and energy field, the individual is capable of taking in energy and information from the environment and releasing energy and information to the environment. Because of this exchange, the individual is an open system—an underlying assumption and building block.

General system theory is a general science of wholeness. It is concerned with the problems of organization, phenomena that are not resolvable to individual events, and dynamic interactions manifested in the difference of the behavior of the parts when isolated. As a result, order and behavior are not understandable by investigation of the respective parts in isolation (von Bertalanffy, 1968). Thus, the assumption of wholeness and the building block of pattern result.

The principle of hierarchial order is applicable (von Bertalanffy, 1968). The individual as an open system attempts to move toward a higher order by progressive differentiation, as for example, the differentiation of the cells of the zygote to form a human being. Within the order of the universe, the human being is of a higher order than other two-legged animals. Characteristic of higher order is Rogers's fifth assumption of human beings as sentient thinking beings, and congruent with it is the building block of pattern.

Using these five assumptions and building blocks as a base, the life process in human beings becomes a phenomenon of wholeness, of continuity, and of dynamic and creative change. It has its own unity. It is inseparable from the environment and occurs in pandimensionality. Because the individual is the recipient of nursing services, life processes of humanity are the *core* around which nursing revolves. According to Rogers (1970, 1988, 1992), the science of nursing is the study of human and environmental fields and is directed toward describing the life process of humanity and explaining and predicting the nature and direction of its development.

ROGERS'S THEORY: PRINCIPLES OF HOMEODYNAMICS

Although Rogers offers no theoretical statement, she grounds her *principles of homeodynamics* in the five basic assumptions and four building blocks discussed earlier. The principles of homeodynamics are composed of three separate principles—integrality, resonancy, and helicy (Rogers, 1970, 1988, 1992). By combining the principles of homeodynamics with the concept of humanity from her definition of nursing, a theoretical statement can be postulated. Using the definition that a theory interrelates concepts in such a way as to create a different way of looking at a particular phenomenon, an appropriate theoretical statement might be that nursing is the use of the principles of homeodynamics for the service of humanity.

Integrality

The first principle is that of *integrality*. Because of the inseparability of human beings and their environment, sequential changes in the life process are continuous revisions occurring from the interactions between human beings and their environment. Between the two entities, there is a constant mutual interaction and mutual change whereby simultaneous molding is taking place in both at the same time. This molding is one of association, not causality. Thus, integrality is the continuous, mutual, simultaneous interaction process between human and environmental fields.

Resonancy

The next principle, *resonancy,* speaks to the nature of the change occurring between human and environmental fields. The change in the pattern of human beings and environments is propagated by waves that move from longer waves of lower frequency to shorter waves of higher frequency. The life process in human beings is a symphony of rhythmical vibrations oscillating at various frequencies. Human beings experience their environments as a resonating wave of complex symmetry uniting them with the rest of the world. Resonancy, then, is the identification of the human field and the environmental field by wave patterns manifesting continuous change from longer waves of lower frequency to shorter waves of higher frequency.

Helicy

Finally, the principle of *helicy* deals with the nature and direction of change in the human-environment field. The human-environment field is a dynamic, open system in which change is continuous due to the constant interchange between the human and the environment. This change is also innovative. Because of the constant interchange, an open system is never exactly the same at any two moments; rather, the system is continually new or different. The difference cannot be predicted since open systems have choices about the matter, energy, and information which they accept as input and send out as output; thus, the change is unpredictable. Finally, the direction of change is toward ever increasing diversity and complexity. The life process evolves through a constant series of change in a rhythmical manner. The rhythms are not repeated although they may appear to be similar over time. The changes incorporate the past and lead to new patterns. This process and these patterns are unpredictable, dynamic, and increasingly diverse. Helicy encompasses the concepts of rhythmic change, evolutionary influence, and unitary human-environment fields. Helicy proposes that the direction of change which occurs between human and environment fields is toward ever increasing diversity and complexity and is seen in rhythms which are not precisely repeated.

Consequently, the principles of homeodynamics are a way of viewing human beings in their wholeness. Changes in the life process of humans are irreversible, nonrepeatable, rhythmic, and present a growing diversity of pattern. Change proceeds by continuous repatterning of both human and environmental fields by resonating oscillations of longer waves of lower frequency to shorter waves of higher frequency. Change reflects the mutual simultaneous interaction between the two fields in pandimensionality.

COMPARISON WITH OTHER THEORIES

The principles of homeodynamics are closely aligned to selected principles of general system theory. The homeodynamic principle of helicy can be compared to the principles of equifinality and negentropy. *Equifinality* means that an open system may attain a time-independent state independent of initial conditions and determined only by the system parameters. Thus, the system has a goal. The *negentropic* principle provides that open systems have mechanisms that can slow down or arrest the process of movement toward less efficiency and growth. Environmental exchange can provide support for such mechanisms.

For example, growth and development in the individual are equifinal. The same final state can be reached from different initial states and by means of different pathways. The various phases or stages along the way are maintained for an interval until spontaneous transition toward a higher order evokes new developments. The evolution toward an increase of order and organization at a higher level is made possible by negentropy. Thus, growing diversity and evolutionary emergence are made possible.

Consider the case of identical twins Susie and Joanie. Shortly after their two-month birthday, one of the twins, Susie, spent six weeks in bilateral leg casts to correct a congenital deformity. As a result of this experience, Susie is maintained at a developmental plateau, and Joanie continues to develop along the sequential axis. Consequently, Susie experiences an altered developmental pattern, the extent of which is depicted in Figure 14–1. At four months, the difference in development between the twins is substantial, whereas at eight months the difference has been greatly reduced. The equifinal state of this development will be achieved despite the increased time required.

Because of the evolutionary nature of this framework, many developmental theories are consistent with it. Infants are born with many capabilities. They have a repertoire of reflexes and behaviors with which they communicate with the world. The fetus evolves from a complex of cells into an organism that cues and responds to the environment, both inanimate and animate.

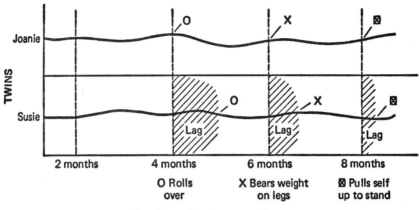

Figure 14–1. Pictorial representation of the altered developmental pattern experienced by one twin, Susie, as a result of leg-casting for six weeks following her second-month birthday.

Developmental theorists have demonstrated that the innate competence of the infant evolves through time.

For example, Erikson's (1963) psychosocial stages of development, beginning with trust versus mistrust and autonomy versus shame and doubt, through generativity versus self-absorption and ego integrity versus despair, profess a forward growth of an increasingly complex individual. Havinghurst's (1972) developmental tasks support the same philosophy of growth and development as Erikson. Development is an ongoing process from learning the first basic tasks of walking, eating, and talking to control of bodily functions to adjusting to retirement, and/or death of a spouse.

Another example is Piaget's (Piaget & Inhelder, 1969) concepts of intellectual development. From sensorimotor to preoperational to concrete operational to formal operational thought, a nonreversible growth occurs. Kohlberg (1973) validates Piaget's work in his findings that moral development begins when thought processes shift from preoperational to concrete operations. Again, Kohlberg found that males develop through a series of stages, from a premoral punishment and obedience orientation to a principled morality and a universal ethical principle orientation. Gilligan (1982) has challenged the developmental theorists and their exclusion of women's thought and development in the presentations of their work. Gilligan's thought-provoking observations are supportive of Rogers's conceptual model of the uniqueness of unitary human beings. In all these developmental theories, what has happened in the past in the individual's life will always affect the future.

Biologically, the individual also develops, moving from simple reflex responses and gross motor movements to complex control over fine motor movements. Such progressive differentiation is characteristic of the human organism. Specific biological functions such as the menstrual cycle have an ongoing effect on the body. With the onset of puberty, changes in the body structure, such as increased breadth of the hips and breast development, begin. Such changes persist past the menopause. Although the functioning of the body before puberty and following menopause may be said to be similar, the persistence of the identified changes mandates that the postmenopausal functioning be viewed differently from prepuberty functioning, thus illustrating the principle of helicy.

Components of Roy's (Roy & Andrews, 1991) adaptation model may also be viewed as consistent with Rogers's abstract system. Roy's model postulates that the individual's adaptation level is a function of the interaction between adaptation mechanisms and the environment. The physiological adaptation to the environmental stimulus of altitude change such as that experienced by mountain climbers demonstrates the mutual interaction between the individual and the environment. The simultaneous change in the mountain climber and in the altitude is consistent with the principle of integrality.

According to Roy (Roy & Andrews, 1991), the individual's adaptation of self-concept is affected by social experience, which reflects the external stimuli that surround the person and the processes of perception and social learning. Rogers's principle of helicy postulates that each new mutual interaction promotes continuous innovative changes. For example, a woman who is a wife and mother has developed a self-concept consistent with her perceptions of her interactions with her husband and children. When that same woman becomes a college student, interactions with faculty, students, and the college environment promote changes and adaptations in her self-concept.

This mother–wife–student has a change in her environment and therefore a change in her interaction with that environment. This is representative of integrality. The new environment of a university includes new faculty, new peers, new books, and new learning experiences in laboratories; and the new environment causes changes in the old environment—the home—and how the woman interacts with the environment there. At specified points in time the changes caused by the new environment create changes in the life pattern in which she has been functioning.

As the mother–wife–student grows and changes because of her interaction with faculty, peers, and the college environment, she integrates the material presented and is herself altered—emerging from the program as a different woman. This change affects the rhythms that have related to her former life style. Before entering the program, the mother of the family always cooked the meals; after she enters the program, another member of the family may assume the cooking role, thus changing the rhythms of family functioning. Rogers's principle of helicy can be used in the changes of rhythms occurring because of the change in the environment.

Resonancy examines the variations occurring during the life process of the "whole" person. Experiences as a student mandate changes in the wife–mother. Because of the progression in space–time, the wife–mother–student can never return to the wife–mother unaffected by the experience of being a student.

ROGERS'S THEORY AND NURSING'S METAPARADIGM

Martha Rogers (1992) speaks to nursing's metaparadigm. She presents five assumptions about *human beings*. Each human is assumed to be a *unified* being with individuality. The human is in continuous exchange of energy with the environment. The life processes of a human evolve irreversibly and unpredictably in pandimensionality. There is pattern to life. Finally, the human is capable of abstraction, imagery, language, thought, sensation, and emotion. Humans are irreducible, indivisible, pandimensional energy fields identified by pattern and manifesting characteristics and behaviors that are different from those of the parts and that cannot be predicted from knowledge of the parts.

Environment consists of the totality of patterns existing external to the individual. Both the individual and the environment are considered to be open systems. Environment is an irreducible, indivisible, pandimensional energy field identified by pattern and integral with the human field (Rogers, 1992).

Nursing is an art and science that is humanistic and humanitarian. It is directed toward the unitary human and is concerned with the nature and direction of human development. The goal of nurses is to participate in the process of change so that people may benefit (Rogers, 1992).

Health is not specifically addressed and indeed, if viewed as a state, is not appropriate to Rogers's theory. Malinski (1986) quoted personal communication with Rogers in which Rogers stated that she viewed health as a value term. This communication confirms previous inferences that disease, pathology, and health are value terms. Value terms change and, when discussed in terms of the dynamics of the behaviors manifested by the human field, need to be individually defined.

USE OF ROGERS'S PRINCIPLES IN THE NURSING PROCESS

If the profession of nursing is viewed as concerned with unitary human beings, the principles of homeodynamics provide guidelines for predicting the nature and direction of the individual's development as responses to health-related problems are made. Using these guidelines, the professional practice of nursing would then seek to promote symphonic integration of human beings and their environments, to strengthen the coherence and integrity of the human field, and to direct and redirect patterning of the human and environmental fields for the realization of maximum health (Rogers, 1992). These goals would be reflected in the nursing process.

To successfully use the principles of homeodynamics, there needs to be a consideration of the nurse and an involvement of both the nurse and the client in the nursing process. If anything or anyone external to the individual is part of the environment, then the nurse would be part of the client's environment. Because of the mutual interaction of the individual and the environment, it is implied that the client is a willing, integral participant in the nursing process. Consequently, individualized nursing care results, which Rogers

(1992) maintains is necessary if the client is to achieve maximum potential in a positive fashion. Nursing, then, is working *with* the client, not *to* or *for* the client. This involvement in the nursing process by the nurse demonstrates concern for the total person rather than one aspect, one problem, or a limited segment of need fulfillment.

In the nursing assessment phase of the nursing process, all facts and opinions about the individual and the environment are collected. Because of our limited measuring devices and data-collection tools, the information collected in the assessment is frequently of an isolate or particulate nature. However, to implement the guidelines, the analysis of the data must be in such a fashion as to reflect wholeness, which may be achieved by asking several questions and seeking the responses from the collected data.

The first series of questions reflect the principle of integrality. What is the interaction between the person and the environment? How has one adjusted to the other? Are there any maladjustment factors present? Are they able to work together? What factors support or undermine this working relationship? If the individual is in an environment that is not the normal one, how are the two environments different? Based on the differences, what kind of predictions can be made about the individual's interaction with this new environment?

The next series of questions would reflect the principle of resonancy. How has the life process of the individual progressed? What kind of variations have occurred during the course of this life process? What factors have influenced these variations? What role has the environment played in these variations? How would a strange environment affect the individual's life process?

The last series of questions would be influenced by the principle of helicy. What kinds of rhythms are reflected in the collected data? How complex are these rhythms? Are they old established rhythms or new emerging ones? How does the environment support these rhythms? If the individual is in a strange environment, how will these rhythms be affected by the new environment? What sequential stages of development has the individual passed through? What were the effects? How has the environment supported or retarded the progress of the individual? How will a new environment affect this progress? What kinds of goals does the individual have? How have these goals affected development? Where do the individuals wish to go as reflected by their goals? What kinds of new vistas are sought?

To reflect the idea of patterning, additional questions for the principle of helicy would be considered. What kinds of patterns characterize the individual? How have the patterns developed? What kinds of past experience have influenced the development of specified patterns? How has the environment promoted certain patterns? How complex are the patterns? How has time affected the patterns? Although these questions may be answered, it must be remembered that the responses reflect a specific point in space-time. Consequently, the identified patterns are not static but ever-changing, reflecting both a change in time and additional new past experiences. By no means are these questions all inclusive, but using them as a reference will help provide the nurse with a view of the whole individual. It will identify individual differences and the sequential cross-sectional patterning in the life process. It will also show the total pattern of events for the person in pandi-mensionality (Lutjens, 1991). The nursing assessment, then, is an assessment of the whole human being and not an assessment of only physical or mental status. It is an assessment of health and health potential for the individual and not an assessment of an illness or a disease process. As a result, the indi-vidual is paramount, not the disease.

As a result of the nursing assessment, a conclusion is drawn about the indi-vidual. This conclusion is the nursing diagnosis, the second step in the nurs-ing process, and it reflects the principles of homeodynamics. Rhythms, pat-terns, diversity, interactions, and life-process variations become evident. The nursing diagnosis seeks to identify sequential, cross-sectional patterns in the life process and encompasses human–environment relationships (Rogers, 1970). Such a nursing diagnosis is not consistent with the problem-oriented system for providing care. In the problem-oriented system, a problem is iden-tified and is stated as a symptom, finding, or (medical) diagnosis. As such, the problem reflects a piece of the individual and not the whole human being. Although also imperfect, nursing diagnoses based on Gordon's functional health patterns have greater potential for usefulness with Rogers's framework because they tend to reflect a more unitary view of the individual. Given the static nature and outdatedness of the term *diagnosis,* its use in this dynamic abstract system may not even be appropriate (Smith, 1988). Rogers did not discuss nursing process in her later writings (Fawcett, 1989).

With the nursing diagnosis providing direction for the rest of the nursing care plan, the thrust of the nursing diagnosis depends on its focus. The focus on integrality requires implementation within the environment as well as within the individual. It can be expected that change in one will be associated with simultaneous change in the other. Because of the individual's integration with the environment, health problems cannot be separated from the world's social ills. Therefore, these problems cannot be dealt with effectively by means of the commonly accepted, transitional, disease-oriented measures (Rogers, 1992). Creativity and imagination become essential.

Resonancy requires that the nursing plan be geared toward supporting or modifying variations in the life process of the whole human being. Because the human life process is a unidirectional phenomenon, the intervention cannot be aimed at returning the individual to a former level of existence; rather, the nurse helps the individual move forward to a higher, more diverse level of existence.

Nursing planning in the area of helicy requires an acceptance of individual differences as an expression of evolutionary emergence. The strategies are geared to supporting or modifying rhythms and life goals. To do this requires the informed and active participation of the client in the nursing process. The concept of the unitary human and a recognition of the human being's capac-ity to feel and to reason enables the nurse to assist the individual in the reso-lution of the health problem and in the setting of goals directed toward achieving health (Rogers, 1992). Health will not be achieved by promoting homeostasis and equilibrium but, rather, by taking steps to enhance dynamism and diversity within the individual.

Additionally, helicy requires that the nursing plan be geared toward promoting dynamic repatterning of the whole human being. This repatterning includes the individual's relationship to self and to the environment so that the total potential as a human being can be developed. This repatterning is aimed at assisting people to develop patterns of living that coordinate with environmental changes rather than conflict with them (Rogers, 1992). Although the pattern may be altered or maintained, it must be remembered that this is an evolving, ever-changing pattern rather than a static, constant phenomenon.

Regardless of the focus, the aim of the nursing plan is the attainment of an optimum state of health for the individual. This state of health may not be the ideal but will be the maximum health that is potentially possible for the individual. Generally, implementation strategies seek to strengthen the integrity of the individual–environment relationship and to give direction to humanity's struggle to achieve new levels of well-being. By assisting individuals to mobilize their resources, consciously and unconsciously, their integrity is heightened (Rogers, 1992).

If attainment of an optimum state of health is the aim of the nursing plan, then it becomes the focus for nursing evaluation, the final phase of the nursing process. Has the integrity of the individual–environment relationship been strengthened? Have resources been mobilized? Has the patterning of the human and environmental fields been directed toward the realization of maximum health potential? Only when the nursing goal of the highest possible health state has been realized can nursing interventions be evaluated as effective.

A schematic representation of the relationship between the principles of homeodynamics and the elements of the nursing process is presented in Table 14–1. As can be seen, there is no absolute distinction between the areas covered by the various principles. Table 14–2 attempts to apply the generalities to the specific situation of Janie who is hospitalized. In no way is either table designed to be all inclusive. Rather, they are offered as an attempt to make abstract ideas more concrete and operational.

Although the examples given focus on the individual, the Rogerian model can also be applied to families. An "irreducible, four-dimensional [now pandimensional], negentropic family energy field becomes the focus of study" or practice (Rogers, 1983, p. 226). The definition of the family can be left open to the situation at hand. Families may include nuclear families, extended families, homosexual families, single-person families, or any other structure that the client regards as family.

Johnston (1986) has taken Rogers a step further than family care by using Rogerian theory as an approach for family therapy intervention. Health and family health are viewed as manifestations of family and environment. The interrelationships between the family and environmental fields preclude

TABLE 14-1. RELATIONSHIP OF THE PRINCIPLES OF HOMEODYNAMICS TO THE NURSING PROCESS

Components of the Nursing Process	Principles of Homeodynamics		
	Integrality	Resonancy	Helicy
Nursing assessment component	Look at the interaction of the individual and the environment—how they work together rather than what they are like in isolation.	Look at the variation occurring during the life process of the whole human being.	Look at the rhythmic life patterns of the individual and the environment. Progression of time of necessity creates change in the rhythmic life patterns of the whole human being. Look at life goals. Be aware of growing complexity of the whole human being.
Nursing diagnosis component	Reflects integration of the individual and environmental fields	Reflects the variations in the life process of the whole individual.	Reflects the rhythmic pattern of the individual and environmental fields.
Nursing plan for implementation component	Intervene in the environment as well as in the individual. Change promoted in one area will cause simultaneous change in the other—simultaneous molding.	Support or modify variations in the life process of the whole individual.	Promote dynamic rhythmic repatterning of both the individual and the environment. Accept differences as an expression of evolutionary emergence. Promote dynamism and complexity rather than homeostasis and equilibrium. Support or modify life goals.
Nursing evaluation component	Evaluate changes in the integration that have occurred.	Evaluate the modification made in the variations of the life process of the whole human being.	Evaluate rhythmic repatterning of the individual and the environment. Evaluate goal-directedness. Evaluate relationship of goal to the whole individual.

TABLE 14–2. RELATIONSHIP OF THE PRINCIPLES OF HOMEODYNAMICS TO THE NURSING PROCESS FOR JANIE

Components of the Nursing Process	Principles of Homeodynamics		
	Integrality	Resonancy	Helicy
Nursing assessment component	1. How does Janie see her environment? 2. What kind of differences are there between the hospital and her home? 3. How is she reacting to the changes in her environment? 4. How do her health problem and the environment affect each other?	1. What is Janie's past history? 2. What kinds of deviations from the expected norms have there been? 3. Were these deviations individually or environmentally related? 4. What is the reason for the hospitalization? 5. How will this affect her life?	1. What are Janie's normal behavior patterns and routines? 2. Were the behaviors or routines undergoing a change prior to her admission? 3. What kinds of activities can she perform? 4. What kinds of past experiences has she had? 5. How might those experiences influence her current situation? 6. What is Janie's developmental level? 7. Will the hospital environment support or retard developmental progress? 8. What are Janie's goals?
Nursing diagnosis component	1. What is the nature of the interaction between Janie and the hospital?	1. What is the interference this hospitalization will make in Janie's life?	1. What are the rhythmic patterns that are being exhibited?

Nursing plan for implementation component	1. How can the hospital environment be modified to reduce the differences identified? 2. How can Janie be helped to understand the differences that cannot be eliminated? 3. How can her health potential be improved by manipulating the environment?	1. How can Janie's normal development be promoted? 2. How can the effects of the interferences be minimized?	1. How can Janie's normal behavioral patterns and routines be promoted in the hospital? 2. What kind of modifications can be made to promote her normal behavioral patterns and routines? 3. What kind of provisions can be made to promote her normal growth and development? 4. How can Janie be helped to develop successful rhythmic behavioral patterns within the hospital environment? 5. How can Janie be helped to reach her goals?
Nursing evaluation component	1. Has Janie's behavior changed as a result of environmental modification? 2. What kind of new reactions are now taking place?	1. Is Janie developing normally, based on theories? 2. Has the interference with development been minimized?	1. What kind of rhythmic repatterning has taken place? 2. Is Janie's development being supported? 3. Is she moving toward her goals?

looking at family members as individual units and their actions in isolation. Changes occur in the energy field of the entire family.

LIMITATIONS OF ROGERS'S PRINCIPLES OF HOMEODYNAMICS

Although the principles of homeodynamics are consistent with the universally accepted aims and goals of nursing, there are major limitations to the universal implementation of the principles. Many persons have difficulty understanding the principles. Even though basic assumptions are provided and the principles are defined, the system remains abstract. Terms have not been sufficiently operationalized to provide for clear understanding. By "operationalizing terms" is meant the description of a set of physical procedures that must be carried out in order to assign to every case a value for the concept. For example, to operationalize the concept of width is to place an instrument consisting of the units of inches or centimeters along the edge of the item to be measured and then to count the units. Difficulties with operationalizations of the concepts as well as with bringing the abstractness of the concepts and the relationships to an empirical level for testing are plaguing many nurse scientists (Kim, 1986).

Because of the lack of operational definitions, research done to support or verify the principles provides questionable results. Operational definitions are needed for the development of hypotheses that test the theoretical concepts and for the selection of instruments that will adequately measure the concepts involved (Hardy, 1974). Without such definitions just what was confirmed or not confirmed by these studies is in doubt.

At this stage in the development of nursing science, instruments that will adequately assess human beings in their totality are nonexistent. For example, it is difficult to measure the individual as a unity or to measure energy fields and wave patterns (Burns & Grove, 1987). The issue of measurement is at a critical juncture, and in-depth discussions of ways to address this issue are greatly needed (Parse, 1987). Without such instruments, the ability to use or test the abstract system fully is virtually impossible. Furthermore, the inability to adequately use or test the system makes successful nursing implementation difficult. Thus, the use of principles of homeodynamics in its totality is limited. At best, varying aspects of the principles can be applied to nursing practice in a very limited fashion.

ROGERS'S WORK AND THE CHARACTERISTICS OF A THEORY

1. Theories can interrelate concepts in such a way as to create a **different way of looking at a particular phenomenon.** Rogers's abstract system clearly creates an alternative view of people and their world. The theoretical statement that nursing is the use of the principles of homeodynamics for the service of humanity compels one to look at nursing in a very different way. An excellent example is the principle of helicy with its emphasis on pattern and rhythmicity.

2. **Theories must be logical in nature.** There is definitely a logical development of the major constructs. This logical development proceeds from the identification of assumptions, through the building blocks, to the principles of homeodynamics.

3. **Theories should be relatively simple yet generalizable.** The theory is generalizable because it is not dependent on any given setting. It has been stated that Rogers's conception of man is elegant in its simplicity (Fawcett, 1989). However, the theory is far from simple in that its level of abstraction and the nature of the terminology contribute to difficulties in understanding. In addition, the theory is based on the use of open systems that are inherently complex.

4. **Theories can be the bases for hypotheses that can be tested or for theory to be expanded, and**

5. **Theories contribute to and assist in increasing the general body of knowledge within the discipline through the research implemented to validate them.** It is clear that the abstract level of the system leads to the generation of a plethora of research questions. Barrett (1990), Fawcett (1989), Ference (1989), Malinski (1986), Madrid and Winstead-Fry (1986), and Rogers (1989) all cite numerous studies ostensibly designed to test this framework. However, research is hampered by the lack of simplicity, operational definitions, and valid instruments to measure outcomes. The complex interrelationships involved in the framework contribute to these difficulties. Qualitative research approaches have been suggested as an effective method for minimizing these problems (Reeder, 1984; Wilson & Fitzpatrick, 1984). These and other efforts designed to minimize these research problems need to be continued so that nursing can truly benefit from Rogers's abstract system.

6. **Theories can be used by practitioners to guide and improve their practice.** Rogers's ideas can be applied to practice. When these ideas are applied to nursing practice, the understanding of the client's behavior takes on new dimensions. Such dimensions include accepting diversity as the norm, empowering both nurse and client, viewing change as positive, and accepting the integral connectedness of life (Malinski, 1986). This changed understanding results in alterations in the focus of nursing actions. The case study of Janie presented in this chapter provides an example. In addition, nursing interventions such as therapeutic touch and the use of light, color, music, and movement have been derived from Rogers's tenets. However, evidence of positive effects of nursing interventions derived from this model is needed.

7. **Theories must be consistent with other validated theories, laws, and principles but will leave open unanswered questions that need to be investigated.** Rogers's work is consistent with other validated theories, laws, and principles. The abstract nature of the system provides great potential for generating questions for further study and deriving interventions for nursing practice. Rogers's abstract system has also been instrumental in the

development of other theories. Newman's (1994) and Parse's (1992) works are two such examples.

SUMMARY

Building on a broad theoretical base from a variety of disciplines, Rogers developed the principles of homeodynamics. Inherent in the principles are five basic assumptions: (1) the human being is a unified whole, possessing individual integrity and manifesting characteristics that are more than and different from the sum of the parts; (2) the individual and the environment are continuously exchanging matter and energy with each other; (3) the life process of human beings evolves irreversibly and unidirectionally along a space–time continuum; (4) patterns identify human beings and reflect their innovative wholeness; and (5) the individual is characterized by the capacity for abstraction and imagery, language and thought, sensation and emotion. The principles of integrality, helicy, and resonancy are compared to general system theory, developmental theories, and adaptation theories. Ways to use the principles in the nursing process are explored. The difficulty in understanding the principles, the lack of operational definitions, and inadequate instruments for measurement are the major limitations to the effective use of this theory.

REFERENCES

Barrett, E. A. M. (Ed.). (1990). *Visions of Rogers's science–based nursing.* New York: National League for Nursing.

Burns, N., & Grove, S. K. (1987). *The practice of nursing research: Conduct, critique, and utilization.* Philadelphia: Saunders.

Erikson, E. (1963). *Childhood and society* (2nd ed.). New York: Norton. [out of print]

Fawcett, J. (1989). *Analysis and evaluation of conceptual models of nursing* (2nd ed.). Philadelphia: Davis.

Ference, H. M. (1989). Comforting the dying: Nursing practice according to the Rogerian model. In J. Riehl-Sisca (Ed.), *Conceptual models for nursing practice* (3rd ed.) (pp. 197–205). Norwalk, CT: Appleton & Lange.

Gilligan, C. (1982). *In a different voice: Psychological theory and women's development.* Cambridge, MA: Harvard University Press.

Hardy, M. E. (1974). Theories: Components, development, evaluation. *Nursing Research, 23,* 100–107.

Havinghurst, R. (1972). *Developmental tasks and education* (3rd ed.). New York: McKay. [out of print]

Johnston, R. L. (1986). Approaching family intervention through Rogers's conceptual model. In A. L. Whall (Ed.), *Family therapy theory for nursing: Four approaches.* Norwalk, CT: Appleton-Century-Crofts.

Kim, H. S. (1986). *The nature of theoretical thinking in nursing.* Norwalk, CT: Appleton-Century-Crofts.

Kohlberg, L. (1973). *Collected papers on moral development and moral education.* Cambridge, MA: Moral Education and Research Foundation. [out of print]

Lutjens, L. R. J. (1991). *Martha Rogers: The science of unitary human beings.* Newbury Park, CA: Sage.

Madrid, M., & Winstead-Fry, P. (1986). Rogers's conceptual model. In P. Winstead-Fry (Ed.), *Case studies in nursing theory* (pp. 73–102). New York: National League for Nursing.

Malinski, V. M. (Ed.). (1986). *Explorations on Martha Rogers's science of unitary human beings.* Norwalk, CT: Appleton-Century-Crofts.

Newman, M. A. (1994). *Health as expanding consciousness* (2nd ed.). NY: National League for Nursing.

Parse, R. R. (1987). *Nursing science: Major paradigms, theories, and critiques.* Philadelphia: Saunders.

Parse, R. R. (1992). Human becoming: Parse's theory of nursing. *Nursing Science Quarterly, 5,* 35–42.

Piaget, J., & Inhelder, R. (1969). *The psychology of the child.* New York: Basic Books. [out of print]

Reeder, F. (1984). Philosophical issues in the Rogerian science of unitary human beings. *Advances in Nursing Science, 6,* 14–23.

Rogers, M. E. (1970). *The theoretical basis of nursing.* Philadelphia: Davis. [out of print]

Rogers, M. E. (1971). *Accountability.* Convention address, University of Utah College of Nursing, June 5, 1971.

Rogers, M. E. (1983). Science of unitary human beings: A paradigm for nursing. In I. W. Clements, & F. B. Roberts (Eds.), *Family health: A theoretical approach to nursing care.* New York: Wiley Medical.

Rogers, M. E. (1988). Nursing science and art: A prospective. *Nursing Science Quarterly, 1,* 99–102.

Rogers, M. E. (1989). Nursing: A science of unitary human beings. In J. Riehl-Sisca (Ed.), *Conceptual models for nursing practice* (3rd ed.) (pp. 181–188). Norwalk, CT: Appleton & Lange.

Rogers, M. E. (1990). Space-age paradigm for new frontiers in nursing. In M. E. Parker (Ed.), *Nursing theories in practice* (pp. 105–113). New York: National League for Nursing.

Rogers, M. E. (1992). Nursing science and the space age. *Nursing Science Quarterly, 5,* 27–34.

Roy, C., & Andrews, H. A. (1991). *The Roy Adaptation Model: The definitive statement.* Norwalk, CT: Appleton & Lange.

Smith, M. J. (1988). Perspectives on nursing science. *Nursing Science Quarterly, 1,* 80–85.

von Bertalanffy, L. (1968). *General system theory.* New York: Braziller. [out of print]

Wilson, L. M., & Fitzpatrick, J. J. (1984). Dialectic thinking as a means of understanding systems-in-development: Relevance to Rogers's principles. *Advances in Nursing Science, 6,* 24–41.

BIBLIOGRAPHY

Madrid, M., & Barrett, E. A. M. (Eds.). (1994). *Rogers' scientific art of nursing practice.* New York: National League for Nursing.

Malinski, V. M., & Barrett, E. A. M. (1994). *Martha E. Rogers: Her life and her work.* Philadelphia: Davis.

Meleis, A. I. (1985). *Theoretical nursing: Development and progress.* Philadelphia: Lippincott.

Rogers, M. E. (1992). Nightingale's *Notes on nursing:* A prelude to the 21st century. In F. Nightingale. *Notes on nursing: What it is, and what it is not* (Com. ed.). Philadelphia: Lippincott.

Sarter, B. (1988). *The stream of becoming: A study of Martha Rogers's theory.* New York: National League for Nursing.

JOYCE FITZPATRICK'S LIFE PERSPECTIVE RHYTHM MODEL

Julia B. George

Joyce Fitzpatrick (b. 1944) received her BS in nursing from Georgetown University, Washington, DC; her MS in psychiatric–mental health nursing, with additional course work in community health nursing from The Ohio State University, Columbus, Ohio; and her PhD in nursing from New York University. She has proposed a life perspective rhythm model, based upon the work of Martha Rogers and derived from her own research on individuals' abilities to integrate crisis situations into their life perspectives. Fitzpatrick (1989) presents this model in *Conceptual models of nursing*.

Fitzpatrick draws upon Rogers's (1970, 1980) conceptualizations of unitary man. These conceptions are the following:

1. Man is greater than the sum of his parts.
2. Man and environment are open systems that continually exchange matter and energy with each other.
3. The life process develops unidirectionally and irreversibly along the space–time continuum.
4. Man's wholeness is reflected in pattern and organization.
5. Man has the ability to sense, experience emotion, think and use language, deal with abstraction and imagery.

The life perspective rhythm model, a developmental model, proposes that human development is a process that is characterized by rhythms and based in personal meaning. This development occurs within the context of continuous interaction between person and environment. Patterns of rhythm include those dealing with time, motion, consciousness, and perception. The rhythm of development has high and low points with an overall progression toward an increase in the speed of the rhythms. For example, one's perception of time moves from time progressing very slowly to time passing quickly and eventually to timelessness. Not only can the overall life process of development be described but also changes within an individual's life pattern can be identified. The life perspective rhythm view of the person and the environment is consistent with Rogers's belief that the human and the environment are open systems that are in continuous interaction. Within this model, health is viewed as "a continuously developing characteristic of humans with the full life potential that may characterize the process of dying—the heightened awareness of the meaningfulness of life—representing a more fully developed dimension of health (humanness)" (Fitzpatrick, 1989, pp. 405–406).

Life perspective is viewed as a dimension of health or humanness, and the meaning attached to life is of central concern to nursing. Thus, nursing care based upon the life perspective model focuses on enhancing the developmental process in moving toward health, in encouraging individuals to develop their potential as human beings.

REFERENCES

Fitzpatrick, J. (1989). A life perspective rhythm model. In J. Fitzpatrick, & A. Whall (Ed.), *Conceptual models of nursing: Analysis and application* (2nd ed.) (pp. 401–407). Norwalk, CT: Appleton & Lange.

Rogers, M. E. (1970). *An introduction to the theoretical basis of nursing.* Philadelphia: Davis.

Rogers, M. E. (1980). Nursing: A science of unitary man. In J. Riehl, & C. Roy, (Eds.), *Conceptual models for nursing practice* (2nd ed.) (pp. 329–337). New York: Appleton-Century-Crofts.

CALLISTA ROY

Julia Gallagher Galbreath

■ ■ ■

*Callista Roy, RN, PhD (b. 1939) is a nurse theorist at Boston College,
Massachusetts. Before this appointment, Roy was a Post-Doctoral Fellow and
Robert Wood Johnson Clinical Nurse Scholar at the University of California, San
Francisco. Roy has served in many positions, including Chair of the Department
of Nursing, Mount Saint Mary's College, Los Angeles; Adjunct Professor,
Graduate Program, School of Nursing, University of Portland; and Acting
Director and Nurse Consultant, Saint Mary's Hospital, Tucson, Arizona. Roy
earned her BS in nursing in 1963 from Mount Saint Mary's College, Los Angeles;
her MS in nursing in 1966 and doctorate in sociology in 1977 from the University
of California, Los Angeles. She is a Fellow of the American Academy of Nursing
and active in many nursing organizations including Sigma Theta Tau and the
North American Nursing Diagnosis Association (NANDA). She is the author or
co-author of a number of works including* Introduction to nursing: An adaptation
model; Essentials of the Roy Adaptation Model; Theory construction in nursing:
An Adaptation Model; *and* The Roy Adaptation Model: The definitive statement.

The Roy Adaptation Model has evoked much interest and respect since its
inception in 1964 by Roy as part of her graduate work at the University of
California, Los Angeles, under the guidance of Dorothy E. Johnson. In 1970,
the faculty of Mount Saint Mary's College in Los Angeles adopted the Roy
Adaptation Model as the conceptual framework of the undergraduate nursing curriculum. A text was written by Roy and fellow faculty describing the
Roy Adaptation Model and presenting nursing assessment and intervention
reflective of the distinctive focus of the Model. In 1991 Roy and Andrews
wrote a clinical practice text, *The Roy adaptation model: The definitive
statement.* It presents the collective experiences of several contributing
authors who have taught and practiced using the Roy model for the past 20
years. Based upon four earlier books, it includes the diagrammatic conceptualizations of the model developed at the Royal Alexandra Hospitals School
of Nursing, Edmonton, Alberta, Canada, and published in *Essentials of the
Roy adaptation model* (Andrews & Roy, 1986).

Further, Roy and Roberts (1981) wrote *Theory construction in nursing:
An adaptation model* to discuss the use of the Roy model to construct nursing theory. The reader who is excited by the model will find that a rich

251

response has been made and continues to be made by nurse practitioners, educators, and researchers in the analysis, testing, and application of the model for nursing (Gaertzen, 1991; Rambo, 1983; Randell, Tedrow, & Van Landingham, 1982; Riehl-Sisca, 1989).

THE ROY ADAPTATION MODEL

Roy credits the works of von Bertalanffy's (1968) general system theory and Helson's (1964) adaptation theory as forming the basis of the scientific assumptions underlying the Roy model. The philosophic assumptions flow, according to Roy, from humanism and veritivity. The term *veritivity* was coined by Roy to identify the common purposefulness of human existence (Roy & Andrews, 1991). Table 15–1 identifies the assumptions underlying the Roy Model.

The four essential elements of the Roy Adaptation Model are the following:

1. The person who is the recipient of nursing care
2. The concept of environment
3. The concept of health
4. Nursing (Roy & Andrews, 1991, pp. 5–6).

The model presents concepts related to these four areas, clarifying each and defining their interrelationships.

TABLE 15–1. ASSUMPTIONS UNDERLYING THE ROY ADAPTATION MODEL

Scientific	
Systems Theory	Adaptation-Level Theory
Holism	Behavior as adaptive
Interdependence	Adaptation as a function of stimuli and adaptation level
Control processes	
Information feedback	Individual, dynamic adaptation levels
Complexity of living systems	Positive and active processes of responding

Philosophic	
Humanism	Veritivity
Creativity	Purposefulness of human existence
Purposefulness	Unity of purpose
Holism	Activity, creativity
Interpersonal process	Value and meaning of life

(From Roy, C., & Andrews, H. A. (Eds.). (1991). The Roy adaptation model: The definitive statement (p. 5). Norwalk, CT: Appleton & Lange. Used with permission.)

The Person

The first area of concern is the identity of the recipient of nursing care. Roy (1984) states that the recipient of nursing care may be the person, a family, a group, a community, or a society. Each is considered by the nurse as a holistic adaptive system. The idea of an adaptive system combines the concepts of system and adaptation.

System. First, consider the concept of a system as applied to an individual. Roy conceptualizes the person in a holistic perspective. Individual aspects of parts act together to form a unified being. Additionally, as living systems, persons are in constant interaction with their environments. Between the system and the environment occurs an exchange of information, matter, and energy. Characteristics of a system include inputs, outputs, controls, and feedback. Figure 15–1 illustrates a simple system.

Dunn (1971), a system theorist, calls our attention to the smallest unit of life, the cell. The cell is a living open system. The cell has its inner and outer worlds. From its outer world, it must draw forth the substances it needs to survive. Within itself, the cell must maintain order over its vast numbers of molecules. System openness, therefore, implies the constant exchanging of information, matter, and energy between the system and the environment. These system qualities are held by the person.

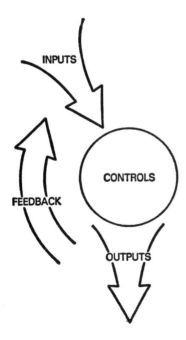

Figure 15-1. Diagrammatic representation of a simple system. *(From Roy, C., & Andrews, H. A. (Eds.). (1991). The Roy adaptation model: The definitive statement (p. 7). Norwalk, CT: Appleton & Lange. Used with permission.)*

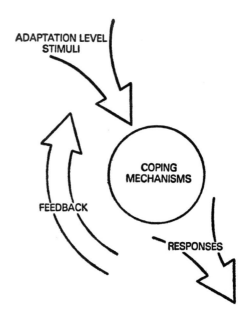

Figure 15-2. The person as a system. *(From Roy, C., & Andrews, H. A. (Eds.). (1991). The Roy adaptation model: The definitive statement (p. 8). Norwalk, CT: Appleton & Lange. Used with permission.)*

Adaptation. Figure 15–2 is used by Roy to represent the adaptive system of a person. The adaptive system has inputs of stimuli and adaptation level, outputs as behavioral responses that serve as feedback, and control processes known as coping mechanisms (Roy & Andrews, 1991). The adaptive system has input coming from the external environment as well as from the person. Roy identifies inputs as stimuli and adaptation level. Stimuli are conceptualized as falling into three classifications: focal, contextual, and residual. The stimulus most immediately confronting the person is the *focal stimulus.* The focal stimulus normally constitutes the greatest degree of change impacting upon the person. *Contextual stimuli* are all other stimuli of the person's internal and external world that can be identified as having a positive or negative influence on the situation. *Residual stimuli* are those internal or external factors whose current effects are unclear.

Along with stimuli, the adaptation level of the person acts as input to that person as an adaptive system. The focal, contextual, and residual stimuli combine and interface to set the adaptation level of the person at a particular point in time. This range of response is unique to the individual; each person's adaptation level is constantly changing. Significant stimuli that comprise the focal, contextual, and residual stimuli include factors such as the degree of change, past experiences, knowledge level, strengths, and/or limitations. Roy used Helson's (1964) work to develop this construct.

Outputs of the person as a system are the responses of the person (see Fig. 15–2). Output responses can be both external and internal. Thus, these responses are the person's behaviors. They can be observed, intuitively perceived by the nurse, measured and subjectively reported by the person. Output responses become feedback to the person and to the environment. Roy has categorized outputs of the system as either adaptive responses or ineffective responses. *Adaptive responses* are those that promote the integrity of the person. The person's integrity, or wholeness, is behaviorally demonstrated when the person is able to meet the goals in terms of survival, growth, reproduction, and mastery. *Ineffective responses* do not support these goals (Roy & Andrews, 1991).

Roy has used the term *coping mechanisms* to describe the control processes of the person as an adaptive system. Some coping mechanisms are inherited or genetic, such as the white blood cell defense system against bacteria that seek to invade the body. Other mechanisms are learned, such as the use of antiseptics to cleanse a wound. Roy presents a unique nursing science concept of control mechanisms that are called the *regulator* and the *cognator*. Roy's model considers the regulator and cognator coping mechanisms to be subsystems of the person as an adaptive system.

The *regulator subsystem* has the components of input, internal process, and output. Input stimuli may originate externally or internally to the person. The transmitters of the regulator system are chemical, neural, or endocrine in nature. Autonomic reflexes, which are neural responses originating in the brain stem and spinal cord, are generated as output responses of the regulator subsystem. Target organs and tissues under endocrine control also produce regulator output responses. Finally, Roy presents psychomotor responses originating from the central nervous system as regulator subsystem responses (Roy & Roberts, 1981). Many physiological processes can be viewed as regulator subsystem responses. For example, several regulatory feedback mechanisms of respiration have been identified. One of these is increased carbon dioxide, the end product of metabolism, which stimulates chemoreceptors in the medulla to increase the respiratory rate. Strong stimulation of these centers can increase ventilation six- to sevenfold (Guyton, 1971).

An example of a regulator process is when a noxious external stimulus is visualized and transmitted via the optic nerve to higher brain centers and then to lower brain autonomic centers. The sympathetic neurons from these origins have multiple visceral effects, including increased blood pressure and increased heart rate. Roy's schematic representation of the regulator processes is seen in Figure 15–3.

The other control subsystem original to the Roy model is the *cognator subsystem* (Roy & Andrews, 1991). Stimuli to the cognator subsystem are also both external and internal in origin. Output responses of the regulator subsystem can be feedback stimuli to the cognator subsystem. Cognator control processes are related to the higher brain functions of perception or information processing, judgment, and emotion. Perception, or information processing, is related to the internal processes of selective attention, coding, and memory. Learning is correlated to the processes of imitation, reinforcement, and insight. Problem solving and decision making are the internal processes related to judgment; and finally, emotion has the processes of defense to seek relief, affective appraisal, and attachment. A schematic presentation by Roy of the cognator subsystem is presented in Figure 15–4.

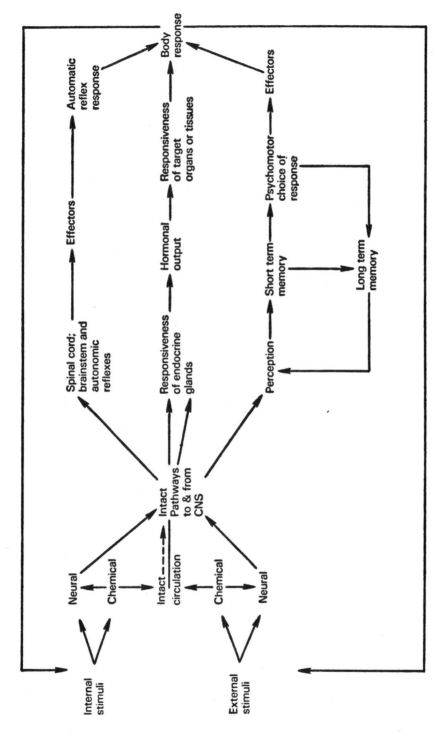

Figure 15-3. The Regulator *(From Roy, C., & McLeod, D. (1984). Theory of the person as an adaptive system. In Roy, C., & Roberts, S. L. Theory construction in nursing: An adaptation model (p. 61). Englewood Cliffs, NJ: Prentice-Hall. Used with permission.)*

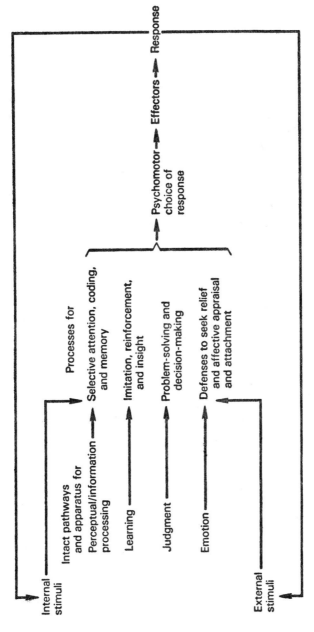

Figure 15-4. The Cognator. *(From Roy, C., & McLeod, D. (1981). The theory of the person as an adaptive system. In Roy, C., & Roberts, S. L., Theory construction in nursing: An adaptation model (p. 64). Englewood Cliffs, NJ: Prentice-Hall. Used with permission.)*

In maintaining the integrity of the person, the regulator and cognator are postulated as frequently acting together. The adaptation level of the person as an adaptive system is influenced by the individual's development and use of these coping mechanisms. Maximal use of coping mechanisms broadens the adaptation level of the person and increases the range of stimuli to which the person can positively respond.

Situation. A decrease in the oxygen supply to Albert Smith's heart muscle stimulates pain receptors that transmit the message of pain along sympathetic afferent nerve fibers to his central nervous system. The autonomic centers of his lower brain then stimulate the sympathetic efferent nerve fibers, and there is an increase in heart and respiratory rates. The result is an increase in the oxygen supply to the heart muscle. This increase can be viewed as regulator subsystem action.

The cognator subsystem also receives the internal pain stimuli as input. Mr. Smith has learned from past experiences that the left chest and arm pain is related to his heart. His judgment is activated in deciding what action to take. He decides to go inside to air conditioning, to sit with his legs elevated, and to take slow, deep breaths. He also decides not to call for emergency help. Certainly, he believes an adaptive response secondary to these actions will occur. However, he may be increasingly alert for further regulator subsystem output responses that might cause him to question his decision. This represents the cognator process of selective attention and coding. Following the episode of pain, Mr. Smith may attempt to gain further insight into the cause of the episode. He may decide that the 90°F weather was causal and remember to limit his activities during extreme heat. In this example, Mr. Smith used the cognator subsystem processes of perception, learning, and judgment.

Although cognator and regulator processes are essential to the adaptive response of the person, these processes are not directly observable. Only the responses of the person can be observed, measured, or subjectively reported. Roy has identified four *adaptive modes* or categories for assessment of behavior that results from the regulator and cognator mechanism responses. These *adaptive modes* are the physiological, self-concept, role function, and interdependence modes (Roy & Andrews, 1991). Behavior related to the modes is the manifestation of the *stimuli*: the person's adaptation level and coping processes. By observing the person's behavior in relation to the adaptive modes, the nurse can identify adaptive or ineffective responses in situations of health and illness. Figure 15–5 diagrammatically conceptualizes the person as an adaptive system that includes the four adaptive modes for assessment.

The four adaptive modes require further explanation. They are as follows.

Physiological Mode. The physiological mode represents physical response to environmental stimuli and primarily involves the regulator subsystem. The basic need of this mode is physiologic integrity and is composed of the needs associated with oxygenation, nutrition, elimination, activity and rest, and

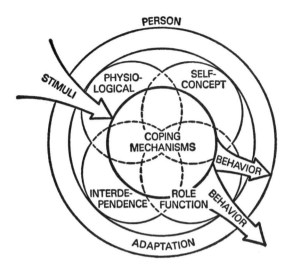

Figure 15-5. The person as an adaptive system. *(From Roy, C., & Andrews, H. A. (Eds.). (1991).* The Roy adaptation model: The definitive statement *(p. 17). Norwalk, CT: Appleton & Lange. Used* **with permission.)**

protection. The complex processes of this mode are associated with the senses, fluid and electrolytes, neurological function, and endocrine function (Andrews & Roy, 1991). These needs and processes may be defined as follows:

- *Oxygenation:*   The pattern of oxygen use related to respiratory and cardiovascular physiology and pathophysiology (Thompson, 1991).

- *Nutrition:*   Patterns of nutrient use for maintaining human functioning, promoting growth, and repairing injured tissue (Servonsky, 1991b).

- *Elimination:*   Patterns of elimination of waste products (Servonsky, 1991a).

- *Activity and Rest:*   Patterns of activity and rest (Roy, 1991a).
- *Protection:*   Patterns related to skin integrity and immunity (Sato, 1991).

- *Senses:*   The input channel of the person through which sensory-perceptual information is processed (Roy, 1991c).

- *Fluids and Electrolytes:*   The complex process of maintaining body fluids and electrolytes in balance for the person (Jensen, 1991).

- *Neurological function:* Key neural processes and the complex relationship of neural function to regulator and cognator coping mechanisms (Roy, 1991b).
- *Endocrine function:* Patterns of endocrine control and regulation that aet in conjunction with the nervous system to maintain control of body processes (Chalifoux, 1991).

Self-Concept Mode. The self-concept mode relates to the basic need for psychic integrity. Its focus is on the psychological and spiritual aspects of the person. Attention is given to the subcategories of physical self and personal self. The physical self has the components of body sensation and body image. The personal self has the components of self-consistency, self-ideal, and moral-ethical-spiritual self. Body sensation is how the person experiences the physical self, and body image is how the person views the physical self. Self-consistency represents the person's efforts to maintain self-organization and to avoid disequilibrium. Self-ideal represents what the person expects to be and do, and the moral-ethical-spiritual self represents the person's belief system and self-evaluator (Andrews, 1991b).

Role Function Mode. The role function mode identifies the patterns of social interaction of the person in relation to others reflected by primary, secondary, and tertiary roles. The basic need met is social integrity (Andrews, 1991a). The primary role determines the majority of a person's behaviors and is defined by the person's sex, age, and developmental stage. Secondary roles are assumed to carry out the tasks required by the stage of development and primary role. Tertiary roles are temporary, freely chosen, and may include activities related to hobbies. Behaviors in this mode are described as instrumental or expressive. Instrumental behaviors are usually physical, have a long-term orientation, and focus on role mastery. Expressive behaviors represent feelings or attitudes, are usually emotional, and seek immediate response.

Interdependence Mode. The interdependence mode is where affectional needs are met. Strongly reflective of the humanistic values held by Roy, the interdependence mode identifies patterns of human value, affection, love, and affirmation. These processes occur through interpersonal relationships on both individual and group levels (Tedrow, 1991).

Environment

Stimuli from within the person and stimuli from around the person represent the element of environment, according to Roy. Environment is specifically defined by Roy as "all conditions, circumstances, and influences that surround and affect the development and behavior of persons and groups" (Roy & Andrews, 1991, p. 18).

Commonly occurring internal and external stimuli of the environment are an area of study for nursing. For example, when an elderly client is institutionalized, significant external environmental stimuli have impinged upon him or her. The study of this environmental condition aids nurses in promoting adaptation to this change or, perhaps more ideally, defining interventions that minimize the risk of institutionalization for the elderly. Similarly, nurses are increasing their involvement in the institutions of our nation: health, education, industry, and politics. By their involvement, they are altering the environmental stimuli related to situations of health and illness in a broad and often far-reaching manner at a community system level.

Health

Previously, the Roy model defined health as a continuum from death to high-level wellness. This continuum is not used in the present model. Instead, Roy defines health as "a state and a process of being and becoming an integrated and whole person" (Roy & Andrews, 1991, p. 19). The integrity of the person is expressed as the ability to meet the goals of survival, growth, reproduction, and mastery. The aim of the nurse practicing under the Roy model is to promote the health of the person by promoting adaptive responses.

Goal of Nursing

Roy defines the *goal of nursing* as the promotion of adaptive responses in relation to the four adaptive modes. *Adaptive responses* are those that positively affect health. Stimuli and the person's adaptation level are inputs to the person as an adaptive system. The person's adaptation level determines whether a positive response to internal or external stimuli will be elicited. Nursing seeks to reduce ineffective responses and promote adaptive responses as output behavior of the person. The nurse, therefore, promotes health in all life processes, including dying with dignity (Roy & Andrews, 1991).

In the example of the person experiencing chest pain, the stimulus immediately confronting Albert Smith, the focal stimulus is the deficit of oxygen supply to his heart muscle. The contextual stimuli include the 90°F temperature, the sensation of pain, and Mr. Smith's age, weight, blood sugar level, and degree of coronary artery patency. The residual stimuli include his history of cigarette smoking and work-related stress.

For Mr. Smith, the stimuli, adaptation level, and coping processes have resulted in an ineffective response. The deficit of oxygen to his heart is a threat to his physiologic integrity and will not maintain his survival. This response became feedback to the system and a focal stimulus. Mr. Smith used the cognator mechanism to adjust the total stimuli by going indoors to a cooler room and decreasing his oxygen needs by sitting down and elevating his legs. After the adjustment of the stimuli, the oxygen needs of his heart muscle were met, and the pain stopped.

A person's ability to cope varies with the state of the person at different times. For example, the person who has suffered major trauma has a narrowed zone of adaptation and may not survive exposure to a bacterial infection. That same person before the injury may have tolerated exposure to the same bacteria without developing any symptoms of illness.

Nursing activities or intervention are delineated by the model as those that promote adaptive responses in situations of health and illness. As a rule, these approaches are identified as actions taken by the nurse to manage the focal, contextual, or residual stimuli impinging on the person. By making these adjustments, the total stimuli fall within the adaptation level of the person. Whenever possible, the focal stimulus—that which represents the greatest degree of change—is the focus of nursing activity. For a person with chest pain, the focal stimulus is the imbalance between the demand for oxygen by the body and the supply of oxygen that the heart can provide. To alter the focal stimuli, the nurse manages the stimuli of demand so that an adaptive response can be made. In turn, when focal stimuli cannot be altered, the nurse promotes an adaptive response by altering contextual stimuli (Roy & Andrews, 1991).

Additionally, the nurse may anticipate that the person has a potential for ineffective responses secondary to stimuli likely to be present in a particular situation. The nurse acts to prepare the person for the anticipated changes through strengthening regulator and cognator coping mechanisms. Plans that broaden the person's adaptation level correlate with the ideas of health promotion currently found in the literature. Finally, nursing actions suggested by the model include approaches aimed at maintaining adaptive responses that support the person's efforts to creatively use his or her coping mechanisms.

THE NURSING PROCESS

The Roy Adaptation Model offers guidelines to the nurse in application of the nursing process. The elements of the Roy nursing process include assessment of behavior, assessment of stimuli, nursing diagnosis, goal setting, intervention, and evaluation (Roy & Andrews, 1991). The six elements of Roy's nursing process parallel the five phases of the nursing process identified in Chapter 2.

Behavioral Assessment

Behavioral assessment is considered to be the gathering of responses or output behaviors of the person as an adaptive system in relation to each of the four adaptive modes: physiological, self-concept, role function, and interdependence. The specific data are gathered by the nurse through the processes of observation, careful measurement, and skilled interview techniques.

Assessment of the client in each of the four adaptive modes enhances a systematic and holistic approach. Such assessment clarifies the focus that the nurse or nursing team will take in caring for the client. Ideally, thoroughly conducted and recorded nursing assessment in the four adaptive modes sets the tone of understanding for an entire health care team of the particular situation of a client. Proficiency in the practice of nursing requires skilled assessment of behaviors and the knowledge to compare the person to specific criteria to evaluate behavioral response as adaptive or ineffective. Figure 15–6 shows a Nursing History/Assessment developed by the nurses at Upper Valley Medical Center in Piqua, Ohio. This form uses the four adaptive modes of

UPPER VALLEY MEDICAL CENTERS
PMMC STOUDER
ADMISSION NURSING ASSESSMENT

INSTRUCTIONS: Check all boxes that apply. For Surgical Admissions: complete white area at P.A.T. and grey area day of admission. *See Care Plan / 24 HR Nursing Assessment & Care Record. N/A-Not Applicable

INTERDEPENDENCE – ROLE FUNCTION – SELF-CONCEPT

Date	Time	Received From: ☐ ER ☐ ☐ admitting ☐ doctor's office	VIA ☐ w/c ☐ ambulatory ☐ cart	Room	Family Physician	☐ male ☐ female	Age

Temp.	Pulse ☐ Regular ☐ Irregular ☐ Regular ☐ Irregular	Resp.	BP (LA)	BP (RA)	Height	Weight

Informant: ☐ patient ☐ family member ☐ friend ☐ transfer form ☐ prior medical record / date: ______ ☐ interview per phone ☐ current ER record ☐ other ______

History and present status of chief complaint: ______

Pain Present: ☐ no ☐ yes / location	Intensity Scale 1 (mild) – 10 (severe)	When did pain start?	How was pain managed at home?

Allergies: (describe reaction) ☐ Medications ☐ food ☐ environment ☐ None — Allergy band on? ☐ yes ☐ N/A

PATIENT HISTORY:

No Yes
☐ ☐ Heart disease (MI, angina, CHF, arrhythmia, murmur, mitral valve, prolapse, pacemaker)
☐ ☐ High Blood Pressure
☐ ☐ Stroke
☐ ☐ Respiratory (asthma, emphysema, bronchitis)
☐ ☐ Kidney (stones, infection, hemodialysis)
☐ ☐ Liver (hepatitis, mono, jaundice)
☐ ☐ Cancer
☐ ☐ Blood Disorder (bleeding, clots, anemia, phlebitis)

No Yes
☐ ☐ Blood Transfusion
☐ ☐ Diabetes
☐ ☐ Thyroid Disease
☐ ☐ Seizures/Fainting
☐ ☐ Muscle Disease
☐ ☐ Neck/Back Disorder, Arthritis
☐ ☐ Depression, Mental Illness
☐ ☐ Alcohol/Drug Abuse
☐ ☐ Communicable disease (TB, STD, ...)
☐ ☐ Other ______

Past Surgeries: ☐ none Pt/Family Reactions to anesthesia: ☐ N/A ☐ no ☐ yes ______

Past Medical Hospitalizations: ☐ none Recent xrays: ☐ no ☐ yes ______ Recent lab: ☐ no ☐ yes

FAMILY HEALTH HISTORY: (Check conditions that apply) ☐ none
☐ cancer ☐ diabetes ☐ stroke ☐ high blood pressure ☐ heart disease ☐ muscle disease ☐ other ______

Medications: (prescription, O.T.C., recreational) Include dose and frequency. Admission Nurse, note time last dose taken.
☐ None

Are medications taken as prescribed: ☐ yes ☐ no ☐ N/A

Home Situation: (marital status, children, significant others, living environment – stairs, etc.)

NSG-001 **Admission Nursing Assessment** (page 1) UVMC 3/88 Rev. 3/92

Figure 15-6. Upper Valley Medical Center Admission Nursing Assessment. *C. Mikolajewski, J. Frantz, C. Garber, J. Snyder, J. Boles, S. Deslich, L. Enz, R. A. Kuntz, C. Strawser, M. Langenkamp. Used with permission.*

INTERDEPENDENCE ROLE-SELF CONCEPT (cont.)

Occupation: _____

Social History: (education, special learning needs, religion, hobbies) _____

Utilization of community resources: ☐ no ☐ home care ☐ hospice ☐ Meals on Wheels ☐ church group ☐ support groups ☐ other _____
Personal Concerns: _____
Do you have any religious special requests? ☐ no ☐ yes _____
Emotional Status: ☐ calm ☐ anxious ☐ angry ☐ quiet ☐ talkative ☐ sad ☐ agitated ☐ other _____

Life changes in past 1-2 years? ☐ none ☐ change in health ☐ new baby ☐ marriage / divorce ☐ death someone close
☐ job / business related change ☐ other _____
Do you feel you deal successfully with stress? ☐ yes ☐ no ☐ depends on circumstance Describe: _____

NEUROLOGICAL

Mental Status: ☐ alert ☐ oriented ☐ disoriented ☐ restless ☐ drowsy ☐ unresponsive ☐ memory loss
☐ other _____

Speech ☐ clear ☐ slurred ☐ garbled ☐ aphasic ☐ hoarse   barriers/ ☐ foreign language _____

2 3 4 5 6 7 8 9   + Reactive
                     − Nonreactive
                     ± Sluggish

Ability to Move Extremities to Command
0 (no movement)   1 (weak)   2 (strong)
RA: LA: RL: LL:

Right Eye: ___ mm   Left Eye: ___ mm

SENSES

Vision Impairment: ☐ no ☐ yes   ☐ glasses / contacts   ☐ artificial eye   ☐ cataracts   ☐ glaucoma ☐ blind ☐ R ☐ L

Hearing Impairment: ☐ no ☐ yes   partial deaf ☐ R ☐ L   total deaf ☐ R ☐ L   hearing aid ☐ R ☐ L

ACTIVITY / REST

Sleep: (Usual time of day and hours) _____
Sleep problems: ☐ none ☐ unrested after sleep ☐ insomnia ☐ nightmares ☐ other _____

SELF-CARE ABILITY (Check appropriate column)						
ACTIVITY	0	1	2	3	4	5
Eating / Drinking						
Bathing						
Dressing / Grooming						
Toileting						
Bed mobility						
Transferring						
Ambulating						
Stair Climbing						
Shopping						
Cooking						
Home Maintenance						

0 - Independent
1 - Assistive Device
2 - Assistance from person
3 - Assistance from person & equipment
4 - Dependent/ unable
5 - Change in last week

FALL RISK EVALUATION

Age <3 or >75	10 points	
Confused and disoriented, hallucinating, senile	15 points	
History of falls	15 points	
Recent history of loss of consciousness, seizure disorder	15 points	
Unsteady on feet / amputation	10 points	
Poor eyesight	5 points	
Poor hearing	5 points	
Drug / alcohol problem, sedatives	5 points	
Postop condition / sedated	5 points	
Language barrier	5 points	
Attitude (resistant, belligerent, combative, fearful)	10 points	
Postural hypotension	5 points	
15 or more indicates risk. Fall precautions started:	TOTAL POINTS	

Fall Band on ☐

Assistive Devices: ☐ none ☐ crutches ☐ bedside commode ☐ walker ☐ cane ☐ splint / brace ☐ wheelchair ☐ prosthesis
☐ other _____
Activity Tolerance: ☐ no problem ☐ weakness ☐ vertigo ☐ unsteady gait ☐ angina ☐ dyspnea ☐ dyspnea at rest
☐ other _____

Admission Nursing Assessment (page 2)

Figure 15–6. (Continued)

264

OXYGENATION - SKIN INTEGRITY

Skin: ☐ Warm ☐ Hot ☐ Cool ☐ Dry ☐ Diaphoretic ☐ Clammy   Skin Color: ☐ Normal ☐ Pale ☐ Cyanotic ☐ Jaundiced ☐ Mottled ☐ Flushed

Edema: ☐ none ☐ yes / location:

Pedal Pulses: ☐ Present ☐ Abnormal / Explain:

Skin Lesions: (mark location of skin lesions by number on diagram)
☐ none ☐ scar (1) ☐ rash (2) ☐ wound or open area (3) ☐ bruise (4) ☐ incision (5) ☐ sutures / staples (6)
☐ abrasions (7) ☐ discolorations (8) ☐ other (9)

Describe

Dressings: ☐ no ☐ yes / location:

Monitor pattern: ☐ N/A

Respirations: ☐ nonlabored ☐ labored ☐ rapid ☐ shallow

Heart sounds: ☐ audible ☐ abnormal

Cough: ☐ no ☐ yes ☐ non-productive
☐ productive / color:

Oxygen: ☐ no ☐ yes - method / amt.:

Tobacco Use: ☐ no ☐ yes / type: _____
_____ pkg/day x _____ years

Breath Sounds: ☐ clear ☐ abnormal / describe:

BRADEN SCALE

RISK PREDICTORS FOR SKIN BREAKDOWN*

SENSORY PERCEPTION	1. COMPLETELY LIMITED	2. VERY LIMITED	3. SLIGHTLY LIMITED	4. NO IMPAIRMENT
MOISTURE	1. CONSTANTLY MOIST	2. VERY MOIST	3. OCCASIONALLY MOIST	4. RARELY MOIST
ACTIVITY	1. BEDFAST	2. CHAIRFAST	3. WALKS OCCASIONALLY	4. WALKS FREQUENTLY
MOBILITY	1. COMPLETELY IMMOBILE	2. VERY LIMITED	3. SLIGHTLY LIMITED	4. NO LIMITATIONS
NUTRITION	1. VERY POOR	2. PROBABLY INADEQUATE	3. ADEQUATE	4. EXCELLENT
SHEAR & FRICTION	1. PROBLEM	2. POTENTIAL PROBLEM	3. NO APPARENT PROBLEM	

* Refer to Braden Scale for description of each subscale category.
Score of 15 or less indicates that patient is a risk. Refer to SKIN CARE DECISION TREE.   **TOTAL**

ELIMINATION

Abdomen: ☐ soft ☐ firm ☐ distended / girth _____ ☐ non-distended ☐ tender / location:

Bowel Sounds: ☐ present ☐ absent   Last BM / color / character:

Bowel Pattern: ☐ diarrhea ☐ constipation ☐ blood in stool ☐ hemorrhoids
☐ no problem ☐ incontinence ☐ laxative / enema Use/List:

Bladder Pattern: ☐ burning ☐ nocturia (No. times/night   ) ☐ difficulty starting flow ☐ frequency
☐ no problem ☐ incontinence - ☐ total ☐ daytime ☐ night time ☐ occasional ☐ urgency ☐ hematuria

Drainage Tubes: ☐ none ☐ indwelling catheter (1) ☐ intermittant catheterization (2) _____ ☐ N/G (3) ☐ G-tube (4)
☐ chest tube (5) ☐ T-tube (6) ☐ penrose (7) ☐ ostomy (8) type: _____
☐ other (9)

Describe Drainage:

LYTES - NUTRITION

Current Diet/Restrictions: ☐ Regular   Is diet followed: ☐ yes ☐ no   Last fluid / food intake   Appetite: ☐ good ☐ fair ☐ poor

Recent weight change last 6 months: ☐ no ☐ yes / describe:

Fluid Intake: ☐ restricted ☐ 0 - 5 glasses / day ☐ 5 - 10 glasses / day ☐ > 10 glasses / day

☐ Caffeine use: Amt. _____   ☐ Alcohol use: Type/Amt. _____

Eating disorders: ☐ none ☐ nausea ☐ emesis ☐ chewing / swallowing difficulty ☐ sore mouth ☐ taste alterations ☐ mouth ulcers
☐ indigestion ☐ ulcer ☐ mouth-white patches ☐ erythema ☐ other

Dentures: ☐ no ☐ yes/ ☐ upper: ☐ full ☐ partial ☐ lower: ☐ full ☐ partial ☐ caps ☐ bridges ☐ loose teeth ☐ retainer ☐ crowns

IV ☐ no ☐ yes -- solution - rate - site - cath no.   ☐ IML   ☐ vascular access device

Admission Nursing Assessment (page 3)

Figure 15–6. (Continued)

ADMISSION NURSING ASSESSMENT

ENDOCRINE	□ N/A	Last Menstrual Period	Problems: □ none □ abnormal bleeding □ breast lump history □ vaginal drainage □ other □ breast feeding	Breast self-exam done: □ no □ yes Frequency
		Pap smear requested during hospitalization: □ no □ yes* *See sticker on front of chart		Last Pap Exam:
	□ N/A	Last Rectal Exam Rectal exam requested during hospitalization □ no □ yes* *see sticker on front chart		

Concerns about current or future effects of illness / surgery / treatment on:
□ appearance □ male / female roles □ other _____

NOTES: _____

Admission Nursing Assessment (page 4)

Figure 15–6. (Continued)

266

TABLE 15–2. INDICATIONS OF ADAPTATION DIFFICULTY

Signs of pronounced regulator activity:
1. increase in heart rate or blood pressure
2. tension
3. excitement
4. loss of appetite
5. increase in serum cortisol

Signs of cognator ineffectiveness include:
1. faulty perception/information processing
2. ineffective learning
3. poor judgment
4. inappropriate affect

(From Roy, C., & Andrews, H. A. (Eds.). (1991). The Roy adaptation model: The definitive statement (p. 32). Norwalk, CT: Appleton & Lange. Used with permission.)

the Roy model. Guide questions related to each adaptive mode can be developed to reflect the age or acuity of the client population being assessed. Information collected includes subjective, objective, and measurement data. Behavior that varies from expectations, norms, and guidelines frequently represents ineffective responses. Roy has identified frequently occurring signs of pronounced regulator activity and cognator ineffectiveness (see Table 15–2). The presence of these behaviors also suggests ineffective responses.

Assessment of Stimuli

After a behavioral assessment, the nurse analyzes the emerging themes and patterns of client behavior to identify ineffective responses or adaptive responses requiring nurse support. When ineffective behaviors or adaptive behaviors requiring support are present, the nurse makes an assessment of internal and external stimuli that may be affecting behavior. In this phase of assessment, the nurse collects data about the focal, contextual, and residual stimuli impacting on the client. This process clarifies the etiology of the problem and identifies significant contextual and residual factors. Common influencing stimuli have been identified by Roy and her colleagues and are listed in Table 15–3.

TABLE 15–3. COMMON STIMULI AFFECTING ADAPTATION

Culture—Socioeconomic status, ethnicity, belief system

Family—Structure, tasks

Developmental stage—Age, sex, tasks, heredity, and genetic factors

Integrity of adaptive modes—Physiological (including disease pathology), self-concept, role function, interdependence

Cognator effectiveness—Perception, knowledge, skill

Environmental considerations—Change in internal or external environment, medical management, use of drugs, alcohol, tobacco

(From Roy, C., & Andrews, H. A. (Eds.). (1991). The Roy adaptation model: The definitive statement (p. 32). Norwalk, CT: Appleton & Lange. Used with permission.)

TABLE 15–4. TYPOLOGY OF COMMONLY RECURRING ADAPTATION PROBLEMS

Physiological Mode

1. Oxygenation
   hypoxia/shock
   ventilatory impairment
   inadequate gas exchange
   inadequate gas transport
   altered tissue perfusion
   poor recruitment of compensatory processes
     for changing oxygen need

2. Nutrition
   weight 20/25% above/below average
   nutrition more/less than body requirements
   anorexia
   nausea and vomiting
   ineffective coping strategies for altered means
     of ingestion

3. Elimination
   diarrhea
   bowel/bladder incontinence
   constipation
   urinary retention
   flatulence
   ineffective coping strategies for altered
     elimination

4. Activity and Rest
   inadequate pattern of activity and rest
   restricted mobility, gait, and/or coordination
   activity intolerance
   immobility
   disuse consequences
   potential for sleep pattern disturbance
   fatigue
   sleep deprivation

5. Protection
   disrupted skin integrity
   pressure sores
   itching
   delayed wound healing
   infection
   potential for ineffective coping with allergic
     reaction
   ineffective coping with changes in immune
     status

6. Senses
   impairment of a primary sense
   potential for injury/loss of self-care abilities
   potential for distorted communication
   stigma
   sensory monotony/distortion
   sensory overload/deprivation
   acute pain
   chronic pain
   perceptual impairment
   ineffective coping strategies for sensory
     impairment

7. Fluid and Electrolytes
   dehydration
   edema
   intracellular water retention
   shock
   hyper or hypo calcemia, kalemia, or natremia
   acid/base imbalance
   ineffective buffer regulation for changing pH

8. Neurological Function
   decreased level of consciousness
   defective cognitive processing
   memory deficits
   instability of behavior and mood
   ineffective compensation for cognitive deficit
   potential for secondary brain damage

9. Endocrine Function
   ineffective hormone regulation, reflected in
     fatigue, irritability, heat intolerance
   ineffective reproductive development
   instability of hormone system loops
   instability of internal cyclical rhythms
   stress

(Continued)

TABLE 15–4. (CONTINUED)

Self-Concept Mode

1. Physical Self	2. Personal Self
body image disturbance	anxiety
sexual dysfunction	powerlessness
rape trauma syndrome	guilt
loss	low self-esteem

Role Function Mode

role transition
role distance
role conflict
role failure

Interdependence Mode

ineffective pattern of giving and receiving
    nurturing
Ineffective pattern of aloneness and relating
separation anxiety

loneliness

(From Roy, C., & Andrews, H. A. (Eds.). (1991). The Roy adaptation model: The definitive statement (pp. 41–42). Norwalk, CT: Appleton & Lange. Used with permission.)

Nursing Diagnosis

Roy describes three methods of making a nursing diagnosis (Roy & Andrews, 1991). One method is to use a typology of diagnoses developed by Roy and related to the four adaptive modes. Table 15–4 is a list of common adaptation problems using this typology. In applying this method of diagnosis to the example of Albert Smith, the diagnosis would be: "Hypoxia."

The second method is to make a diagnosis by stating the observed response within one mode along with the most influential stimuli. Using this method, a diagnosis for Mr. Smith could be stated as: "Chest pain caused by a deficit of oxygen to the heart muscle associated with an overexposure to hot weather."

The third method summarizes responses in one or more adaptive modes related to the same stimuli. For example, if the person experiencing chest pain is a farmer, working outside in hot weather is necessary for success in his or her work. In this case, an appropriate diagnosis might be: "Role failure associated with limited physical (myocardial) ability to work in hot weather."

On the other hand, a nursing diagnosis using any of the foregoing methods can also be a statement of adaptive responses that the nurse wishes to support. For example, if Mr. Smith is seeking help through vocational counseling to adapt to his physical limitation, the nurse may diagnose a need to support this behavior. In this case, an appropriate diagnosis would be: "Adaptation to role failure by seeking an alternative career." Roy and others also have developed a typology of indicators of positive adaptation (see Table 15–5).

Goal Setting

Goals are the end-point behaviors that the person is to achieve. They are recorded as client behaviors indicative of resolution of the adaptation problem. The goal statement includes the behavior, the change expected, and a time frame. Long-term goals reflect resolution of adaptive problems and the availability of energy to meet other goals (survival, growth, reproduction, and mastery). Short-term goals identify expected client behaviors after management of focal or contextual stimuli. As well, they state client behaviors

TABLE 15–5. TYPOLOGY OF INDICATORS OF POSITIVE ADAPTATION

Physiological Mode

1. Oxygenation
   stable processes of ventilation
   stable pattern of gas exchange
   adequate transport of gases
   adequate processes of compensation
2. Nutrition
   stable digestive processes
   adequate nutritional pattern for body
     requirements
   metabolic and other nutritive needs met
     during altered means of ingestion
3. Elimination
   effective homeostatic bowel processes
   stable pattern of bowel elimination
   effective processes of urine formation
   stable pattern of urine elimination
   effective coping strategies for altered
     elimination
4. Activity and Rest
   integrated processes of mobility
   adequate recruitment of compensatory
     movement processes during inactivity
   effective pattern of activity and rest
   effective sleep pattern
   effective environmental changes for altered
     sleep conditions
5. Protection
   intact skin
   effective processes of immunity
   effective healing response
   adequate secondary protection for changes
     in skin integrity and immune status

6. Senses
   effective processes of sensation
   effective integration of sensory input into
     information
   stable patterns of perception, ie, interpreta-
     tion and appreciation of input
   effective coping strategies for altered
     sensation
7. Fluid and Electrolytes
   stable processes of water balance
   stability of salts in body fluids
   balance of acid/base status
   effective chemical buffer regulation
8. Neurological Function
   effective processes of arousal/attention;
     sensation/perception; coding, concept
     formation, memory, language; planning,
     motor response
   integrated thinking and feeling processes
   plasticity and functional effectiveness of
     developing, aging, and altered nervous
     system
9. Endocrine Function
   effective hormonal regulation of metabolic
     and body processes
   effective hormonal regulation of reproductive
     development
   stable patterns of closed loop negative
     feedback hormone systems
   stable patterns of cyclical hormone rhythms
   effective coping strategies for stress

(Continued)

TABLE 15–5. (CONTINUED)

Self-Concept Mode

1. Physical Self
   positive body image
   effective sexual function
   psychic integrity with physical growth
   adequate compensation for bodily changes
   effective coping strategies for loss
   effective process of life closure

2. Personal Self
   stable pattern of self-consistency
   effective integration of self-ideal
   effective processes of moral-ethical-spiritual
     growth
   functional self-esteem
   effective coping strategies for threats to self

Role Function Mode

effective processes of role transition
integration of instrumental and expressive role
  behaviors
integration of primary, secondary, and tertiary
  roles
stable pattern of role mastery
effective processes for coping with role changes

Interdependence Mode

stable pattern of giving and receiving nurturing
affectional adequacy
effective pattern of aloneness and relating
effective coping strategies for separation and
  loneliness

(From Roy, C., & Andrews, H. A. (Eds.). (1991). The Roy adaptation model: The definitive statement (pp. 41–42). Norwalk, CT: Appleton & Lange. Used with permission.)

that indicate cognator or regulator coping. Whenever possible, goals are set mutually with the person. Mutual goal setting respects the privileges and rights of the person (Roy & Andrews, 1991).

Plans for Implementation

Nursing interventions are planned with the purpose of altering or managing the focal or contextual stimuli. Implementation may also focus on broadening the person's coping ability, or adaptation level, so that the total stimuli fall within that person's ability to adapt. The nurse plans specific activities to alter the selected stimuli appropriately (Roy & Andrews, 1991).

Evaluation

The nursing process is completed by evaluation. Goal behaviors are compared to the person's output responses, and movement toward or away from goal achievement is determined. Readjustments to goals and interventions are made on the basis of evaluation data (Roy & Andrews, 1991).

The Roy Nursing Process Applied to Nursing in a Recovery Room

The Roy model can be applied to nursing assessment and interventions in various clinical situations. In the following case study, the Roy model is applied to a person during the period of immediate recovery from surgery and anesthesia.

Behavioral assessment focuses on the physiological mode responses during the first hour of recovery time after a person experiences surgery and general anesthesia. By applying the Roy model, significant behaviors can be conceptualized as regulator output responses. Increased sympathetic or parasympathetic system activity can signal regulator system activity. Regulator output responses that vary from baseline values determined for the person may be the first warning of an ineffective response to postoperative stimuli. Key baseline values are the person's presurgery measures of heart rate, blood pressure, and respiratory rate. Immediately upon observation of changes from the baseline, assessment of stimuli is done. Goals are set with the basic survival of the person as a priority. Interventions are taken so that focal and contextual stimuli are altered and adaptation is promoted. The evaluation of goal achievement is made, and further actions are taken as necessary.

Situation. Mrs. Reed is received from surgery after a major abdominal operation. Before surgery, her baseline vital signs were: heart rate, 80 beats per minute; blood pressure, 120/80 mm Hg; and respiratory rate, 16 per minute. After 45 minutes in recovery, her vital signs are: heart rate, 150 beats per minute; blood pressure, 90/60 mm Hg; respiratory rate, 32 per minute. Increased regulator output response is signaled by sympathetic nervous system stimulation of the heart in response to decreased blood pressure. The nurse decides that Mrs. Reed is showing an ineffective response. Therefore, assessment of stimuli is done.

The focal stimulus is a decrease of arterial blood pressure secondary to an unknown underlying cause. The contextual stimuli are: age 45 years, cool extremities, poor nail blanching, no food or drink for 12 hours, intravenous infusion (IV) of dextrose 5 percent in water with lactated Ringer's solution at 100 cc per hour. Also, contextual stimuli include 200 cc of IV fluids infused during surgery, 10 cc of urine excreted during the first 45 minutes in recovery, $1\frac{1}{2}$ hours of general anesthesia, estimated blood loss of 500 cc during surgery, no operative site bleeding, and level of consciousness slow to respond to tactile stimuli after 45 minutes in recovery. The residual stimuli include history of renal infections.

The nursing diagnosis of a decreased arterial blood pressure secondary to fluid volume deficit is made. A fluid volume loss is suggested both by the contextual data and by the changes in the baseline heart rate, blood pressure, and urine output. The nurse then intervenes by altering contextual stimuli so that an adaptive response is promoted. The goal of a circulatory volume adequate to maintain a blood pressure of plus or minus 20 mm Hg of baseline levels within 15 minutes is set. The nurse plans and then takes the following intervention steps. The IV rate is increased to 300 cc per hour. The foot of the bed is elevated to increase venous return. Forty percent oxygen is given by mask. Mrs. Reed is verbally and tactilely stimulated and told to take slow deep breaths. The nurse prepares vasopressor medications for immediate use and applies an external continuous blood pressure cuff for constant blood pressure monitoring. The nurse also consults with other team members as to Mrs. Reed's clinical presentation.

A constant evaluation of the effectiveness of the nursing actions is made. The nurse holds Mrs. Reed in recovery until the goal of adequate circulation volume is met. Evaluation criteria include urine output greater than 30 cc per hour, mental alertness, rapid nail bed blanching, blood pressure plus or minus 20 mm Hg of presurgery levels, pulse plus or minus 20 beats per minute of baseline, and respirations plus or minus 5 per minute of presurgery levels.

ROY'S WORK AND THE CHARACTERISTICS OF A THEORY

1. Theories can interrelate concepts in such a way as to create a different way of looking at a particular phenomenon. The Roy model does interrelate concepts in such a way as to present a new view of the phenomenon being studied. It identifies the key concepts relevant to nursing: the person, environment, health, and nursing. The person is viewed as constantly interacting with internal and external stimuli. The person is active and reactive to these stimuli. Stimuli are defined as focal, that which invokes the greatest degree of change; contextual; and residual. The theory suggests the influence of multiple causes in a situation, which is a strength when dealing with multifaceted human beings. Adaptation is a positive response made by the person to the experience being encountered. Adaptation is facilitated by the use of the regulator and cognator coping mechanisms. The adaptation level represents the range of stimuli that the person can tolerate and continue to maintain adaptive responses. The areas of response where the effects of coping are evidenced include the four adaptive modes: physiological, self-concept, role function, and interdependence. Thus, by a quick review of the concept of the person who is the recipient of nursing care, one sees that a very specific perspective or image has been defined by the Roy model. Beginning work in the development of theory related to these concepts has been done by Roy, Roberts, and others (Roy & Roberts, 1981). The view suggests a holistic framework as opposed to a view of the ill person as a biological entity with a disease process. It reflects a view of nursing that is concerned with many aspects of the person—physiological, self-concept, role function, and interdependence.

2. Theories must be logical in nature. The sequence of concepts in the Roy model follows logically. In the presentation of each of the key concepts there is the recurring idea of adaptation to maintain integrity. The definition of health is based on the idea of integrity, which in turn is operationalized to mean responses that meet the person's goals of survival, growth, reproduction, and mastery. Promoting adaptive responses in situations of health and illness is the goal of nursing. The person is conceptualized as a holistic, adaptive system.

3. Theories should be relatively simple yet generalizable. The concepts of the Roy model are stated in relatively simple terms. However, the concept of the person as an adaptive system does present a challenging use of specific terms, including cognator and regulator mechanisms and adaptation level. The four adaptive modes may be the first aspect of the model that the student or nurse is able to assimilate. Based upon nursing tradition, assessment of fluid and electrolytes, elimination, oxygenation, roles, and such evoke familiar images. As one nurse studying the theory stated, "It's what we've always done. I don't know what the big deal is!" Perhaps she failed to realize that such a statement was complimentary of the model's fit to clinical practice.

Let us also consider the generalizability of the model in various settings. Use of the Roy model to organize curriculum has been demonstrated by the faculty at Mount Saint Mary's College in Los Angeles. Similarly, extensive use of the model as well as pictorial representations of it have been made by the faculty and students of the Royal Alexandra Hospitals School of Nursing (Andrews & Roy, 1986). Use of the model for the care of various client populations is exemplified by the works of Farkas (1981), Giger, Bower, & Miller (1987), and Janelli (1980). Research studies examining the use of the model in nursing practice include the work of Fredrickson et al., (1991), Hoch (1987), Limandri (1986), and Pollock (1993).

4. Theories can be the bases for hypotheses that can be tested or for theory to be expanded, and

5. Theories contribute to and assist in increasing the general body of knowledge of a discipline through the research implemented to validate them. The testing of a theory in practice is the basis for scientific development of a profession. Because Roy presents her work as a model, subtheorizing is present when application of the model is made for predictive understanding in a clinical situation. The model must be able to clearly identify the connecting relationships between underlying theories. Testable hypotheses are thus generated. Hill and Roberts (1981) discuss "relevant theory derivations" in their study of nursing interventions to promote the health of children with birth defects who are in need of habilitation. Developmental and social learning concepts related to the Roy premises and hypotheses for testing are proposed (see Table 15–6). Multiple examples of hypotheses for testing are generated by Roy and Roberts (1981). Because the model is an umbrella that can link theories, its contributions in the future to the body of nursing knowledge may be considerable.

6. Theories can be used by practitioners to guide and improve their practice. Perhaps the most important aspect of a theory is its usefulness in practice. How does application of the Roy model guide and improve the work of the practitioner? A major strength of the model is that it guides nurses to use observation and interviewing skills in doing an individualized assessment of each person. Behavior related to the four adaptive modes is collected during behavioral assessment. In considering all the adaptive modes—physiological,

TABLE 15-6. RELEVANT THEORY DERIVATIONS

Roy's Premises	Developmental Unit—Child Habilitation	Social Learning Unit—Maternal Locus of Control
Man is an adaptive being.	Habilitation is an adaptation problem.	Generalized expectancy of control is directional towards internality or externality.
If man is an adaptive being, he has an adaptation level. The adaptation level is a function of the interaction between adaptation mechanisms and the environment.	The greater the adaptation level, the greater the habilitation level. The habilitation level is a function of the interaction between adaptation mechanisms and the environment.	
	The greater the deficits in habilitation, the greater the impairment of adaptation level. The greater the impairment of adaptation level, the greater the impairment in activities of daily living.	
	The greater the impairment of adaptation level, the greater the significance of the environment.	A significant stimulus in a child's environment is the mother.
		The greater the maternal internal locus of control, the greater the parenting patterns fostering independence of a child.
		The greater the maternal external locus of control, the less the parenting patterns fostering independence of a child.
Nursing intervention is directed towards manipulation of the environment.	The less the habilitation level of the child, the greater the need for nursing intervention.	The less the parenting patterns foster independence of a child, the less the habilitation level of the child.

(From Roy, C., & Roberts, S. L. (1981). Theory construction in nursing: An adaptation model (pp. 36–37). Englewood Cliffs, NJ: Prentice-Hall. Used with permission.)

self-concept, role function, and interdependence—the nurse is likely to have a comprehensive view of the person.

The concepts of the Roy model are applicable within many practice settings of nursing. Literature cited throughout this chapter reflects application of the model by nurse educators, practitioners, and researchers in a variety of educational and clinical settings.

The use of the model may demand a change in the allocation of time and resources. Painstaking application of the model requires significant input of time and effort. The benefit to the client of complete assessment and implementations in areas of concern, however, justifies the effort and allocation of resources. Even in practice settings that require quick action, the elements of the model are still compatible with quality care. Especially useful is the guide for the assessment of stimuli which helps identify focal, contextual, and residual stimuli. The development by Roy of a typology of nursing diagnoses of common adaptation problems is an exciting outflow of the model. Further integration of Roy's work with that of NANDA is to be seen. Compatibility of the model to the work related to nursing diagnosis by NANDA is discussed in many chapters in the latest text (Roy & Andrews, 1991).

Goal setting and achievement in nursing are likely to be facilitated by application of commonly defined concepts and direction of focus. Because the model encourages identification of the focal, contextual, and residual stimuli within a situation, it immediately indicates the course of nursing action. Nursing actions are geared to altering these stimuli. This aspect of the model helps the practitioner in making specific decisions about what actions to take. In another way, practitioners can see the importance of their actions in influencing the adaptation of the person. For example, the nurse can view nursing actions such as maintaining bed rest or relieving pain or fears as significant in maintaining an adaptive response for the person.

7. Theories must be consistent with other validated theories, laws, and principles but will leave open unanswered questions that need to be investigated. By its structure, the Roy model requires the integration of further theorizing for explanatory and predictive information in clinical situations. The concept of adaptation as developed by the model appears to have good linkage qualities. Theory development has been undertaken by Roy, her coauthors, and others as cited throughout this chapter. Future nursing research and field application will continue to validate and adjust the Roy model.

SUMMARY

The Roy model consists of the four elements of person, environment, health, and nursing. Persons are viewed as living adaptive systems whose behaviors may be classified as adaptive responses or ineffective responses. These responses are derived from the regulator and cognator mechanisms. The assessment of behavior is done in the four adaptive modes: physiological, self-concept, role function, and interdependence. The environment consists of the person's internal and external stimuli. Health is a process of becoming integrated and able to meet the goals of survival, growth, reproduction, and mastery. The goal of nursing is to promote adaptive responses in relation to the four adaptive modes, using information about the person's adaptation level and focal, contextual, and residual stimuli. Nursing activities involve the manipulation of these stimuli to promote adaptive responses.

These elements are in a nursing process that consists of assessment of behaviors and stimuli, nursing diagnosis, goal setting, intervention, and evaluation. Behavioral assessment deals with the four adaptive modes, whereas assessment of stimuli focuses on focal, contextual, and residual stimuli. Nursing diagnosis consists of stating the problem. Goals are set in relation to the problem and are written in behavioral terms. Interventions are planned to manipulate the stimuli, and evaluation compares the person's output responses with the desired behaviors established in the goals.

Roy's model is seen as applicable in the nursing process presented in Chapter 2. The characteristics of a theory are also met. There is need for continued research that centers on hypotheses generated by the model.

REFERENCES

Andrews, H. A. (1991a). Overview of the role function mode. In C. Roy, & H. A. Andrews (Eds.), *The Roy adaptation model: The definitive statement* (pp. 347–361). Norwalk, CT: Appleton & Lange.

Andrews, H. A. (1991b). Overview of the self-concept mode. In C. Roy, & H. A. Andrews (Eds.), *The Roy adaptation model: The definitive statement* (pp. 269–279). Norwalk, CT: Appleton & Lange.

Andrews, H. A., & Roy, C. (1986). *Essentials of the Roy adaptation model.* Norwalk, CT: Appleton-Century-Crofts.

Andrews, H. A., & Roy, C. (1991). Overview of the physiological mode. In C. Roy, & H. A. Andrews (Eds.), *The Roy adaptation model: The definitive statement* (pp. 57–66). Norwalk, CT: Appleton & Lange.

Chalifoux, Z. (1991). Endocrine function. In C. Roy, & H. A. Andrews (Eds.), *The Roy adaptation model: The definitive statement* (pp. 237–259). Norwalk, CT: Appleton & Lange.

Dunn, H. L. (1971). *High level wellness.* Arlington, VA: Beatty.

Farkas, L. (1981). Adaptation problems with nursing home application for elderly persons: An application of the Roy adaptation nursing model. *Journal of Advanced Nursing, 6,* 363–368.

Fredrickson, K., Jackson, B. S., Strauman, T., & Strauman, J. (1991). Testing hypotheses derived from the Roy adaptation model. *Nursing Science Quarterly, 4,* 168–174.

Gaertzen, I. E. (Ed.). (1991). *Differentiating nursing practice into the twenty-first century.* Kansas City, MO: American Academy of Nursing.

Giger, J. A., Bower, C. A., & Miller, S. W. (1987). Roy adaptation model: ICU adaptation model: ICU application. *Dimensions of Critical Care Nursing, 6,* 215–224.

Guyton, A. C. (1971). *Basic human physiology: Normal function and mechanisms of disease*. Philadelphia: Saunders.

Helson, H. (1964). *Adaptation level theory*. New York: Harper & Row.

Hill, B. J., & Roberts, C. S. (1981). Formal theory construction: An example of the process. In C. Roy, & S. L. Roberts, *Theory construction in nursing: An adaptation model* (pp. 30–39). Englewood Cliffs, NJ: Prentice-Hall.

Hoch, C. C. (1987). Assessing delivery of nursing care. *Journal of Gerontological Nursing, 13,* 10–17.

Janelli, L. M. (1980). Utilizing Roy's adaptation model from a gerontological perspective. *Journal of Gerontological Nursing, 6,* 140–150.

Jensen, K. (1991). Fluids and electrolytes. In C. Roy, & H. A. Andrews (Eds.), *The Roy adaptation model: The definitive statement* (pp. 191–204). Norwalk, CT: Appleton & Lange.

Limandri, B. J. (1986). Research and practice with abused women: Use of the Roy adaptation model as an explanatory framework. *Advances in Nursing Science, 8,* 52–61.

Pollock, S. E. (1993). Adaptation to chronic illness: A program of research for testing nursing theory. *Nursing Science Quarterly, 6,* 86–92.

Rambo, B. (1983). *Adaptation nursing: Assessment and intervention*. Philadelphia: Saunders.

Randell, B., Tedrow, M. P., & Van Landingham, J. (1982). *Adaptation nursing: The Roy conceptual model applied*. St. Louis: Mosby.

Riehl-Sisca, J. P. (1989). *Conceptual models for nursing practice* (3rd ed.). New York: Appleton & Lange.

Roy, C. (1976). *Introduction to nursing: An adaptation model*. Englewood Cliffs, NJ: Prentice-Hall. [out of print]

Roy, C. (1984). *Introduction to nursing: An adaptation model* (2nd ed.). Englewood Cliffs, NJ: Prentice-Hall.

Roy, C. (1991a). Activity and rest. In C. Roy, & H. A. Andrews (Eds.), *The Roy adaptation model: The definitive statement* (pp. 117–147). Norwalk, CT: Appleton & Lange.

Roy, C. (1991b). Neurological function. In C. Roy, & H. A. Andrews (Eds.), *The Roy adaptation model: The definitive statement* (pp. 205–235). Norwalk, CT: Appleton & Lange.

Roy, C. (1991c). Senses. In C. Roy, & H. A. Andrews (Eds.), *The Roy adaptation model: The definitive statement* (pp. 165–189). Norwalk, CT: Appleton & Lange.

Roy, C., & Andrews, H. A. (1991). *The Roy adaptation model: The definitive statement*. Norwalk, CT: Appleton & Lange.

Roy, C., & Roberts, S. (1981). *Theory construction in nursing: An adaptation model*. Englewood Cliffs, NJ: Prentice-Hall.

Sato, M. K. (1991). Protection. In C. Roy, & H. A. Andrews (Eds.), *The Roy adaptation model: The definitive statement* (pp. 149–164). Norwalk, CT: Appleton & Lange.

Servonsky, J. (1991a). Elimination. In C. Roy, & H. A. Andrews (Eds.), *The Roy adaptation model: The definitive statement* (pp. 99–116). Norwalk, CT: Appleton & Lange.

Servonsky, J. (1991b). Nutrition. In C. Roy, & H. A. Andrews (Eds.), *The Roy adaptation model: The definitive statement* (pp. 81–98). Norwalk, CT: Appleton & Lange.

Tedrow, M. P. (1991). Overview of the interdependence mode. In C. Roy, & H. A. Andrews (Eds.), *The Roy adaptation model: The definitive statement* (pp. 385–403). Norwalk, CT: Appleton & Lange.

Thompson, C. (1991). Oxygenation. In C. Roy, & H. A. Andrews (Eds.), *The Roy adaptation model: The definitive statement* (pp. 67–79). Norwalk, CT: Appleton & Lange.

von Bertalanffy, L. (1968). *General system theory*. New York: Braziller.

BETTY NEUMAN

Julia B. George

■ ■ ■

Betty Neuman was born in 1924 on a 100-acre farm in Ohio; she was the middle of three children and the only daughter. When she was 11, her father died after six years of intermittent hospitalizations for treatment of chronic kidney disease. His praise of his nurses influenced Neuman's view of nursing and her commitment to becoming an excellent bedside nurse. Her mother's work as rural midwife was also a significant influence.

After graduation from high school, Neuman could not afford nursing education. She worked as an aircraft instrument repair technician, as draftsperson for an aircraft contracting company, and as a short-order cook in Dayton, Ohio, while saving for her education and helping support her mother and younger brother. The creation of the Cadet Nurse Corps Program expedited her entrance into a hospital school of nursing.

In 1947 Neuman graduated from the diploma program of Peoples Hospital (now General Hospital Medical Center), Akron, Ohio. She received a BS in public health nursing (1957) and an MS as a public health–mental health nurse consultant (1966) from the University of California, Los Angeles. In 1985 she was granted a PhD in clinical psychology by Pacific Western University. She has practiced bedside nursing as a staff, head, and private duty nurse in a wide variety of hospital settings. Her work in community settings has included school and industrial nursing, office nurse in her husband Kree's private practice in obstetrics; and counseling and crisis intervention in community mental health settings. In 1967, six months after completion of her MS degree, she became the faculty chair of the program from which she graduated and began her contributions as teacher, author, lecturer, and consultant in nursing and interdisciplinary health care.

In 1973 she and her family returned to Ohio. Since then she has worked as a state mental health consultant, provided continuing education programs, and continued the development of her model. She was one of the first California Nurse Licensed Clinical Fellows of the American Association of Marriage and Family Therapy and has maintained a limited private counseling practice. She is also a licensed real estate agent and obtained a private pilot's license in California. In addition to her professional activities, she has exercised her interest in personal property management and other investments.

The Neuman Systems Model was originally developed in 1970 in response to the request of graduate students at the University of California, Los Angeles, for an introductory course that would provide an overview of the physiological, psychological, sociocultural, and developmental aspects of human beings (Neuman, 1995). The model was developed to provide structure for the integration of this material in a wholistic manner. After a two-year evaluation, the model was first published in *Nursing Research* (Neuman & Young, 1972).

Neuman (1982, 1989, 1995) has published three editions of *The Neuman Systems Model*. She has also had chapters in all editions of *Conceptual models for nursing practice,* the latest being the third edition edited by Riehl-Sisca (1989), and in Parker's (1990) *Nursing theories in practice.* Neuman continues work on the model but also incorporated The Neuman Systems Model Trustees Group in 1988. Neuman (1995) states that the trustees group was established for the perpetuation, preservation, and protection of the integrity of the model. Any future permanent changes in the original Neuman Systems Model diagram (see Fig. 16–1), other than those made by Neuman herself, must have unanimous approval from the trustees.

DEVELOPMENT OF THE NEUMAN SYSTEMS MODEL

Neuman (1995) says that her personal philosophy of *helping each other live* was supportive in developing the wholistic systems perspective of the Neuman Systems Model. She drew upon her clinical experiences from a variety of health care and community settings and the theoretical perspectives of stress and systems. Caplan's (1964) levels of prevention were also incorporated into the model. Others whose works were drawn upon include de Chardin (1955), Cornu (1957), Edelson (1970), Emery (1969), Laszlo (1972), Lazarus (1981), Selye (1950), and von Bertalanffy (1968).

Nursing is considered a system because nursing practice contains elements in interaction with one another (Neuman, 1995). Advantages of an open systems perspective in nursing include the use of systems as a unifying force across various scientific fields as well as the increasing complexity of nursing, which calls for an organizational system that can respond to change. A systems perspective supports recognition of the complex whole while valuing the importance of the parts. The relationships between the parts and the interactions of the parts or the whole with the environment provide a mechanism for viewing the system–environment exchanges, which support the dynamic and constantly changing nature of the system.

Neuman (1995) views wholism as both a philosophical and a biological concept. Wholism includes relationships that arise from wholeness, dynamic freedom, and creativity as the system responds to stressors from the internal and external environments.

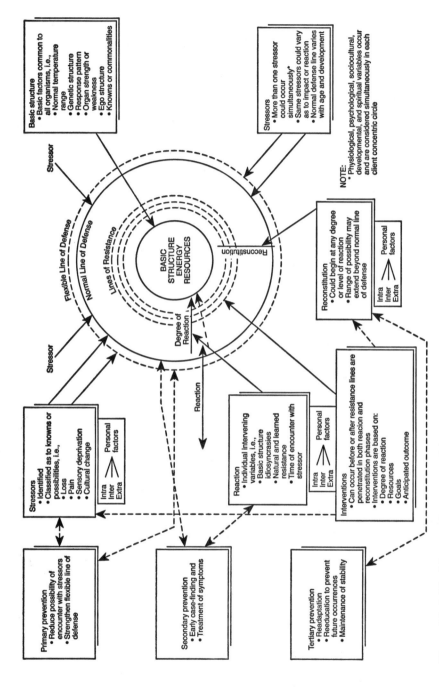

Figure 16–1. The Neuman Systems Model. *(From Neuman, B. (1995). The Neuman Systems Model (3rd ed) (p. 17). Norwalk, CT: Appleton & Lange.)*

THE NEUMAN SYSTEMS MODEL

The Neuman Systems Model's two major components are stress and the reaction to stress (Neuman, 1995). The client in the Neuman Systems Model is viewed as an open system in which repeated cycles of input, process, output, and feedback constitute a dynamic organizational pattern. Using the systems perspective, the client may be an individual, a group, a family, a community, or any aggregate. In their development toward growth and survival, open systems continuously become more differentiated and elaborate or complex. As they become more complex, the internal conditions of regulation become more complex. Exchanges with the environment are reciprocal; both the client and the environment may be affected either positively or negatively by each other. The system may adjust to the environment or adjust the environment to itself. The environmental influences are identified as intra-, inter-, and extrapersonal.

The ideal is to achieve optimal system stability. Neuman agrees with Heslin (1986) that when a system achieves stability a revitalization occurs. As an open system, the client system has a propensity to seek or maintain a balance among the various factors, both within and outside the system, that seek to disrupt it (Neuman, 1995). Neuman labels these forces as stressors and views them as capable of having either positive or negative effects. Reactions to the stressors may be possible, or not yet occurring, or actual, with identifiable responses and symptoms.

The Neuman Systems Model diagram (see Fig. 16–1) presents the major aspects of the model: the *physiological, psychological, sociocultural, developmental, and spiritual variables; basic structure and energy resources; lines of resistance; normal line of defense; flexible line of defense; stressors; reaction; primary, secondary, and tertiary prevention; intra-, inter-, and extrapersonal factors; and reconstitution.* The *environment, health,* and *nursing* are inherent parts of the model, although they are not labeled within the model. The client system is represented in the diagram by a basic structure surrounded by a series of concentric circles.

Basic Structure and Energy Resources

The basic structure, or central core, is made up of those basic survival factors common to the species (Neuman, 1995). These factors include the system variables, genetic features, and strengths and weaknesses of the system parts. If the client system is a human being, the basic structure contains such features as the ability to maintain body temperature within a normal range, genetic characteristics such as hair color and response to stimuli, and the functioning of various body systems and their interrelationships. There are also the baseline characteristics associated with each of the five variables, such as physical strength, cognitive ability, and value systems.

Neuman (1995) identifies system stability or homeostasis as occurring when the amount of energy that is available exceeds that being used by the system. This stability preserves the character of the system. Since the system is an open system, the stability is dynamic. As output becomes feedback and input, the system seeks to regulate itself. A change in one direction is countered by a compensating movement in the opposite direction. When the system is disturbed from its normal, or stable, state there is a rapid surge in the amount of energy needed to deal with the disorganization that results from the disturbance.

Client Variables

Neuman (1995) views the individual client wholistically and considers the variables (physiological, psychological, sociocultural, developmental, and spiritual) simultaneously and comprehensively. In the ideal situation, these variables function in harmony with stability in relation to internal and external environmental stressors. Each of the variables should be considered when assessing system reaction to stressors for each of the concentric circles in the model diagram. It is vital to avoid fragmentation if optimum stability of the client system is to be promoted through nursing care.

The *physiological* variable refers to the structure and functions of the body. The *psychological* variable refers to mental processes and relationships. The *sociocultural* variable refers to system functions that relate to social and cultural expectations and activities. The *developmental* variable refers to those processes related to development over the lifespan. The *spiritual* variable refers to the influence of spiritual beliefs.

Neuman (1995) indicates that the first four variables are commonly understood by nursing. Because the spiritual variable has been more recently added to the model, she discusses it in more detail. This variable is viewed as an innate component of the basic structure that may or may not be acknowledged or developed by the client. Neuman views it as permeating all the other variables of the client system and existing on a developmental continuum from complete unawareness of the presence and potential of the variable to a highly developed spiritual understanding that supports optimal wellness. The continuum includes denial of the existence of the spiritual variable.

Lines of Resistance

The lines of resistance protect the basic structure and become activated when the normal line of defense is invaded by environmental stressors. An example of a response involving lines of resistance is the activation of the immune system mechanisms. If the lines of resistance are effective in their response, the system can reconstitute; if the lines of resistance are not effective, the resulting energy depletion may lead to death.

Normal Line of Defense

In terms of system stability, the normal line of defense represents stability over time (Neuman, 1995). It is considered to be the usual level of stability for the system or the normal wellness state and is used as the baseline for determining deviation from wellness for the client system. The normal line of defense has changed over time as a result of coping with a variety of stressors. The stability represented by the normal line of defense is actually a range of responses to the environment.

Any stressor may invade the normal line of defense when the flexible line of defense offers inadequate protection. When the normal line of defense is invaded or penetrated, the client system reacts. The reaction will be apparent in symptoms of instability or illness and may reduce the system's ability to withstand additional stressors.

Flexible Line of Defense

The flexible line of defense is represented in the model diagram as the outer boundary and initial response, or protection, of the system to stressors. The flexible line of defense serves as a cushion and is described as accordionlike as it expands away from or contracts closer to the normal line of defense (Neuman, 1995). It protects the normal line of defense and acts as a buffer for the client system's usual stable state. Ideally, the flexible line of defense prevents stressors from invading the system. As the distance between the flexible and normal lines of defense increases, so does the degree of protection available to the system.

The flexible line of defense is dynamic rather than stable and can be altered over a relatively short period by factors such as inadequate nutrition or sleep. Either single or multiple stressors may invade the flexible line of defense.

Environment

Neuman (1995) defines environment as all the internal and external factors or influences that surround the client or client system. The influence of the client on the environment and the environment on the client may be positive or negative at any time. Variations in both the client system and the environment can affect the direction of the reaction. For example, individuals who experience sleep deprivation are more susceptible to viruses of the common cold from the environment than those who are well rested.

The *internal* environment exists within the client system. All forces and interactive influences that are solely within the boundaries of the client system make up this environment.

The *external* environment exists outside the client system. Those forces and interactive influences that are outside the system boundaries are identified as external.

Neuman (1989, 1990, 1995) identifies a third environment, the *created environment*. The created environment is developed unconsciously by the client and is symbolic of system wholeness. It represents the open system exchange of energy with both the internal and external environments. It is dynamic and depicts the unconscious mobilization of all system variables but particularly the psychological and sociocultural variables. The purpose of this mobilization is the integration, integrity, and stability of the system. Based on Lazarus's (1981) work, its function is seen as a protective coping shield that encompasses both the internal and external environments. Because it serves as an insulator, the created environment may change the client system's response to stressors. A major objective of the created environment is to provide a positive stimulus toward health for the client. The created environment is developed to be protective but may have a negative effect on the system if it uses energy needed to react to environmental stressors.

To assess the created environment, the caregiver needs to identify three aspects. First, what has been created, what is the nature of the created environment? Second, to what extent is it used and what value does the client place upon it, what are the outcomes? Third, what protection is needed or is possible, what is the ideal that is yet to be created? The created environment is a process-based concept of perpetual adjustment that may increase or decrease the client's state of wellness (Neuman, 1995).

Stressors

Neuman (1995) defines stressors as stimuli that produce tensions and have the potential for causing system instability. The system may need to deal with one or more stressors at any given time. It is important to identify the type, nature, and intensity of the stressor; the time of the system's encounter with the stressor; and the nature of the system's reaction or potential reaction to that encounter, including the amount of energy needed. The reaction may occur in one or more subparts of the system. A reaction in one subsystem may in turn affect the original stressor. Outcomes may be positive with the potential for beneficial system changes that may be temporary or permanent.

Stressors are present both within or outside of the system. Neuman (1995) classifies stressors as intra-, inter-, or extrapersonal in nature. *Intrapersonal* stressors are those that occur within the client system boundary and correlate with the internal environment. An example for the individual client system is the autoimmune response. *Interpersonal* stressors occur outside the client system boundary, are proximal to the system, and have an impact on the system. An example is role expectations. *Extrapersonal* stressors also occur outside the system boundaries but are at a greater distance from the system than are interpersonal stressors. An example is social policy. Interpersonal and extrapersonal stressors correlate with the external environment. The created environment includes intra-, inter-, and extrapersonal stressors.

Health

Neuman (1995) identifies health as optimal system stability, or the optimal state of wellness at a given time. Health is seen as a continuum from wellness to illness (see Fig. 16–2). Health is also described as dynamic, with changing levels occurring within a normal range for the client system over time. The levels vary because of basic structure factors and the client system's response and adjustment to environmental stressors. Wellness may be determined by identifying the actual or potential effects of invading stressors on the system's available energy levels. The client system moves toward illness and death (entropy) when more energy is needed than is available and toward wellness (negentropy) when more energy is available, or can be generated, than is needed.

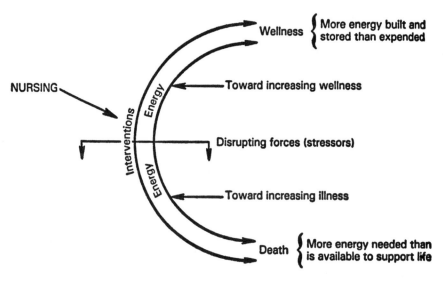

Figure 16–2. Wellness–illness based on the systems concept. *(Adapted from Neuman, B., (1982). The Neuman systems model: Applications to nursing education and practice (p. 11). Norwalk, CT: Appleton-Century-Crofts. Used with permission.)*

Reaction

Although reaction is identified within Figure 16–2, Neuman does not discuss it separately. She points out that reactions and outcomes may be positive or negative, and she discusses system movement toward negentropy or entropy.

Prevention

Primary, secondary, and tertiary prevention as interventions are used to retain, attain, and maintain system balance. More than one prevention mode may be used simultaneously.

Primary prevention occurs before the system reacts to a stressor; it includes health promotion and maintenance of wellness. Primary prevention focuses on strengthening the flexible line of defense through preventing stress and reducing risk factors. This intervention occurs when the risk or hazard is identified but before a reaction occurs. Strategies that might be used include immunization, health education, exercise, and life style changes.

Secondary prevention occurs after the system reacts to a stressor and is provided in terms of existing symptoms. Secondary prevention focuses on strengthening the internal lines of resistance and, thus, protects the basic structure through appropriate treatment of symptoms. The intent is to regain optimal system stability and to conserve energy in doing so. If secondary prevention is unsuccessful and reconstitution does not occur, the basic structure will be unable to support the system and its interventions, and death will occur.

Tertiary prevention occurs after the system has been treated through secondary prevention strategies. Its purpose is to maintain wellness or protect the client system reconstitution through supporting existing strengths and continuing to conserve energy. Tertiary prevention may begin at any point after system stability has begun to be reestablished (reconstitution has begun). Tertiary prevention tends to lead back to primary prevention.

Reconstitution

Reconstitution begins at any point following initiation of treatment for invasion of stressors. Neuman (1995) defines reconstitution as the increase in energy that occurs in relation to the degree of reaction to the stressor. Reconstitution may expand the normal line of defense beyond its previous level, stabilize the system at a lower level, or return it to the level that existed before the illness. It depends on successful mobilization of client resources to prevent further reaction to the stressor, and it represents a dynamic state of adjustment.

Nursing

Neuman (1995) also discusses nursing as part of the model. The major concern of nursing is to help the client system attain, maintain, or retain system stability. This may be accomplished through accurate assessment of both the actual and potential effects of stressor invasion and assisting the client system to make those adjustments necessary for optimal wellness. In supporting system stability, the nurse provides the linkage between the client system, the environment, health, and nursing.

Propositions of the Neuman Systems Model

Neuman (1974) presented the assumptions that she identified as underlying the Neuman Systems Model. She has now labeled these as propositions (Neuman, 1995). These propositions follow:

1. Although each individual client or group as a client system is unique, each system is a composite of common known factors or innate characteristics within a normal, given range of response contained within a basic structure.

2. Many known, unknown, and universal environmental stressors exist. Each differs in its potential for disturbing a client's usual stability level, or normal line of defense. The particular interrelationships of client variables—physiological, psychological, sociocultural, developmental, and spiritual—at any point in time can affect the degree to which a client is protected by the flexible line of defense against possible reaction to a single stressor or a combination of stressors.

3. Each individual client/client system has evolved a normal range of response to the environment that is referred to as a normal line of defense, or usual wellness/stability state. It represents change over time through coping with diverse stress encounters. The normal line of defense can be used as a standard from which to measure health deviation.

4. When the cushioning, accordion-like effect of the flexible line of defense is no longer capable of protecting the client/client system against an environmental stressor, the stressor breaks through the normal line of defense. The interrelationships of variables—physiological, psychological, sociocultural, developmental, and spiritual—determine the nature and degree of the system reaction or possible reaction to the stressor.

5. The client, whether in a state of wellness or illness, is a dynamic composite of the interrelationships of variables—physiological, psychological, sociocultural, developmental, and spiritual. Wellness is on a continuum of available energy to support the system in an optimal state of system stability.

6. Implicit within each client system is a set of internal resistance factors known as lines of resistance, which function to stabilize and return the client to the usual state of wellness (normal line of defense) or possibly to a higher level of stability following an environmental stressor reaction.

7. Primary prevention relates to general knowledge that is applied to client assessment and intervention in identification and reduction or mitigation of possible or actual risk factors associated with environmental stressors to prevent possible reaction. The goal of health promotion is included in primary prevention.

8. Secondary prevention relates to symptomatology following a reaction to stressors, appropriate ranking of intervention priorities, and treatment to reduce their noxious effects.

9. Tertiary prevention relates to the adjustive processes taking place as reconstitution begins and maintenance factors move the client back in a circular manner toward primary prevention.

10. The client as a system is in dynamic, constant energy exchange with the environment (pp. 20–21).

THE NEUMAN SYSTEMS MODEL AND NURSING'S METAPARADIGM

The four major concepts in nursing's metaparadigm are identified by Neuman as part of her model and have been discussed. A brief summary of each follows.

The *human being* is viewed as an open system that interacts with both internal and external environmental forces or stressors. The human is in constant change, moving toward a dynamic state of system stability or toward illness of varying degrees.

The *environment* is a vital arena that is germane to the system and its function; it includes internal, external, and created environment (Neuman, 1995). The environment may be viewed as all factors that affect and are affected by the system.

Health is defined as the condition or degree of system stability and is viewed as a continuum from wellness to illness (Neuman, 1995) (see Fig. 16–2).

Stability occurs when all the system's parts and subparts are in balance or harmony so that the whole system is in balance. When system needs are met, optimal wellness exists. When needs are not satisfied, illness exists. When the energy needed to support life is not available, death occurs.

The primary concern of *nursing* is to define the appropriate action in situations that are stress-related or in relation to possible reactions of the client or client system to stressors. Nursing interventions are aimed at helping the system adapt or adjust and to retain, restore, or maintain some degree of stability between and among the client system variables and environmental stressors with a focus on conserving energy.

THE NEUMAN SYSTEMS MODEL AND THE NURSING PROCESS

Neuman (1982, 1995) presents a three step nursing process format (see Table 16–1). The first step is entitled "Nursing Diagnosis" and includes the use of a data base to identify variances from wellness and development of hypothetical interventions. The second step, "Nursing Goals," includes caregiver–client negotiation of intervention strategies to retain, attain, or maintain system stability. The third step, "Nursing Outcomes," includes nursing intervention using the prevention modes, confirming that the desired change has occurred or reformulating the nursing goals, using the outcomes of short-term goals to determine longer-term goals, and validating the nursing process through client outcomes. Neuman's first step parallels the assessment and diagnosis phases of the five-phase nursing process. Her second step equates to the planning phase, and her third step equates to the implementation and evaluation phases.

Using the Neuman Systems Model in the *assessment* phase of the nursing process, the nurse focuses on obtaining a comprehensive client data base to determine the existing state of wellness and the actual or potential reaction to environmental stressors. A more specific guide to assessment is presented in Table 16–2, "An Assessment and Intervention Tool." The collected data are prioritized and compared to, or synthesized with, relevant theories to explain the client's condition. Variances from the usual state of wellness are identified and a summary of impressions developed. The summary includes intra-, inter-, and extrapersonal factors.

The synthesis of data with theory also provides the basis for the *nursing diagnosis*. In the Neuman model, the diagnostic statement should reflect the entire client condition.

Planning involves negotiation between the caregiver and the client, or recipient of care. The overall goal of the caregiver is to guide the client to conserve energy and to use energy as a force to move beyond the present, ideally in a way that preserves or enhances the client's wellness level. More specific goals will be derived from the nursing diagnoses. The perceptions of both the client and the caregiver must be considered in setting goals.

According to Neuman (1995), nursing actions (*implementation*) are based on the synthesis of a comprehensive data base about the client and the theory(ies)

TABLE 16–1. THE NEUMAN NURSING PROCESS FORMAT

Nursing Diagnosis

	Variances from wellness are determined by correlations and constraints	I. Nursing Diagnosis

Data base

Variances from wellness are determined by correlations and constraints

Hypothetical interventions are determined for prescriptive change

I. Nursing Diagnosis
A. Data base—determined by
1. Identification and evaluation of potential or actual stressors that pose a threat to the stability of the client/ client systems.
2. Assessment of condition and strength of basic structure factors and energy resources.
3. Assessment of characteristics of the flexible and normal lines of defense, lines of resistance, degree of potential reaction, reaction, and/or potential for reconstitution following a reaction.
4. Identification, classification, and evaluation of potential and/or actual intra-, inter-, and extra-personal interactions between the client and environment, considering all five variables.
5. Evaluation of influence of past, present, and possible future life process and coping patterns on client system stability.
6. Identification and evaluation of actual and potential internal and external resources for optimal state of wellness.
7. Identification and resolution of perceptual differences between caregivers and client/client system.
Note: In all the above areas of consideration the caregiver simultaneously considers five variables (dynamic interactions in the client/ client system)—physiological, psychological, sociocultural, developmental, and spiritual.

(Continued)

TABLE 16–1. (CONTINUED)

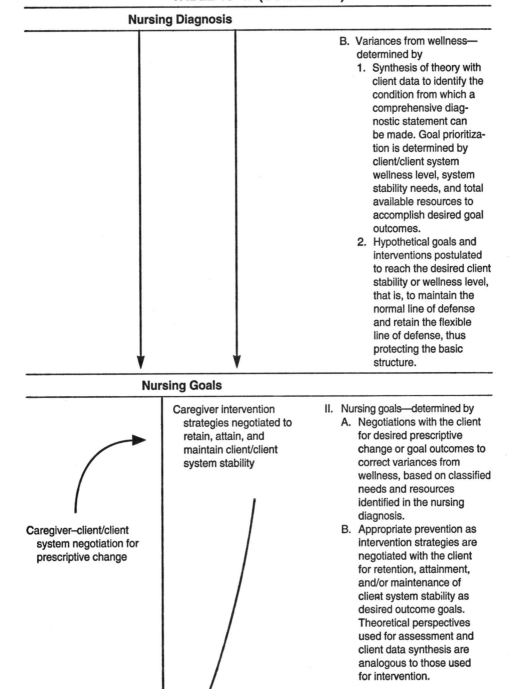

Nursing Diagnosis

B. Variances from wellness—determined by
1. Synthesis of theory with client data to identify the condition from which a comprehensive diagnostic statement can be made. Goal prioritization is determined by client/client system wellness level, system stability needs, and total available resources to accomplish desired goal outcomes.
2. Hypothetical goals and interventions postulated to reach the desired client stability or wellness level, that is, to maintain the normal line of defense and retain the flexible line of defense, thus protecting the basic structure.

Nursing Goals

Caregiver intervention strategies negotiated to retain, attain, and maintain client/client system stability

Caregiver–client/client system negotiation for prescriptive change

II. Nursing goals—determined by
A. Negotiations with the client for desired prescriptive change or goal outcomes to correct variances from wellness, based on classified needs and resources identified in the nursing diagnosis.
B. Appropriate prevention as intervention strategies are negotiated with the client for retention, attainment, and/or maintenance of client system stability as desired outcome goals. Theoretical perspectives used for assessment and client data synthesis are analogous to those used for intervention.

(Continued)

TABLE 16–1. (CONTINUED)

Nursing Outcomes

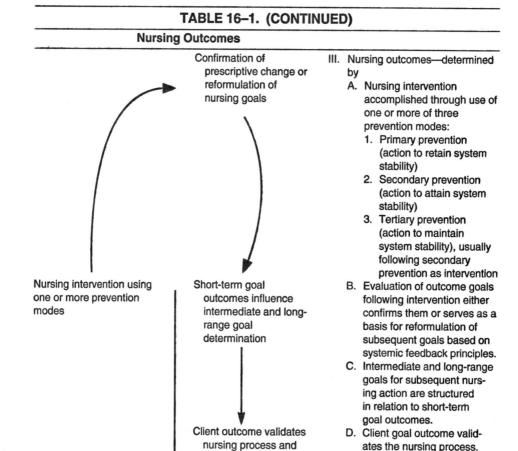

Confirmation of prescriptive change or reformulation of nursing goals

Nursing intervention using one or more prevention modes

Short-term goal outcomes influence intermediate and long-range goal determination

Client outcome validates nursing process and acts as feedback for further system input as required

III. Nursing outcomes—determined by
   A. Nursing intervention accomplished through use of one or more of three prevention modes:
      1. Primary prevention (action to retain system stability)
      2. Secondary prevention (action to attain system stability)
      3. Tertiary prevention (action to maintain system stability), usually following secondary prevention as intervention
   B. Evaluation of outcome goals following intervention either confirms them or serves as a basis for reformulation of subsequent goals based on systemic feedback principles.
   C. Intermediate and long-range goals for subsequent nursing action are structured in relation to short-term goal outcomes.
   D. Client goal outcome validates the nursing process.

that are appropriate in light of the client's perceptions and possibilities for functional competence within the environment. The modes for identifying these actions are the levels of prevention as intervention. Table 16–3 presents a guide to nursing actions using prevention as intervention.

Evaluation is implied in the discussion of reassessment in Table 16–2. It is more explicitly identified in the "Nursing Outcomes" step of Neuman's three-step nursing process (see Table 16–1). According to this third step, evaluation confirms that the anticipated or prescribed change has occurred. If this is not true, then goals are reformulated. Immediate and long-range goals are then structured in relation to the short-range outcomes.

TABLE 16–2. AN ASSESSMENT AND INTERVENTION TOOL

A. Intake Summary
1. Name _____
   Age _____
   Sex _____
   Marital status _____
2. Referral source and related information __
   _____

B. Stressors as Perceived by Client
   (If client is incapacitated, secure data from
   family or other resources.)
1. What do you consider your major stress
   area, or areas of health concern? (Identify
   these areas.)
2. How do present circumstances differ from
   your usual pattern of living? (Identify life-
   style patterns.)
3. Have you ever experienced a similar
   problem? If so, what was that problem
   and how did you handle it? Were you
   successful? (Identify past coping
   patterns.)
4. What do you anticipate for yourself in the
   future as a consequence of your present
   situation? (Identify perceptual factors,
   that is, reality versus distortions—
   expectations, present and possible future
   coping patterns.)
5. What are you doing and what can you do
   to help yourself? (Identify perceptual
   factors, that is, reality versus distortions—
   expectations, present and possible future
   coping patterns.)
6. What do you expect caregivers, family,
   friends, or others to do for you? (Identify
   perceptual factors, that is, reality versus
   distortions—expectations, present and
   possible future coping patterns.)

C. Stressors as Perceived by Caregiver
1. What do you consider to be the major
   stress area, or areas of health concern?
   (Identify these areas.)
2. How do present circumstances seem to
   differ from the client's usual pattern of
   living? (Identify life style patterns)
3. Has the client ever experienced a similar
   situation? If so, how would you evaluate
   what the client did? How successful do
   you think it was? (Identify past coping
   patterns.)
4. What do you anticipate for the future as
   a consequence of the client's present

situation? (Identify perceptual factors, that
is, reality versus distortions—expectations,
present and possible future coping patterns.)
5. What can the client do to help him- or
   herself? (Identify perceptual factors, that
   is, reality versus distortions—
   expectations, present and possible future
   coping patterns.)
6. What do you think the client expects from
   caregivers, family, friends, or other
   resources? (Identify perceptual factors,
   that is, reality versus distortions—
   expectations, present and possible future
   coping patterns.)

Summary of Impressions
Note any discrepancies or distortions between
   the client's perception and that of the
   caregiver related to the situation.

D. Intrapersonal Factors
1. Physical (examples: degree of mobility,
   range of body function)
2. Psycho-sociocultural (examples: attitudes,
   values, expectations, behavior patterns,
   and nature of coping patterns)
3. Developmental (examples: age, degree
   of normalcy, factors related to present
   situation)
4. Spiritual belief system (examples: hope
   and sustaining factors)

E. Interpersonal Factors
   Examples are resources and relationship
   of family, friends, or caregivers that either
   influence or could influence Area D.

F. Extrapersonal Factors
   Examples are resources and relationship of
   community facilities, finances, employment,
   or other area which either influence or could
   influence Areas D and E.

G. Formulation of a Comprehensive Nursing
   Diagnosis
   This is accomplished by identifying and
   ranking the priority of needs based on total
   data obtained from the client's perception,
   the caregiver's perception, or other
   resources, such as laboratory reports, other
   caregivers, or agencies. Appropriate theory is
   related to the above data.
   With this format, reassessment is a
   continuous process and is related to the
   effectiveness of intervention based upon the

(Continued)

TABLE 16–2. (CONTINUED)

prior stated goals. Effective reassessment would include the following as they relate to the total client situation:

1. Changes in nature of stressors and priority assignments
2. Changes in intrapersonal factors
3. Changes in interpersonal factors
4. Changes in extrapersonal factors

In reassessment it is important to note the change of priority of goals in relation to the primary,

secondary, and tertiary prevention as intervention categories. An assessment tool of this nature should offer a current, progressive, and comprehensive analysis of the client's total circumstances and relationship of the five client variables (physiological, psychological, sociocultural, developmental, and spiritual) to environmental influences.

From Neuman, B. (1995). The Neuman Systems Model. (pp. 59–61). Norwalk, CT: Appleton & Lange.

TABLE 16–3. FORMAT FOR PREVENTION AS INTERVENTION

Nursing Action

Primary Prevention	Secondary Prevention	Tertiary Prevention
1. Classify stressors that threaten stability of the client/client system. Prevent stressor invasion.	1. Following stressor invasion, protect basic structure.	1. During reconstitution, attain and maintain maximum level of wellness or stability following treatment.
2. Provide information to retain or strengthen existing client/client system strengths.	2. Mobilize and optimize internal/external resources to attain stability and energy conservation.	2. Educate, reeducate, and/or reorient as needed.
3. Support positive coping and functioning.	3. Facilitate purposeful manipulation of stressors and reactions to stressors.	3. Support client/client system toward appropriate goals.
4. Desensitize existing or possible noxious stressors.	4. Motivate, educate, and involve client/client system in health care goals.	4. Coordinate and integrate health service resources.
5. Motivate toward wellness.	5. Facilitate appropriate treatment and intervention measures.	5. Provide primary and/or secondary preventive intervention as required.
6. Coordinate and integrate interdisciplinary theories and epidemiological input.	6. Support positive factors toward wellness.	
7. Educate or reeducate.	7. Promote advocacy by coordination and integration.	
8. Use stress as a positive intervention strategy.	8. Provide primary preventive intervention as required.	

Note: *A first priority for nursing action in each of the areas of prevention as intervention is to determine the nature of stressors and their threat to the client/client system. Some general categorical functions for nursing action are initiation, planning, organization, monitoring, coordinating, implementing, integrating, advocating, supporting, and evaluating. An example of a limited classification system for stressors is illustrated by the following four categories: (1) deprivation, (2) excess, (3) change, and (4) intolerance. Copyright © 1980 by Betty Neuman. Revised 1987 by Betty Neuman.*

STRENGTHS AND WEAKNESSES
OF THE NEUMAN SYSTEMS MODEL

The major strength of the Neuman Systems Model is its flexibility for use in all areas of nursing—administration, education, and practice. The third edition of *The Neuman Systems Model* includes many chapters that discuss the use of the model in all of these areas throughout the United States and in Australia, Canada, England, Holland, Sweden, and Wales. This widespread acceptance supports the essentially universal applicability of the model.

Neuman (1995) reports that the model was designed for nursing but can be used by other health disciplines, which can be viewed as either a strength or weakness. As a strength, if multiple health disciplines use the model, a consistent approach to client care would be facilitated. If all disciplines use similar data collection techniques based upon the assessment tool presented by Neuman, perhaps the client would not have to tell his or her story so many different times—at least once to each health care discipline. As a weakness, if the model is useful to a variety of disciplines, it is not specific to nursing and thus may not differentiate the practice of nursing from that of other disciplines.

The major weakness of the model is the need for further clarification of terms used. Interpersonal and extrapersonal stressors need to be more clearly differentiated. It may be that interpersonal stressors occur between two people and extrapersonal stressors occur between a group or society and the person. This differentiation is not clearly made. Other areas that require greater specification are how to identify variances of wellness and levels of wellness. Reaction also needs to be defined.

THE NEUMAN SYSTEMS MODEL
AND THE CHARACTERISTICS OF A THEORY

1. Theories can interrelate concepts in such a way as to create a different way of looking at a particular phenomenon. Neuman has presented a view of the client that is equally applicable to an individual, a family, a group, a community, or any other aggregate. The systems view she presents, in conjunction with the prevention modalities as intervention, are a unique way of viewing health care phenomena. The interaction of the client system and its environments as they relate to health provide a useful view of the world. The emphasis on primary prevention, including health promotion, is specific to this model and increasingly important in today's health care environment.

2. Theories must be logical in nature. The Neuman Systems Model, particularly as presented in the model diagram, is logically consistent. The three-step nursing process is also logical, with its emphasis on a comprehensive data base, mutual decision making between caregiver and client system, and use of outcomes. However, there are some inconsistencies between the diagram and the verbal presentation of the model. The diagram includes reaction that is not specifically discussed in the text. Conversely, the verbal presentation incorporates health, environment, and nursing, which do not appear in the diagram. It is inferred that the diagram is considered to be the most important representation of the model because it is changes in the diagram that require unanimous agreement of the Neuman Trustees. Logically, based upon this inference, the concepts in the verbal presentation should be derived from the diagram.

Other inconsistencies relate to Neuman's emphasis on a wholistic approach and a comprehensive view of the client system and her discussion of health and illness. The wholistic and comprehensive view is associated with an open system. Health and illness are presented on a continuum with movement toward health described as negentropic and toward illness as entropic. Entropy is a characteristic of a closed, rather than an open, system. She does speak of levels of wellness, rather than levels of illness, but does not make it clear if health and illness are dichotomous.

3. Theories should be relatively simple yet generalizable. Once understood, the Neuman Systems Model is relatively simple, and has readily acceptable definitions of its components. Its generalizability is supported by the more than three dozen chapters in the third edition of *The Neuman Systems Model* that discuss the use of the model in curriculum, nursing practice, and nursing administration in the United States and internationally. Neuman (1995) also indicates that although the model was designed for nursing, it can be used by other health care providers.

An initial drawback to simplicity is the diagram of the model (see Figure 16–1). In its efforts to represent multiple relationships and components, the diagram has become awesome. With a guide to the diagram, the components can be clearly understood, and the initial sense of overwhelming complexity overcome.

4. Theories can be the bases for hypotheses that can be tested or for theory to be expanded, and

5. Theories contribute to and assist in increasing the general body of knowledge within the discipline through the research implemented to validate them. Hypotheses can be and have been derived from the Neuman Systems Model and the relationships within the model. The third edition of *The Neuman Systems Model* cites multiple published research articles, doctoral dissertations, and masters theses that have reported research based on the model. The areas of research have included client systems of individuals, families, and groups of practicing nurses and nursing students in educational settings, hospitals, and the community.

6. Theories can be used by practitioners to guide and improve their practice. Neuman has provided tools that are specifically designed to assist practitioners in using the model in practice (see Table 16–2 and Table 16–3). The model is congruent with the increasing emphases on home health care and health promotion. It has been widely used by practitioners in nursing education, practice, and administration nationally and internationally.

7. Theories must be consistent with other validated theories, laws, and principles but will leave open unanswered questions that need to be investigated. Neuman identifies the theories upon which she drew to develop the systems model. Her work appears to be consistent with these theories, and there is no apparent conflict with other theories. There are many questions yet to be answered, including: Does the created environment more often have a positive or negative system outcome? Does the use of the Neuman Systems Model increase the effectiveness of communication with other health care providers? What is the most effective way to identify a client system's optimal level of wellness?

The Neuman Systems Model does not fully meet all the characteristics of a theory. Since it is presented as a model, this is not surprising. Neuman (1995) reports that she and A. Koertvelyessy have found that the major theory of the model is that of optimal client system stability. This theory is that the health of the client system is represented by stability. Neuman cites an unpublished paper as the only reference for the theory.

SUMMARY

The Neuman Systems Model was developed to help teach graduate students an integrated approach to client care. The model is based in general system theory and views the client as an open system that responds to stressors in the environment. The client variables are physiological, psychological, sociocultural, developmental, and spiritual. The client system consists of a basic or core structure that is protected by lines of resistance. The usual level of health is identified as the normal line of defense that is protected by a flexible line of defense. Stressors are intra-, inter-, and extrapersonal in nature and arise from the internal, external, and created environments. When stressors break through the flexible line of defense, the system is invaded and the lines of resistance are activated and the system is described as moving into illness on a wellness–illness continuum. If adequate energy is available, the system will be reconstituted with the normal line of defense restored at, below, or above its previous level. Nursing interventions occur through three prevention modalities. Primary prevention occurs before the stressor invades the system; secondary prevention occurs after the system has reacted to an invading stressor; and tertiary prevention occurs after secondary prevention as reconstitution is being established.

This model has been widely used in all areas of nursing practice. Its flexibility and universality are documented in the many publications that describe its use in nursing education, research, administration, and direct patient care. Further definition of some of the concepts in the model will serve to strengthen it further.

REFERENCES

Caplan, G. (1964). *Principles of preventive psychiatry*. New York: Basic Books. [out of print]

Cornu, A. (1957). *The origin of Marxist thought*. Springfield, IL: Thomas. [out of print] de Chardin, P. T. (1955). *The phenomenon of man.* London: Collins. [out of print]

Edelson, M. (1970). *Sociotherapy and psychotherapy.* Chicago: University of Chicago. [out of print]

Emery, F. (Ed.). (1969). *Systems thinking.* Baltimore: Penguin Books. [out of print]

Heslin, K. (1986). *A systems analysis of the Betty Neuman model.* Unpublished student paper. University of Western Ontario, London, Ontario, Canada.

Laszlo, E. (1972). *The systems view of the world: The natural philosophy of the new development in the sciences.* New York: Braziller. [out of print]

Lazarus, R. (1981). The stress and coping paradigm. In C. Eisdorfer, D. Cohen, A. Kleinman, & P. Maxim (Eds.), *Models for clinical psychopathology* (pp. 177–214). New York: SP Medical and Scientific Books.

Neuman, B. (1974). The Betty Neuman health-care systems model: A total person approach to patient problems. In J. P. Riehl, & C. Roy (Eds.), *Conceptual models for nursing practice* (pp. 99–114). New York: Appleton-Century-Crofts. [out of print]

Neuman, B. (1982). *The Neuman Systems Model.* Norwalk, CT: Appleton-Century-Crofts. [out of print]

Neuman, B. (1989). *The Neuman Systems Model* (2nd ed.). Norwalk, CT: Appleton & Lange. [out of print]

Neuman, B. (1990). Health on a continuum based on the Neuman Systems Model. *Nursing Science Quarterly, 3,* 129–135.

Neuman, B. (1995). *The Neuman Systems Model* (3rd ed.). Norwalk, CT: Appleton & Lange.

Neuman, B. M., & Young, R. J. (1972). A model for teaching total person approach to patient problems. *Nursing Research, 21,* 264–269.

Parker, M. E. (Ed.). (1990). *Nursing theories in practice.* New York: National League for Nursing.

Riehl-Sisca, J. (1989). *Conceptual models for nursing practice* (3rd ed.). Norwalk, CT: Appleton & Lange.

Selye, H. (1950). *The physiology and pathology of exposure to stress.* Montreal, Quebec, Canada: ACTA. [out of print]

von Bertalanffy, L. (1968). *General system theory.* New York: Braziller. [out of print]

JOSEPHINE E. PATERSON AND LORETTA T. ZDERAD

Susan G. Praeger*

■ ■ ■

Josephine E. Paterson and Loretta T. Zderad's book, Humanistic Nursing, *was published in 1976 and republished in 1988. Josephine Paterson retired in 1985 as a clinical nurse specialist at the Northport Veterans Administration Medical Center at Northport, New York. She is a graduate of Lenox Hill Hospital School of Nursing and St. John's University. She received her master's degree from Johns Hopkins School of Hygiene and Public Health, Baltimore, Maryland. Her Doctor of Nurse Science is from Boston University School of Nursing, Boston, Massachusetts, where she specialized in mental health and psychiatric nursing. Dr. Paterson has conceptualized and taught humanistic nursing to graduate students, faculty, and staff in a variety of settings. She also served on the faculty of the State University of New York at Stonybrook.*

Loretta T. Zderad retired in 1985 as the Associate Chief for Nursing Education at the Northport Veterans Administration Medical Center, Northport, New York. She is a graduate of St. Bernard's Hospital School of Nursing and of Loyola University. She received her Master of Science degree from Catholic University, Washington, DC and a Doctor of Philosophy from Georgetown University, Washington, DC. She has taught in several universities and has led groups on humanistic nursing. Dr. Zderad also served on the faculty of the State University of New York at Stonybrook.

Josephine E. Paterson and Loretta T. Zderad have described what they call a "humanistic nursing practice" theory in several publications and presentations. It is a practice theory because they believe that the theory of a science of nursing develops from the lived experiences of the nurse and the person receiving care. Theory becomes a response to the phenomenological experience. R. D. Laing is quoted as saying that "theory is the articulated vision of experience" (Zderad, 1978, p. 45). This means that nursing practice is the

*Gratitude is expressed to Christina R. Hogarth for her contributions to this chapter in earlier editions.

basis for what we believe about nursing. Our experience in the world of health care is the foundation for understanding the nature of nursing and what it means to be a nurse.

Humanistic nursing is nursing's response to the humanistic movement in psychology, which was seen as an alternative to the two dominant psychological views of the time. Freudian psychology was seen as being too limited in its orientation toward the sick personality, and behavioral psychology was seen as being too mechanistically oriented. The humanistic orientation tries to take a broader view of the potential of human beings, trying to understand them from the context of their experience of living in the world. Rather than trying to supplant other views, its aim is to supplement them (Bugental, 1978).

There is no simple way to define the essence of humanistic nursing because it is concerned with the phenomenological experiences of individuals, the exploration of human experiences. It requires that we enter the nursing situation fully aware of the "lenses" that we wear. We need to know what values, biases, myths, and expectations we bring to the nursing experience. And we need to fully appreciate what values, biases, myths, and expectations others bring to the nursing experience. The combination of these perspectives brings uniqueness to nursing. The practice of humanistic nursing is rooted in existential thought.

Existentialism is a philosophical approach to understanding life. Individuals are faced with possibilities when making choices. These choices determine the direction and meaning of one's life. Like humanistic psychology, existentialism was a response to the dominant philosophies of positivism and determinism. A philosophical approach of the nineteenth century found in the writings of Kierkegaard and Nietzsche, it emerged in popularity during the twentieth century with two world wars and the threat of nuclear destruction as major social concerns. Individuals needed to understand life in personally relevant terms.

The early writings of existentialists provided a basis for viewing human existence in individually meaningful terms. By having the opportunity for choice, each act we choose is significant and gives meaning to our lives. One of the criticisms leveled against existentialism has been that it presents a despairing view of life (Paterson & Zderad, 1976/1988). Since individuals are faced with freedom of choice, there is always the possibility for making errors. Imagine the experience of being an adolescent making career and personal choices while facing developmental needs of autonomy, identity, body image, and peer acceptance. Intimacy, sexual activity, success, independence, contraception, fear of failure, risk taking, and needs for intimacy all play a part in the daily experience of a middle to late adolescent and influence the eventual outcome of this time of life. Consequently, individuals experience dread as well as hope in the possible consequences of their actions.

According to Corey (1991), several propositions can be drawn from existential thought that have relevance for the helping professions. Corey says that existentialism identifies individuals as (1) having the capacity for self-awareness; (2) having freedom and responsibility; (3) striving to find their own identity while being in relationship with others; (4) being involved in a search for meaning in life; (5) having to experience anxiety or dread if they are going to assume responsibility for their own lives; and, finally, (6) being aware of the reality of death in order to experience the significance of living. Consequently, we live in a world of many possibilities, and the responsibility for making the most out of this existence rests within each of us. As a philosophy, existentialism is particularly applicable to nursing within the framework of holistic health because of the emphasis on self-determination, free choice, and self-responsibility.

Phenomenology, the study of the meaning of a phenomenon to a particular individual, is often thought to have had a significant influence on the development of existentialism because existentialism requires an analysis of the human situation from the perspective of the individual's own experience (Shaffer, 1978). When combined with humanism into an existential-phenomenological-humanistic approach, we are referring to a reverence for life that values the need for human interaction in order to determine the meaning that comes from the individual's unique way of experiencing the world. Although we are ultimately alone in choosing the paths our lives will take, we can find meaning in sharing our experiences with others who are also facing the uncertain choices of daily living. This means that we as nurses must acknowledge our own struggles and needs as part of the process of living. Simultaneously, we must acknowledge the importance of the struggles and needs of others. Only by the interaction of sharing with others, of recognizing the human experience that is unique for each of us but also shared, can we really enter into a humanistic nursing practice.

That Paterson and Zderad have been influenced by the writings of existentialists, humanistic psychologists, and phenomenologists is seen in their emphasis on the meaning of life as it is lived, the nature of dialogue, and the importance of the perceptual field. The influence of scholars such as Bergson (1946), Buber (1965), de Chardin (1961), Desan (1972), Hesse (1966), Jung (1933), Marcel (1956, 1965), and Nietzsche (1927a, 1927b) is readily apparent in the writing of Paterson and Zderad. Their work, *Humanistic nursing*, is a result of years of experience in clinical nursing, reflection, and exploration of these experiences as they have been lived with psychiatric clients, students, nurses, and other helping professionals.

HUMANISTIC NURSING THEORY AND NURSING'S METAPARADIGM

Human Beings

In the theory of humanistic nursing practice, human beings are viewed from an existential framework of becoming through choices. "Man is an individual being necessarily related to other men in time and space. As every man is beholden to other men for his birth and development, interdependence is inherent in the human situation, . . . [and] human existence is coexistence" (Paterson & Zderad, 1976/1988, p. 15). Human beings are characterized as being capable, open to options, persons with values, and the unique manifestation of their past, present, and future. It is through relationships with others that the human being becomes, which in turn, allows for each person's unique individuality to become actualized. Implications for nursing practice are clear. People need information. They need options. Individuals and groups need opportunities to make their own choices.

Health

Health is seen as a matter of personal survival, as a quality of living and dying. It is described as being more than the absence of disease. Individuals have the potential for well-being but also for more-being. Well-being implies a steady state, whereas more-being refers to being in the process of becoming all that is humanly possible (Paterson & Zderad, 1978).

By understanding the existential premise of this theory, it becomes apparent that health is a process of finding meaning in life. Health is experienced in the process of living, of being involved in each moment. Paterson and Zderad suggest throughout their text that we become more (more-being) by being in relationships with each other. When we relate authentically to another, we are experiencing health. This conceptualization of health implies that disease, medical diagnosis, or any form of labeling does little to determine a person's capacity for health. Health can be found in a person's willingness to be open to the experiences of life regardless of his or her physical, social, spiritual, cognitive, or emotional status. Implications for nursing practice include being open to a wide range of definitions of health. Diagnostic categories are useful only if agreed to by the person to whom they refer. The importance of relationships is paramount. The relationship that the nurse has with the person receiving care is critical, but even more important is the need for an appreciation of the relationships that exist in daily living.

Nursing

Nursing, then, is seen within the human context. It is a nurturing response of one person to another in a time of need that aims toward the development of well-being and more-being. Nursing works toward this aim by helping to increase the possibility of making responsible choices, since this is how human beings are able to become. "The nursing situation is a particular kind of human situation in which the interhuman relating is purposely directed toward nurturing the well-being or more-being of a person with perceived needs related to the health–illness quality of living" (Paterson & Zderad, 1976/1988, p. 18). Nursing is concerned with the individual's unique being and striving toward becoming. Nursing focuses on the whole and looks beyond the categorizations of the parts. When a person is ill and the body is manifesting certain changes, these changes influence the person's world and the experience of being in the world. The client's perspective of the world is a vital consideration in nursing. As Paterson and Zderad say:

Nursing implies a special kind of meeting of human persons. It occurs in response to a perceived need related to the health–illness quality of the human condition. Within that domain, which is shared by other health professions, nursing is directed toward the goal of nurturing well-being and more-being (human potential). Nursing, therefore does not involve a merely fortuitous encounter but rather one in which there is purposeful call and response. In this vein, humanistic nursing may be considered as a special kind of lived dialogue (Paterson & Zderad, 1976/1988, p. 24).

Nursing is seen as a unique blend of theory and methodology. The theory may be articulated from the open framework that is derived from the human situation. This framework can be used to suggest the possible dimensions of humanistic nursing practice. Theory cannot exist without the practice of nursing, for it depends on the experience of nursing and on the reflecting of that experience. It is this practice of nursing, its methodology, that Paterson and Zderad (1976/1988) describe as a unique blend of art and science. It is suggested that nurses have downplayed the art of nursing in an attempt to be accepted among other empirical disciplines. However, science and art both play critical roles in humanistic nursing. If one thinks of the rules that we follow (thermoregulation, fluid and electrolyte balance, stages of grieving, growth and development) as our science, we can see that these rules guide us. They give direction to our nursing practice, but all those laws, principles, and theories remain meaningless unless they are applied to living situations. How a nurse uses theory in response to knowing a client is the art of nursing. The art of nursing is embodied in the interaction between the nurse and the client. Like all art, that interaction is often meaningful, effective, and capable of leaving a lasting impression. Nursing as an art is being able to use theories within the context of life as people struggle to become all that they are capable of becoming.

The elements of the framework for humanistic nursing, as stated by Paterson and Zderad (1976/1988), may be described as follows:

> Incarnate men (patient and nurse) meeting (being and becoming) in a goal-directed (nurturing well-being and more-being), intersubjective transaction (being with and doing with) occurring in time and space (as measured and as lived by patient and nurse) in a world of men and things (p. 21).

To use this framework for a nursing practice theory, the authors have suggested three concepts that together provide the basis (or components) of nursing: dialogue, community, and phenomenologic nursology. By coming together through dialogue, a community is formed through which nursing strives to nurture and comfort. The model that should come to mind is a visual model, readily accessible from one's many life experiences. The concepts that form this theory should generate mental pictures of people that one has known—people touching, listening, laughing, crying, contemplating, being in the day-to-day world. An appreciation of the importance of these people to ourselves and to those we work with can provide the model of humanistic nursing.

Dialogue. Nursing is a lived dialogue. It is the nurse–nursed relating creatively. Humans need nursing. Nurses need to nurse. Nursing is an intersubjective experience in which there is real sharing. Involved in this dialogue are meeting, relating, presence, and a call and response (Paterson & Zderad, 1976/1988).

Meeting. Meeting is the coming together of human beings and is characterized by the expectation that there will be a nurse and a nursed. Factors that influence this meeting are feelings that are aroused by the anticipation of the meeting, the amount of control that the nurse or client has in coming together, the uniqueness of the nurse and the client, and the decision for disclosure and enclosure with the other.

Relating. The process of nurse–nursed "doing" with each other is relating, being with the other. Two ways of relating are described that distinguish the human situation. We are able to relate as subject to object as well as subject to subject. "Both types of relationships are essential for genuine human existence" (Paterson & Zderad, 1976/1988, p. 26). Subject–object relating refers to how human beings use objects and know others through abstractions, conceptualizations, categorizing, labeling, and so on. Subject–subject relating occurs when two persons are open to each other as fully human. The "I–Thou" relationship described by Martin Buber (1958) provides the opportunity to develop this unique potential. Paterson and Zderad further describe relating as follows:

> Through the scientific objective approach, that is, subject–object relating, it is possible to gain certain knowledge about a person; through intersubjective, that is, subject–subject relating, it is possible to know a person in his unique individuality. Thus, both subject–subject and subject–object relationships are essential to the clinical nursing process. Both are integral elements of humanistic nursing (p. 27).

Presence. The quality of being open, receptive, ready, and available to another person in a reciprocal manner is presence. Presence necessitates being open to the whole of the nursing experience, behavior that is difficult to achieve when the nurse at times is required to focus on specific details of the client's body or behavior. "Man is an embodied being, and the nurse, in nurturing the patient's well-being and more-being, must relate to him and his body in their mysterious interrelatedness" (Paterson & Zderad, 1976/1988, p. 29).

Call and response. The complex nature of the lived dialogue is seen in call and response. Call and response are transactional, sequential, and simultaneous. Nurses and clients call and respond to each other both verbally and nonverbally, and there is the potential to be "all-at-once." Paterson and Zderad (1976/1988) describe the "all-at-once" as nurses being able to relate simultaneously to the subjective and objective aspects of the lived situation. Despite the fact that we can express this experience verbally or in writing in succession only, it is paradoxically occurring simultaneously for the nurse.

It is through nursing acts that the dialogue of nursing is lived. The meaning of those acts to the nurse and to the client may differ and may act as a potential catalyst for effecting change in the dialogue.

When considering nursing as a lived dialogue, it is necessary to take into account the situation in which it occurs—the real world of other human beings and things within a framework of time and space.

Community. The phenomenon of community is the second component critical to humanistic nursing practice theory. It is two or more persons striving together, living-dying all at once. To understand community is to recognize and value uniqueness. Humanistic nursing leads to community; it occurs within a community and is affected by community. It is through the intersubjective sharing of meaning in community that human beings are comforted and nurtured. Community is the experience of persons, and it is through community, persons relating to others, that it is possible to become (Paterson & Zderad, 1976/1988; Praeger, 1980). This component represents the strong humanistic influence of the theory. People find meaning in their existence by sharing and relating to others. Paterson and Zderad consider community as the "We" that occurs with clients, families, professional colleagues, and other health care providers.

Phenomenologic nursology. Nursing, its practice and theory, would not be complete without a methodology. Patterson and Zderad named their methodology phenomenologic nursology. There are five phases in this phenomenologic approach to nursing, as discussed below.

1. *Preparation of the nurse knower for coming to know.* The nurse is ever prepared and striving to be open and caring. This involves learning to take risks, being open to experiences, to one's own view of the world, and to another's perceptual framework. To achieve this, the nurse needs to be exposed to a wide range of experiences. Nurses can be prepared for this by immersing themselves in studies in the humanities, where varying views about the nature of being are expressed. Individual experiences, as a person and a nurse, are valid and important. The wider the range of experiences the nurse has, the wider the possibility for knowing. Relating the experiences of human beings in literature and the other arts to the nurse's experience with clients opens the way for knowing individuals in the nursing situation. Self-knowledge, the "authenticity with self," is important to knowing and can be

facilitated through clinical supervision and different forms of personal growth therapy (Paterson & Zderad, 1976/1988).

2. *Nurse knowing the other intuitively.* This phase is the merging of the self with the rhythmic spirit of the other. Intuitive knowing of the other requires getting "inside" the other, into the rhythm of the other's experience, which results in a special, difficult to express, knowledge of the other. Intuitive knowing presumes the I–Thou relationship described by Buber (1958). It also presumes a phenomenological approach: being open to the meaning of the experience for the other. For the nurse to be able intuitively to grasp the phenomenon of a nursing situation, several steps can be taken to facilitate openness. Paterson and Zderad (1976/1988) suggest that we go into the nursing situation without any preconceived notions, trying to avoid expectations, labeling, and judgments. It is important first to know where one's preconceptions come from by being aware of one's philosophical and theoretical biases. Being aware of nursing routines and how they can dull our sensitivities can enhance one's perspective. For instance, routine testing of urine, blood pressure, and fetal heart tones during prenatal visits can reduce the pregnant woman to feeling like a weigh and check station. When we use closed-end questions or checklists during assessment, we limit in advance the range of responses that a client can give. Openness and a refusal to be lulled by routines help nurses better appreciate how these activities require a conscious effort on the part of the nurse to be self-aware. By doing this, however, nurses can be open to all the nursing situation and will be better able to grasp intuitively the subtle nuances involved in human interaction.

3. *Nurse knowing the other scientifically.* This phase implies a separateness from what is known. It requires taking the all-at-once phenomena that are known intuitively and looking at them, mulling them over, analyzing, sorting, comparing, contrasting, relating, interpreting, giving a name to, and categorizing them. This is taking the I–Thou and reflecting on it as an "it." Paterson and Zderad (1976/1988) say, "The challenge of communicating a lived nursing reality demands authenticity with the self and rigorous effort in the selection of words, phrases, and precise grammar" (p. 73). To achieve this goal, the nurse must be adequately prepared in the liberal arts and sciences. Nurses need to be able to reflect critically on the experience at the same time that they are immersed in the experience. Communication skills are critical as the nurse seeks clarification and verification from the client. For example, when working with adolescents who are struggling with home, school, and relationship problems, the unfolding of their story can be laid out in a genogram and ecomap. These tools can then be used to identify patterns over generations, to visualize recurrent themes, and to help the adolescent recognize areas of strengths as well as areas of risk.

4. *Nurse complementarily synthesizing known others.* This phase involves relating, comparing, and contrasting what occurs in nursing situations to enlarge one's understanding of nursing. The nurse compares and synthesizes multiple known realities and arrives at an expanded view. The nurse allows a dialogue between the realities and permits differences (Paterson & Zderad,

1976/1988). In this phase, the nurse uses not only personal experience but also the rich theoretical foundation of education and practice in order to put the clinical situation in perspective.

5. Succession within the nurse from the many to the paradoxical one. The fifth phase evolves from the descriptive process of a lived phenomenon. It is the articulated vision of experience that becomes expressed in a coherent whole. This phase is the process of refining the intuitive grasp achieved before, struggling with the known realities, and making an intuitive leap toward truth, thus forming a new hypothetical construct. Since the multiple realities and known truths are part of the nurse, the new truth is really an expression of the knower in abstract or conceptual terms beyond the individual data. It is a truth beyond the synthesis of the whole. So, the paradox rests in the fact that the nurse starts with a general notion, an intuitive grasp; then studies it, compares, contrasts, and synthesizes it in order to arrive at a truth that is uniquely personal but has meaning for all: a descriptive theoretical construct of nursing.

These last three phases (analysis, synthesis, and description) involve many of the same techniques. In each of these phases, the nurse might compare and contrast the phenomena. Commonalities in various experiences could be explored as well as the relationship between variables in the clinical situation. It would also be important to determine what distinguishes one phenomenon from another. For example, why do some women respond to menopause with fear and grieving whereas others experience it as a time of joy and renewed energy? Other techniques for analyzing, synthesizing, and describing a nursing phenomenon include stating what it is not, using analogy or metaphor. These techniques help the nurse better understand the meaning of the experience (Paterson & Zderad, 1976/1988).

PHENOMENOLOGIC NURSOLOGY AND THE NURSING PROCESS

Phenomenologic nursology as developed by Paterson and Zderad is a methodology for understanding and describing nursing situations. It is a method of inquiry, as is the problem-solving approach of the nursing process. Phenomenologic nursology is a method of seeking to understand the nurse–nursed experience so that the nurse can be with the nursed in a human and therefore healing manner. The nursing process assumes the presence of a nursing problem that the nurse and client will solve together. Phenomenologic nursology assumes a perceived health need by an individual who is involved in an interaction with a health care provider.

Phenomenology is a descriptive process. It is not concerned specifically with facts; it assumes that facts exist (Owens, 1970). Rather, it is concerned with the nature of the facts and what they mean to the individual. Phenomenology describes phenomena but does not attempt to explain or predict their occurrence.

Nursing process and nursology are similar in many aspects. Both methodologies use a systematic approach to client interaction.

The first step of the nursing process is *assessment*. Assessment includes a collection of subjective and objective data about an individual obtained through observation, interaction with the client, and information from other sources such as laboratory studies. Phenomenologic nursology includes the collection of subjective and objective data but is broader in scope than what is traditionally meant by assessment.

Preparation of the nurse knower for coming to know as the first phase of phenomenologic nursology can be seen as a prerequisite similar to but distinct from the nursing process. Almost all nurses are educated in the humanities and sciences before beginning nursing practice in the clinical situation. The nursing process assumes that the individual undertaking the process is educated in the bio-psycho-social-spiritual needs of the individual. Phenomenologic nursology makes these same assumptions but also assumes that the nurse has a sensitivity to and knowledge of the human condition as well as self-knowledge. The humanistic theory and practice of nursing require that the practitioner be able to subjectively experience the other. As mentioned earlier, the nursing student can be helped to understand another's situation by studying the humanities and fine arts. Experiencing life events through literature, drama, and the arts enriches the student's understanding of human experiences such as love, joy, loneliness, suffering, and death. The use of guided imagery and other exercises are also helpful in developing empathy, the ability to experience the other. The development of self-awareness is important if the nurse expects to encounter others in dialogue. Self-awareness can be enhanced through journaling, working in small groups, and through meditation.

Nurse knowing the other intuitively also occurs before the traditional assessment phase of the nursing process, even though intuition is indeed a kind of initial assessment. This phase is characterized by a "taking in" of the client in the human situation, the empathic encounter, the beginning of the I–Thou relationship wherein the nurse understands the other's experience all-at-once. It is an intuitive grasp of the other's situation (Paterson & Zderad, 1976/1988). The use of intuition is a significant aspect of assessment. Although intuition is not a new tool in nursing, its respectability has often been denied. In the effort to establish itself as a profession, nursing has used an increasingly scientific, objective approach to the study of nursing and the individuals who use nursing services. The humanistic nurse, however, believes that the subjective experience of human beings is as valid as the objective experience that can be measured.

The assessment and early analysis phases of the nursing process can be compared to the *nurse knowing the other scientifically*. This phase of nursology includes the more familiar method of looking at a phenomenon from many aspects: comparing, classifying, and looking for themes in relationships and among the parts. Dividing persons into biological, psychological, social, and spiritual parts is an example of classifying data. It is important to understand in the phenomenologic method of nursology that the call comes first, followed by intuition, then assessment, and then analysis. In the problem-solving method, a problem statement by the client is followed by scientific data collection organized by parts, and intuition is not included in the assessment or analysis.

The later stages of analysis in the nursing process are quite similar to the phase in nursology called *nurse complementarily synthesizing known others.* During the analysis portion of the nursing process, as described earlier, the nurse compares the data with other known realities such as developmental stages, Maslow's hierarchy of needs, and physiologic principles. In nursology, the nurse compares "multiple known realities" with the data and the experience of the client. In other words, the nurse examines the data and experience of the client in light of scientific and subjective knowledge and then compares, contrasts, and ultimately synthesizes to an expanded view (Paterson & Zderad, 1976/1988). Comparisons do occur in the phenomenologic method, but the purpose of the comparisons is directed toward identifying relationships and patterns with much consideration given to opposites and polarities. The phenomenologist synthesizes opposites and patterns into a larger concept, whereas the problem solver chooses a pattern and decides whether it is a problem or not (Oiler, 1982).

Diagnosis refers to the step of the nursing process in which the nurse makes a problem statement. The nurse collects data regarding the client's stated need, then analyzes the data by classifying it, comparing it to known theory and principles, and finally arriving at a conclusion that is a statement of the problem. Succession within the nurse from the many to the paradoxical one can be compared to the stage of identifying a diagnosis. After synthesizing the ideas, data, and experience, the nurse reaches a conclusion that is broader than the classifications and reflects the experience of the client as well as the nurse's initial intuitive grasp of the situation. This conclusion has meaning for all (Paterson & Zderad, 1976/1988).

The *planning* and *implementation* phases of the nursing process describe a goal or outcome to be reached by the client with steps (objectives) to be accomplished toward the goal. Specific nurse and client actions are spelled out in detail. Phenomenologic nursology does not describe the formation of a goal-directed nursing care plan. Humanistic nursing is concerned with being with another who is in need. The goal of more-being or well-being is accomplished through dialogue. In the dialogue between nurse and nursed, there is the *meeting* and the *presence* of the nurse for the other, and the *call* and *response* between the nurse and the nursed, the I–Thou relationship. This is the therapeutic relationship. Paterson and Zderad (1976/1988) say that this relationship takes place in the nursing situation in the real world; however, they do not elaborate on incorporating the "doing" aspects of nursing into the dialogue. The theory evolved from the authors' psychiatric nursing practice and experience where the "doing" is the relationship. However, glimpses of how they have practiced humanistic nursing are available in the rich descriptions of clinical experiences throughout the text. Examples of using touch, participating in a task such as shampooing, and spending time with clients demonstrate that any nursing interaction with a client can be a vehicle for nurturing more-being.

The *evaluation* phase of the nursing process is deciding whether the client's behavior has changed as measured by the goals and objectives. The behavior changes result from the actions of the nurse and client. By nature of being humanistic, the concern is not with the resultant behavior but with the meaning of the experience for the client. The humanistic nurse might see a change in the client's perspective of his or her experience. A client who is able to make choices about health care activities and assume responsibility for those choices would be able to find meaning in life. By doing this with a nurse, the client would have the opportunity to affirm the humanness of the situation from his or her own perspective, resulting in personal growth, more-being, or health. For example, humanistic nursing may involve being-with another who is grieving, rather than using a series of strategies designed to assist a person toward resolution of grief work. Being-with a person who is grieving in an I–Thou relationship expands the individual's opportunities for more-being so that sadness may be shared with another. This may result in the client's feeling more able to make choices and continue with life's demands. An outcome of nursing process, in contrast, may be that the client demonstrates an activity that indicates grieving is progressing—for instance, by returning to school or work.

PATERSON AND ZDERAD'S WORK AND THE CHARACTERISTICS OF A THEORY

1. Theories can interrelate concepts in such a way as to create a different way of looking at a particular phenomenon. Paterson and Zderad (1976/1988) say that nursing is a lived dialogue between the nurse and the nursed directed toward the goal of nurturing well-being and more-being in the everyday world of men and things. The authors have interrelated the four concepts of human beings, health, nursing, and society so that a different way of looking at the phenomenon of nursing has been created for using existential philosophy and phenomenological methodology within a humanistic framework. Nursing is described as an intersubjective transaction that has a new and different description of nursing although it is similar in concept to other nursing theories. Theories describe, explain, or predict phenomena. Humanistic nursing theory is descriptive; the phenomenological approach is a descriptive method.

2. Theories must be logical in nature. Humanistic nursing theory is logical because Paterson and Zderad provide a framework and methodology for nursing practice. Also, the ideas and concepts fit together in a meaningful way.

3. Theories should be relatively simple yet generalizable. Humanistic nursing theory is not simple; indeed it is somewhat difficult to grasp unless the nurse is familiar with existential philosophy and phenomenology. The theory focuses on the dialogue between the nurse and the nursed as a unique encounter between two people. Knowledge gained by repeated study of this encounter provides a generalizable concept. In fact, the final step of nursology is the expression of a concept. Thus the theory is generalizable.

4. Theories can be the bases for hypotheses that can be tested or for theory to be generated, and

5. Theories contribute to and assist in increasing the general body of knowledge within the discipline through the research implemented to validate them. Paterson and Zderad's (1976/1988) theory provides a basis for hypotheses that can be tested. The authors describe several replications of the methodology and present numerous concepts that could be examined. Since it is testable, phenomenologic nursology is an excellent medium for concept and theory development.

6. Theories can be used by practitioners to guide and improve their practice. Humanistic nursing theory, including phenomenologic nursology, can certainly be used by nurses to guide and improve practice. Although nurses may find the concepts new at first, a study of humanistic psychology and existential philosophy facilitates an understanding of the concepts and an appreciation of human potential.

7. Theories must be consistent with other validated theories, laws and principles but will leave open unanswered questions that need to be investigated. Humanistic nursing theory is consistent with existentialism, humanistic psychology, and phenomenology upon which it is based. Because the theory is descriptive and generalizable, it can be applied in any nursing situation and leaves the nursing situation always open for examination.

STRENGTHS AND LIMITATIONS

This theory has several notable strengths. The methodology is well developed and the concepts are fully described within the parameters of existential philosophy, phenomenology, and nursing. This theory broadens the possibilities for explaining and describing nursing. The study of human beings and nursing using this phenomenological method is a valid approach that enhances knowledge of nursing. An important contribution of this theory is that the methodology leads to concept formation, which is the basis of theory and the springboard of new inquiry. The theory provides a unique, unusual approach to the study of nursing. Another strength is the strong nursing focus. The theory developed from the lived experiences of clinical nurses and reflects that nursing perspective.

Reading the text provides an opportunity to experience the authors' own grappling with theory development. The text is written with a readable style that is often poetic in quality. Although the authors tend to combine words into broader hyphenated meanings, they attempt to explain each term in a variety of ways. One of the joys of this text is sitting down to the individual essays and experiencing the possibilities that the authors suggest are available in nursing. Each chapter is inspiring and stimulates creative ideas for clinical practice. Some readers might find the text too intuitive and lacking in concrete imperatives. It is not a handy reference text that can be used to solve clinical practice problems quickly. There are no formulas for successful nursing in their theory. This is as it should be, for the theory posits that nursing is interactive and based on the moment of the interaction.

Unfortunately, some nurses might need to be well read in the humanities, particularly philosophy, in order to understand the language and the existential tone. Another difficulty may occur for new practitioners regarding the functional aspects of nursing. Since it is essentially descriptive, humanistic nursing theory provides challenges for quantitative validation that some may view as a limitation, although this would be of limited concern to a humanistic nurse or philosopher who is concerned with description.

REFERENCES

Bergson, H. (1946). *The creative mind*. New York: The Philosophical Library. [out of print]

Buber, M. (1958). *I and Thou* (2nd ed.). New York: Charles Scribner's Sons. [out of print]

Buber, M. (1965). Distance and relation. In M. Friedman (Ed.), & R. G. Smith (Trans.), *The knowledge of man*. New York: Harper & Row. [out of print]

Bugental, J. F. T. (1978). The third force in psychology. In D. Welch, G. Tate, & F. Richards (Eds.), *Humanistic psychology: A sourcebook*. Buffalo, NY: Prometheus Books. [out of print]

Corey, G. (1991). *Theory and practice of counseling and psychotherapy* (4th ed.). Pacific Grove, CA: Brooks/Cole.

de Chardin, T. (1961). *The phenomenon of man*. New York: Harper & Row. [out of print]

Desan, W. (1972). *Planetary man*. New York: Macmillan. [out of print]

Hesse, H. (1966). *Steppenwolf*. New York: Holt, Rinehart & Winston. [out of print]

Jung, C. G. (1933). *Modern man in search of a soul*. New York: Harcourt, Brace & World. [out of print]

Marcel, G. (1956). *The philosophy of existentialism*. M. Harari (Trans.). New York: Citadel Press. [out of print]

Marcel, G. (1965). *Being and having: An existentialist diary*. New York: Harper Torchbooks, Harper & Row. [out of print]

Nietzsche, F. (1927a). Beyond good and evil. In H. Zimmern (Trans.). *The philosophy of Nietzsche*. New York: Random House. [out of print]

Nietzsche, F. (1927b). Thus spake Zarathustra. In T. Common (Trans.). *The philosophy of Nietzsche*. New York: Random House. [out of print]

Oiler, C. (1982). The phenomenological approach to nursing research. *Nursing Research, 31,* 180.

Owens, T. (1970). *Phenomenology and intersubjectivity*. The Hague, Netherlands: Martinus Nijhoff. [out of print]

Paterson, J., & Zderad, L. (1978, December). *Humanistic nursing.* Paper presented at the 2nd Annual Nurse Educator Conference, New York, NY.

Paterson, J., & Zderad, L. (1988). *Humanistic nursing.* New York: National League for Nursing. (Originally published, 1976, Wiley.)

Praeger, S. G. (1980). *Humanistic nursing education: Considerations and proposals.* Project in lieu of dissertation, University of Northern Colorado.

Shaffer, J. B. P. (1978). *Humanistic psychology.* Englewood Cliffs, NJ: Prentice-Hall. [out of print]

Zderad, L. T. (1978). From here-and-now to theory: Reflections on "How." In *Theory development: What, why, how?* New York: National League for Nursing. [out of print]

JEAN WATSON

Barbara Talento

■ ■ ■

Jean Watson (b. 1940) received her nursing diploma from Lewis Gale Hospital, Roanoke, VA; her BS in nursing from the University of Colorado, Boulder; her MS in psychiatric–mental health nursing from the University of Colorado, Denver; and her PhD in Educational Psychology from the University of Colorado, Boulder. She is currently Distinguished Professor, Director, Center for Human Caring, School of Nursing, University of Colorado Health Science Center, Denver. She has practiced nursing in private practice, as a clinical consultant, nurse researcher, faculty member, and educational administrator. She is a Fellow in the American Academy of Nursing and has received numerous other awards and honors, including a Visiting Kellogg Fellowship at Western Australia Institute of Technology and an International Fulbright Award. She holds honorary doctorates from Assumption College, Worcester, MA, and the University of Akron, OH. Watson has been an invited distinguished lecturer in numerous countries such as Israel, Canada, Japan, Australia, and Taiwan as well as in the United States. She is the author of numerous articles, book chapters, and two books. Her research has been in the area of human caring and loss.

The foundation of Jean Watson's theory of nursing was published in 1979 in *Nursing: The philosophy and science of caring.* In 1985, with a re-release in 1988, her theory was published in *Nursing: Human science and human care.* Watson believes that the main focus in nursing is on carative factors that are derived from a humanistic perspective combined with a scientific knowledge base. For nurses to develop humanistic philosophies and value systems, a strong liberal arts background is necessary. This philosophy and value system, in turn, provides a solid foundation for the science of caring. A liberal arts base can assist nurses to expand their vision and views of the world and to develop critical thinking skills. An expanded world view and critical thinking skills are needed in the science of caring, which focuses on health promotion rather than on cure of disease.

According to Watson (1979), curing disease is the domain of medicine. She asserts that the caring stance that nursing has always held is being threatened by the tasks and technology demands of the curative factors. In Watson's works, one finds reference to existential humanists such as Erikson

(1963), Heidegger (1962), Maslow (1954), and Rogers (1967). In addition, she uses the theories of Selye (1956) and Lazarus (1966) to delineate stress and caring, and the theories of Leininger (1981) and Henderson (1964) for nursing knowledge. Overall, a humanistic value system undergirds her construction of the science of caring.

WATSON'S THEORY

Watson (1979) proposes seven assumptions about the science of caring and ten primary carative factors to form the framework of her theory. The basic assumptions are the following:

1. Caring can be effectively demonstrated and practiced only interpersonally.
2. Caring consists of carative factors that result in the satisfaction of certain human needs.
3. Effective caring promotes health and individual or family growth.
4. Caring responses accept a person not only as he or she is now but as what he or she may become.
5. A caring environment is one that offers the development of potential while allowing the person to choose the best action for himself or herself at a given point in time.
6. Caring is more "healthogenic" than is curing. The practice of caring integrates biophysical knowledge with knowledge of human behavior to generate or promote health and to provide ministrations to those who are ill. A science of caring is therefore complementary to the science of curing.
7. The practice of caring is central to nursing (pp. 8–9).

Watson (1985/1988) views caring as the most valuable attribute nursing has to offer to humanity, yet caring has, over time, received less emphasis than other aspects of the practice of nursing. She states:

> The human care role [in nursing] is threatened by increased medical technology, bureaucratic-managerial institutional constraints in a nuclear age society. At the same time there has been a proliferation of curing and radical treatment cure techniques often without regard to costs (p. 33).

In today's world, nursing seems to be responding to the various demands of the machinery with less consideration of the needs of the person attached to the machine. In Watson's view, the disease might be cured, but illness would remain because without caring health is not attained. Caring is the essence of nursing and connotes responsiveness between the nurse and the person; the nurse co-participates with the person. Watson contends that caring can assist the person to gain control, become knowledgeable, and promote health changes. In Watson's humanistic value system, there is a high regard for autonomy and freedom of choice, which leads to an emphasis on client self-knowledge and self-control and client as the person in charge.

The structure for the science of caring is built upon the following ten carative factors:

1. The formation of a humanistic-altruistic system of values
2. The instillation of faith–hope
3. The cultivation of sensitivity to one's self and to others
4. The development of a helping–trust relationship
5. The promotion and acceptance of the expression of positive and negative feelings
6. The systematic use of the scientific problem-solving method for decision making
7. The promotion of interpersonal teaching–learning
8. The provision for a supportive, protective, and(or) corrective mental, physical, sociocultural, and spiritual environment
9. Assistance with the gratification of human needs
10. The allowance for existential-phenomenological forces (Watson, 1979, pp. 9–10).

Of these ten carative factors, the first three form the "philosophical foundation for the science of caring" (Watson, 1979, p. 10). *The formation of a humanistic-altruistic value system* (carative factor 1) begins developmentally at an early age with values shared with parents. This value system is mediated through one's own life experiences, the learning one gains, and exposure to the humanities. Watson (1979) suggests that caring that is based on humanistic values and altruistic behavior can be developed through examination of one's own views, beliefs, interactions with various cultures, and personal growth experiences. These are all perceived as necessary to the nurse's own maturation, which then promotes altruistic behavior toward others.

Faith–hope (carative factor 2) is essential to both the carative and the curative processes. Nurses need to transcend the push toward acceptance of only Western medicine and assist the person in an understanding of alternatives such as meditation or the healing power of belief in self or in the spiritual (Watson, 1979). Watson's (1985/1988) emphasis on the spiritual, with the inclusion of the soul, is unusual in theory development. When modern science has nothing further to offer the person, the nurse can continue to use faith–hope to provide a sense of well-being through those beliefs that are meaningful to the individual.

Cultivation of sensitivity to self and others (carative factor 3) explores the need of the nurse to begin to feel an emotion as it presents itself. It is only through development of one's own feelings that one can genuinely and sensitively interact with others. As nurses strive to increase their own sensitivity, they become more authentic. Becoming authentic encourages self-growth and self-actualization in both the nurse and those with whom the nurse interacts. A basic premise of Watson's (1985/1988) is that:

> A person's mind and emotions are windows to the soul. Nursing care can be and is physical, procedural, objective, and factual, but at the highest level of nursing the nurses' human care responses, the human care transactions, and the nurses' presence in the relationship transcend the physical material world, bound in time and space, and make contact with the person's emotional and subjective world as the route to the inner self and the higher sense of self (p. 50).

Furthermore, she contends that nurses promote health and higher level functioning only when they form person-to-person relationships as opposed to manipulative relationships (Watson, 1979).

To appreciate the remaining seven carative factors, one needs to understand that they spring from the foundation developed by these first three. Therefore, the nurse develops a humanistic-altruistic value system, believes in the instillation of faith–hope, and cultivates sensitivity to self and to others to develop a helping-trust relationship and the rest of the carative factors. One of the strongest tools the nurse can use in *establishing a helping–trust relationship* (carative factor 4) is a mode of communication that establishes rapport and caring. Watson uses the works of Rogers (1962), Carkhuff (1971), and Gazda (1975) to define the characteristics needed in the helping–trust relationship. These characteristics are congruence, empathy, and warmth. Congruence implies that nurses are genuine in their interactions and do not put up facades; that nurses act in an open and honest manner. Empathy refers to the attempt that nurses make to tune into the feelings of their clients. Empathy may be described as "walking in another's moccasins" in that it allows the nurse to accept the client's feelings without responding defensively with anger or fear. Warmth refers to the positive acceptance of another. It is expressed most often by open body language, touch, and tone of voice.

Communication in this context includes verbal and nonverbal communication and listening in a manner that connotes empathetic understanding. It is through this intense focus on communication that the nurse can center on clues and themes that can lead to an even greater depth of awareness for the person. One barrier in this process is that thoughts are often substituted for feelings, which precludes the ability to reach deeper levels of awareness. *The expression of feelings, both positive and negative* (carative factor 5) ought to be facilitated because, according to Watson (1979), such expression improves one's level of awareness. "Feelings alter thoughts and behavior, and they need to be considered and allowed for in a caring relationship" (p. 44). Indeed, if one can become aware of the feeling, one can often understand the behavior it engenders.

In carative factor 6, the issue of *research and systematic problem solving* is presented. Because nurses are occupied with the tasks of nursing (ie, treatments, procedures, charts), they often fail to address the larger issues of conducting research, defining the discipline, or developing a scientific base for nursing. However, Watson (1979) believes that:

> Without the systematic use of the scientific problem-solving method, effective practice is accidental at best and haphazard or harmful at worst. The scientific problem-solving method is the only method that allows for control and prediction, and that permits self-correction (pp. 55–56).

Watson makes a strong argument for the need for the absolutism of the scientific method, but she also values the relative nature of nursing and makes an equally strong argument for the need to examine and develop other methods of knowing to provide a holistic perspective. The science of caring should not always be neutral and objective, two important characteristics of the scientific method.

Promotion of interpersonal teaching–learning (carative factor 7) is the factor that affords people the most control over their own health because it provides them with both information and alternatives. The caring nurse focuses on the learning process as much as the teaching process, for learning offers the best way to individualize the information to be disseminated. Understanding the person's perceptions of the situation assists the nurse to prepare a cognitive plan that works within the person's framework and alleviates the stress of the event (Watson, 1979).

Carative factor 8 deals with the daily, routine functions that the nurse uses to promote health, restore to health, or prevent illness. It is the factor labeled as *provision for a supportive, protective and(or) corrective mental, physical, sociocultural, and spiritual environment.* Watson (1979) divides these functions into external variables, such as the physical, safety, and environmental factors, and internal variables, such as mental, spiritual, or cultural activities, which the nurse manipulates in order to provide support and protection for the person's mental and physical well-being.

There is an interdependence between the external and the internal environments because it is the person's perceptions that render the environment as threatening or nonthreatening. Although the subjective appraisal of threat can be a distortion of reality, the perception of threat is still a stressful event to the person. Events such as change of job, divorce, illness, and loss of a loved one can arouse a sense of threat. Through assessment, the nurse can determine the person's appraisal of the situation and abilities to cope. Then the nurse can supply situational support, help the person develop a more accurate perception, or provide the cognitive information that can strengthen the patient's own coping mechanisms. Watson (1979) suggests that the nurse also must provide comfort, privacy, and safety as part of this carative factor. In addition, she believes that a basic element is a clean-esthetic environment. While clean, sterile surroundings might not be health promoting, esthetics can improve health through promotion of increased self-worth and dignity. A pleasant environment improves the affective state, facilitates interactions with others, and promotes a sense of satisfaction with life.

Carative factor 9, *assistance with the gratification of human needs,* is grounded in a hierarchy of needs similar to that of Maslow (1954). However, Watson has created a hierarchy that she considers to be relevant to the science of caring in nursing. The following are Watson's (1979) ordering of needs:

1. Lower Order Needs (Biophysical Needs)   **Survival Needs**
   The need for food and fluid
   The need for elimination
   The need for ventilation
2. Lower Order Needs (Psychophysical Needs)   **Functional Needs**
   The need for activity-inactivity
   The need for sexuality
3. Higher Order Needs (Psychosocial Needs)   **Integrative Needs**
   The need for achievement
   The need for affiliation
4. Higher Order Need (Intrapersonal-Interpersonal Need)   **Growth-seeking**
   The need for self-actualization (p. 108).   **Need**

Establishing hierarchical needs does not preclude the necessity to view each person in the context of the whole. Meeting only lower order needs may not assist the complex human being toward self-actualization. Each need is viewed in the context of all the others, and all are valued. Watson (1979) also says:

> Keeping in mind the holistic-dynamic framework for viewing the human needs, the carative factor assistance with the gratification of human needs leads to a more complete development of each human need. Some needs are more familiar and concrete because of the tangible ways in which they manifest themselves. Others are more abstract and elusive. They are equally important for quality nursing care and the promotion of optimal health (pp. 109–111).

Overall, the theme is that, despite the hierarchical nature in which they are presented, the needs all deserve to be attended to and valued.

Research findings have established a correlation between emotional distress and illness. Therefore, an assessment that uses an holistic approach that examines the "dynamic, symbolic aspects of each need" (Watson, 1979, p. 117) provides a more balanced portrait of the person. Watson states:

> The current thinking about holistic care emphasizes (1) that etiological components that have many factors interact and produce change through complex neurophysiological and neurochemical pathways, (2) that each psychological function has a physiological correlate, and (3) that each physiological function has a psychological correlate (pp. 117–118).

TABLE 18–1. HOLISTIC CARE NEEDS IN BULIMIA AND ANOREXIA

Watson's Hierarchy	Application to Bulimia and Anorexia
Higher Order Need (interpersonal)	Self-actualization retarded
	Unrealistic sense of perfection never achieved
Higher Order Needs (psychosocial)	Diminished sense of achievement secondary to distorted body image
	Self-involvement leads to diminished affiliative activity, possibly impaired sexual relationships
Lower Order Needs (psychophysical)	Purge or binge or self-imposed starvation depletes cellular nutrition, leading to decreased activity
	Body image distortion may impair sexuality
Lower Order Needs (biophysical)	Food and fluids restricted

As an example, disturbances found in the biophysical need for food and fluid demonstrate the requirement for holistic care. Bulimia, anorexia, and gastrointestinal ulcers are just a few of the disorders that indicate the complex interaction between the physiological and the psychological. Watson's work delineates the interrelationship in each area of her hierarchy (see Table 18–1).

Allowance for existential phenomenological factors is carative factor 10. Phenomenology is a way of understanding people from the way things appear to them, from their frame of reference (Watson, 1979). Existential psychology is the study of human existence using phenomenological analysis. For the nurse, this factor helps to reconcile and mediate the incongruity of viewing the person holistically while at the same time attending to a hierarchical ordering of needs. Incorporating these factors into the science of nursing assists the nurse to understand the meaning the person finds in life or to help the person find meaning in difficult life events, or both. Because life, illness, and death are basically irrational, the nurse using carative factor 10 may assist the person to find the strength or courage to confront life or death. Watson suggests that each nurse must turn inward to face his or her own existential questions before being able to assist others to cope with the human predicament.

WATSON'S THEORY AND NURSING'S METAPARADIGM

Human Being

Although in Watson's earlier writings she refers to her work as a philosophy and science of nursing, in her later book she clearly states that the work represents a nursing theory (Watson, 1985/1988). In that context, and using nursing's heritage, she adopts a view of the human being as:

. . . a valued person in and of him- or herself to be cared for, respected, nurtured, understood, and assisted; in general a philosophical view of a person as a fully functional integrated self. The human is viewed as greater than, and different from, the sum of his or her parts (p. 14).

She believes that humans are best viewed in a developmental conflicts frame and that "systematic attention to developmental conflicts of individuals and their families is necessary for health care" (Watson, 1979, p. 246). These conflicts, based upon Erikson's model, are primarily psychosocial and represent crises and turning points encountered throughout the human life cycle. Commonly occurring, these conflicts can elicit a stress reaction that requires a coping response. The nurse must understand human beings when they are sick, well, or under stress.

Health

Although acknowledging the World Health Organization's definition of health as the positive state of physical, mental, and social well-being, Watson (1979) believes that other factors need to be included. She adds the following three elements:

1. A high level of overall physical, mental, and social functioning.
2. A general adaptive-maintenance level of daily functioning.
3. The absence of illness (or the presence of efforts that lead to its absence) (p. 220).

Watson states that what has traditionally been called health care is a myth. That which has been called health care, the diagnosing of disease, treatment of illness, and prescription of drugs, is medical care. True health care focuses on life style, social conditions, and environment. Watson (1985/1988) adds:

Health refers to unity and harmony within the mind, body, and soul. Health is also associated with the degree of congruence between the self as perceived and the self as experienced (p. 48).

One major factor affecting health is stress or stress-related activities that are also associated with life style, social conditions, and environment. Illness, on the other hand, may not be disease but may be a disharmony between body, soul, and spirit that may lead to stress. In addition, Watson believes the individual should define his or her own state of health or illness, since she prefers to view health as a subjective state within the mind of the person.

Environment/Society

One of the variables that affects society in today's world is the social environment. Society provides the values that determine how one should behave and what goals one should strive toward. These values are affected by change in the social, cultural, and spiritual arenas, which in turn affects the perception of the person and can lead to stress. People also have an intrinsic need to belong, to be part of a group(s) and of society as a whole. Furthermore, each person has a need for affection, a need to love and be loved. Stress or illness can separate the person from those who meet such affiliative or affectional needs. It is within the practice of caring that nursing can assist in meeting these needs. Watson (1979) states:

> Caring (and nursing) has existed in every society. Every society has had some people who have cared for others. A caring attitude is not transmitted from generation to generation by genes. It is transmitted by the culture of the profession as a unique way of coping with its environment (p. 8).

Nursing

According to Watson (1979), "nursing is concerned with promoting health, preventing illness, caring for the sick, and restoring health" (p. 7). Nursing focuses on health promotion as well as treatment of disease. She sees nursing as having to move educationally in the two areas of stress and developmental conflicts to provide holistic health care, which she believes is central to the practice of caring in nursing. One of Watson's (1985/1988) assumptions is that "nursing's social, moral, and scientific contributions to humankind and society lie in its commitment to human care ideals in theory, practice, and research" (p. 33).

In further writings Watson (1985/1988) defines nursing as ". . . a human science of persons and human health–illness experiences that are mediated by professional, personal, scientific, esthetic, and ethical human care transactions" (p. 54). Nursing in this context is rooted in the humanities as well as in the natural sciences. Nursing's goal, through the caring process, is to help people gain a high degree of harmony within the self in order to promote self-knowledge and self-healing, or to gain insight into the meaning of the happenings in life. Yet nursing is faced with the explosion of technology, the increase in the acuity of patients along with a decrease in the length of hospital stay. All these factors have an impact on the practitioner's ability to focus beyond the *cure* factor to the *care* factor. The relationship between the nurse and the patient/client entails several unique features based upon mutual expectations. The client certainly expects the nurse to follow whatever orders there are for treatment but also expects the nurse to be humane and caring. The nurse values caring but is often willing to sacrifice that valued attribute in order to accomplish the tasks of the technological age. The struggle within the practice of nursing will be that of reinforcing humanistic studies and the knowledge that to be humane, caring practitioners we must believe in the dignity and worth of each patient/client. Nursing must reinforce the values that are held as a profession and insist on those values as the linchpin upon which to build the priorities of patient care.

WATSON'S THEORY AND THE NURSING PROCESS

Watson recommends a broad approach to nursing that searches out connections rather than separations between the parts that make up the whole of the person. To accomplish this, nurses employ a scientific problem-solving method by which they can draw from a data base and basic nursing principles to make nursing judgments and decisions. Watson (1979) points out that the nursing process contains the same steps as the scientific research process. The rationales for these processes are identical in that both try to solve a problem or answer a question. Both try to discover the best solution. However, she believes nurses tend to be frightened by the scientific research processes. If nurses could learn that the processes are basically the same and that they provide a framework for decision making, then nurses would derive comfort from the order established by using the scientific process. This might best be accomplished by teaching the two processes, nursing and research, at the same time, to practice them together, and to recognize that the ultimate goal in nursing is high quality patient care that can be achieved by using this systematic approach.

Watson (1979) further elaborates the two processes as follows (Italics indicate the research process interwoven in the nursing process):

Assessment
- Assessment involves *observation, identification,* and *review* of the *problem; use* of the applicable *knowledge in literature.*
- It includes conceptual knowledge for the *formulation* and *conceptualization* of a *framework* in which to view and assess the problem.
- It also includes the *formulation of hypotheses* about relationships and factors that influence the problem.
- Assessment also includes *defining variables* that will be examined in solving the problem.

Plan
- The plan helps to determine how *variables will be examined* or measured.
- It includes a *conceptual approach* or design for solving problems that is referred to as the nursing care plan.
- It also includes determining what data will be collected and on what person and how the data will be collected.

Intervention
- Intervention is direct action and implementation of the plan.
- It includes the collection of data.

Evaluation
- Evaluation is the method of and the process for *analyzing data* as well as the examination of the effects of intervention based on the data.
- It includes *interpretation* of the *results,* the degree to which a positive outcome occurred, and whether the results can be generalized beyond the situation. (pp. 65–66).

Beyond that, according to Watson, evaluation may also generate additional hypotheses or possibly even lead to the generation of a nursing theory based on the problem studied and the solutions. An application of Watson's work in the nursing process is seen through the case study of Anthony M. (see Table 18–2 on page 328).

Situation. Anthony M. was a 14-year-old with a slender, almost cachectic, appearance. He weighed 85 pounds and was 5 feet 6 inches tall. Both his mother and father were deeply concerned about his weight loss of almost 30 pounds and were upset by daily battles related to eating. Anthony was equally upset since he felt he was at just the right weight. He felt that his parents had no right to control what or how much he ate. He was admitted to an adolescent psychiatric unit where the family's problem could be addressed.

Anthony complained that his parents were demanding and tried to control his life. He felt that they did not understand him and probably did not love him. When discussing his weight, he denied being hungry, so therefore he felt that he was eating enough. He stated, "Look, I'm fat and ugly, can't they see that? Girls don't like me, I've never been invited to a boy–girl party. The guys think I'm O.K., especially since I help with their homework, but I don't hang around with anyone special."

Anthony's weight was not within the norm for his age or height. At his height, his optimal weight should have ranged between 115 and 130 pounds. His skin appeared dry and flaky. His bones were clearly visible; there seemed to be no flesh covering them. He was listless and taciturn. His approach to food was marked by extreme disinterest.

WATSON'S WORK AND THE CHARACTERISTICS OF A THEORY

According to Watson (1985/1988), "a theory is an imaginative grouping of knowledge, ideas, and experience that are represented symbolically and seek to illuminate a given phenomenon" (p. 1). She rejects traditional, quantifiable methodology when such methodology sacrifices the pursuit of new knowledge of human behavior. She sees nursing as being increasingly involved in procedures and variable manipulation while it might best be involved in a search for alternative views to study human caring, health–illness, and health promotion. She states that she views nursing as ". . . both a human science and an art, and as such it cannot be considered qualitatively continuous with traditional, reductionistic, scientific methodology" (p. 2). Watson suggests that nursing might want to develop its own science that would not be related to the traditional sciences but rather would develop its own concepts, relationships, and methodology. Table 18–3 illustrates her ideas of nursing's context as opposed to the traditional view. Yet, her work has been developed within the traditional context and can be compared to the characteristics of a theory as delineated in Chapter 1.

1. Theories can interrelate concepts in such a way as to create a different way of looking at a particular phenomenon. The use of the term *caring* is not

TABLE 18–2. WATSON'S THEORY IN NURSING PROCESS APPLIED TO ANTHONY M.

Nursing Process	Application of Theory
ASSESSMENT	
Lower Order Needs (biophysical)	How does Anthony M. view his body? Is he within norms for his height, weight, and age? Does he consume enough calories to maintain normal growth? Does a physical assessment indicate all systems are functioning at normal levels?
Lower Order Needs (psychophysical)	Is his body image realistic? Is he participating in the usual activities of his age? Does evaluation of laboratory tests indicate nutritional deficiencies?
Higher Order Needs (psychosocial)	Are his relationships with peers satisfactory? How does he view his nascent sexuality? Has starvation retarded puberty? Does his environment appear facilitative of personal growth? Does he feel loved or lovable? Has he established a sense of autonomy from his parents?
Higher Order Needs (intrapersonal)	How does Anthony M. feel about himself? Does he like his world? Does he feel he is accomplishing his goals?
NURSING DIAGNOSES	Disturbances in self-concept related to: Body image disturbance Powerlessness Impaired social interaction Unresolved independence or dependence
PLANNING AND IMPLEMENTATION Use carative factors	Establish a caring environment through empathetic understanding. Develop a helping–trust relationship by encouraging expression of feelings of fear of weight gain, anger at treatment plan, resentment of authority figures. Use warmth, empathy, and congruence to establish open communication. Promote interpersonal teaching–learning by involving patient in nutritional plan. Teach patient how to deal with conflict, issue of autonomy. Facilitate relationships within the family that foster autonomy. Encourage identification of stress factors. Assist in dealing with sexual identity. Encourage Anthony M. to assess his social interactions and develop satisfying ones. Emphasize personal satisfaction rather than perfection.
EVALUATION	Has a trusting relationship been established? Is Anthony M. developing normally in the areas assessed: biophysically, psychophysically, psychosocially, and intrapersonally? Has Anthony M. learned the skills necessary to grow and mature successfully?

unique to Watson. What is unique is her basic assumptions for the science of caring in nursing and the ten carative factors that form the structure for that concept. She describes caring in both philosophical and scientific terms. Caring is placed in a hierarchical context, meeting lower order biophysical needs first and moving toward higher order psychosocial and intrapersonal

TABLE 18–3. DIFFERING PERSPECTIVES BETWEEN TRADITIONAL SCIENCE AND HUMAN SCIENCE

Traditional Medical Natural Science Context	Emerging Alternative Nursing Human Science and Context for Caring
Normative	Ipsative
Reductionistic	Transactional
Mechanistic	Metaphysical
	Humanistic—contextual
Method centered	Phenomena centered
Neutrality of values	Value laden; values acknowledged, clarified
Disease centered on pathology–physiology, the physical body	Person–experience centered
	Human responses to illness and personal meanings of human condition
Ethics of "science"	Human-social ethics-morality
More quantitative	More qualitative
Absolutes, givens, laws	Relativism, probabilism
Human as object	Human as subject
Objective experiences	Subjective—intersubjective experiences
Facts	Experience, meaning
Nomothetic	Idiographic + /nomothetic
Concrete—observable	Abstract—may or may not "be seen"
Analytical	Dialectical, philosophical, metaphysical
Science as product	Science as creative process of discovery
Human = sum of parts ex. (bio-psycho-socio-cultural-spiritual-being)	Human = mind–body–spirit gestalt of whole being (not only more than sum of parts, but different)
Physical, materialistic	Existential—phenomenological-spiritual
"Real" is that which is measurable, observable, and knowable	"Real" is abstract, largely subjective as well as objective, but it may or may not ever be fully known, observable, fully measured, what is "real," holds mystery and unknowns yet to be discovered

Used with permission from Watson, J. (1988). Nursing: Human science and human care (p. 10). New York: National League for Nursing.

needs. Watson also says that the needs are interrelated. For example, food and fluid needs are lower order biophysical needs that must be met, yet intake of food and fluids is strongly related to love, security, culture, and self-concept. The science of caring suggests that the nurse recognize and assist with each of the client's interrelated needs in order to help the client reach the highest order need of self-actualization.

2. Theories must be logical in nature. Watson's work is logical in that the carative factors are based on broad assumptions that provide a supportive framework. She uses these carative factors to help delineate nursing from medicine. The carative factors are logically derived from the assumptions and related to the hierarchy of needs.

3. Theories should be relatively simple yet generalizable. Watson's theory is relatively simple because it does use theories from other disciplines that are familiar to nurses. It becomes more complex when entering the area of existential-phenomenology, for many nurses may not have the liberal arts background to provide the proper foundation for understanding this area. On the other hand, nurses do have the empirical knowledge of human nature, including working with persons who are dealing with pain, loss, and suffering. The theory is relatively simple, but the fact that it de-emphasizes the pathophysiological for the psychosocial diminishes its ability to be generalizable. Watson (1979) discusses this problem in the preface of her book when she speaks of the "trim" and "core" of nursing. She defines trim as the clinical focus, the procedures and techniques. The core of nursing is that which is intrinsic to the nurse–client interaction that produces a therapeutic result. Core mechanisms are the carative factors. Unfortunately, those are the very factors that seem to be most often sacrificed in today's technological world.

4. Theories can be the bases for hypotheses that can be tested or for theory to be expanded. Watson's work is based upon phenomenological studies that generally ask questions rather than state hypotheses. Its purpose is to describe the phenomena, to analyze, and to gain an understanding.

5. Theories contribute to and assist in increasing the general body of knowledge within the discipline through research implemented to validate them. Watson has suggested that the best method for testing her theory is through field study. One example is her work in the area of loss and caring that took place in Cundeelee, Western Australia, and involved a tribe of aborigines. She first had the aborigines describe the phenomena of loss. They then defined what caring meant to them. Through analysis of the descriptive data, Watson (1985/1988) was able to develop a theory of transpersonal caring, which states that loss creates a disharmony in three spheres: mind, body, and spirit. The nurse can enter into the process of transpersonal caring by comforting, listening, and allowing for free expression of feelings based on the culturally relevant norms of the person. Because the carative factors expand on theories learned from other disciplines and mold them into uniquely nursing knowledge, continued research that involves the carative factors should increase the general body of knowledge in nursing.

Since Watson did her early work, many theorists and researchers have extended the concept of caring into the areas of nursing philosophy/ethics, practice, and education. Currently, five categories of caring are being researched or written about: caring as a human trait, caring as a moral imperative, caring as an affect, caring as an interpersonal relationship, and caring as a therapeutic intervention (Morse, Solberg, Neander, Botorff, & Johnson, 1990). Bishop and Scudder (1991), Gadow (1988), Gaut (1993), and Leininger (1988) all discuss caring within the context of one of these categories. Benner and Wrubel (1988) are researching caring as a nursing outcome and find that both patient and nurse benefit. Morse, Botoroff, Neander and Solberg (1991) did a comparative analysis of the newer concepts in the theories of caring and found that further refinement in both theory construction and in research methodology needs to be made. However, while urging continued research, Watson (1990) passionately extols her readers to look beyond traditional methods of knowing. She states, "If our aim for caring knowledge in nursing is higher than achieving machinelike knowledge, if our aim is to express and to reflect life and life forces, it is not enough to be technically correct. Much of nursing contains caring knowledge that enriches the soul. . . . How does any one way to knowledge development exemplify the wonder of humanity and human caring processes of nursing?" (p. 17). In an effort to quantify "caring," researchers may lose sight of the intangibles. Qualitative research methodologies may well capture the ephemeral characteristics of caring but are time intensive. In an era of fiscal stringency, when time on task is valued, nurses need the research to prove that caring is as efficacious, if not more so, as the technology they use.

6. **Theories can be used by practitioners to guide and improve their practice.** Watson's work can be used to guide and improve practice. It can provide the nurse with the most satisfying aspects of practice and can provide the client with the holistic care so necessary for human growth and development.

7. **Theories must be consistent with other validated theories, laws, and principles but will leave open unanswered questions that need to be investigated.** Watson's work is supported by the theoretical work of numerous humanists, philosophers, developmentalists, and psychologists. She clearly designates the theories of stress, development, communication, teaching–learning, humanistic psychology, and existential phenomenology that provide the foundation for the science of caring. She presents these in a way that provides a uniquely nursing view, that leads to further questions to be investigated.

ANALYSIS AND CONCLUSIONS

The strength of Watson's work is that it not only assists in providing the quality of care that clients ought to receive but also provides the soul-satisfying care for which many nurses enter the profession. Because the science of caring ranges from the biophysical through the intrapersonal, each nurse becomes an active co-participant in the client's struggle toward self-actualization. In addition, the client is placed in the context of the family, the community, and the culture. All of this encourages the nurse to make the client, rather than the technology, the focus of practice. Along with that comes the nurse's responsibility and opportunity for personal growth.

The limitations may very well be the same issues. Given the acuity of illness that leads to hospitalization, the short length of stay, and the increasingly complex technology, such quality of care may be deemed impossible to give in a hospital. Bureaucratic structures are not known for their attention to much beyond the cost–benefit ratio. The rewards from within that structure are for the "trim" and not for the "core" of nursing, often placing the practitioner in an untenable position. Nurses who function in any bureaucratic structure that focuses on task accomplishment, whether that structure be in a hospital, home health or official public health agency, visiting nurse association, or any other location, are subject to the same limitations in relation to Watson's theory.

Although Watson acknowledges the need for a biophysical base to nursing, this area receives little attention in her writings. The ten carative factors primarily delineate the psychosocial needs of the person. In addition, while the carative factors have a sound foundation based on other disciplines, they need further research in nursing to demonstrate their application to practice.

SUMMARY

Watson provides many useful concepts for the practice of nursing. She ties together many theories commonly used in nursing education and does so in a manner helpful to practitioners of the art and science of nursing. The detailed descriptions of the carative factors can give guidance to those who wish to employ them in practice or research. Using her theory can add a dimension to practice that is both satisfying and challenging.

REFERENCES

Benner, P., & Wrubel, J. (1988). *The primacy of caring: Stress and coping in health and illness.* Menlo Park: Addison-Wesley.

Bishop, A. H., & Scudder, J. R. (1991). *Nursing: The practice of caring.* New York: National League for Nursing.

Carkhuff, R. (1971). *The development of human resources in education and psychology and social change.* New York: Holt, Rhinehart & Winston.

Erikson, E. (1963). *Childhood and society* (2nd ed.). New York: Norton.

Gadow, S. (1988). Covenant without cure. In J. Watson, & M. Ray (Eds.), *The ethics of care and the ethics of cure.* New York: National League for Nursing.

Gaut, D. A. (1993). *A global agenda for caring.* New York: National League for Nursing.

Gazda, G. (1975). *Basic approaches to group psychotherapy and group counseling.* Springfield, IL: Thomas.

Heidegger, M. (1962). *Being and time.* New York: Harper & Row. [out of print]

Henderson, V. (1964). The nature of nursing. *American Journal of Nursing, 64,* 62–68.

Lazarus, R. S. (1966). *Psychological stress and the coping process.* New York: McGraw Hill. [out of print]

Leininger, M. (Ed.). (1981). *Caring.* Thorofare, NJ: Charles B. Slack.

Leininger, M. (1988). History, issues and trends in discovery and uses of care in nursing. In M. Leininger (Ed.), *Care: Discovery and uses in clinical and community nursing.* Thorofare, NJ: Slack.

Maslow, A. (1954). *Motivation and personality*. New York: Harper & Bros. [out of print]

Morse, J. M., Botorff, J. L., Neander, W., & Solberg, S. (1991). Comparative analysis of conceptualizations and theories of caring. *Image, Journal of Nursing Scholarship, 23,* 199–126.

Morse, J. M., Solberg, S. M., Neander, W. L., Botorff, J. L., & Johnson, J. L. (1990). Concepts of caring and caring as a concept. *Advances in Nursing Science, 13*(1), 1–14.

Rogers, C. (1962). The interpersonal relationship: The core of guidance. *Harvard Educational Review, 32,* 416.

Rogers, C. (1967). *Person to person: The problem of being human*. Lafayette, CA: Real People Press. [out of print]

Selye, H. (1956). *The stress of life*. New York: McGraw Hill. [out of print]

Watson, J. (1979). *Nursing: The philosophy and science of caring*. Boston: Little, Brown.

Watson, J. (1988). *Nursing: Human science and human care, A theory of nursing*. New York: National League for Nursing (Originally published 1985, Appleton-Century-Crofts).

Watson, J. (1990). Caring knowledge and informed moral passion. *Advances in Nursing Science, 13*(1), 15–24.

BIBLIOGRAPHY

Chinn, P. (1988). *Ethical issues in nursing*. Rockville, MD: Aspen.

Gaines, B., Saunders, J., & Watson, J. (1984). Philosophy of nursing: A national survey. *Western Journal of Nursing Research, 6,* 401–404.

Sakalys, J., & Watson, J. (1986). Professional educational post-baccalaureate education for professional nursing . . . Reintegration of the classical liberal arts model. *Journal of Professional Nursing, 2,* 91–97.

Schroeder, C., & Maeve, M. X. (1992). Nursing care partnerships at the Denver Nursing Project in Human Caring: An application and extension of caring theory in practice. *Advances in Nursing Science, 15*(2), 25–38.

Watson, J. (1981). The lost art of nursing. *Nursing Forum, 20,* 244–249.

Watson, J. (1981). Professional identity crisis—Is nursing finally growing up? *American Journal of Nursing, 81,* 1488–1490.

Watson, J. (1985). Nursing's scientific quest. *Nursing Outlook, 29,* 413–416.

Watson, J. (1987). Academic and clinical collaboration: Advancing the art and science of human caring. *Community Nursing Research, 20,* 1–16.

Watson, J. (1987). Nursing on the caring edge—Metaphorical vignettes. *Advances in Nursing Science, 10,* 10–18.

Watson, M. J. (1988). New dimensions of human caring theory. *Nursing Science Quarterly, 1,* 175–181.

ROSEMARIE RIZZO PARSE

Janet S. Hickman

■ ■ ■

Rosemarie Rizzo Parse earned her Bachelor of Science degree in Nursing from Duquesne University, Pittsburgh, and her Master's Degree in Nursing and PhD from the University of Pittsburgh. She holds the Marcella Niehoff Chair in Nursing Research at Loyola University in Chicago and is a Fellow of the American Academy of Nursing. Parse is the founder and editor of Nursing Science Quarterly, *a Chestnut House publication. She is founder and president of Discovery International, Inc., Pittsburgh, Pennsylvania, an organization that sponsors seminars and provides consultation services related to nursing education, research, and practice, as well as health guidance services to individuals, families, and communities.*

In addition to Dr. Parse's (1981, 1987; Parse, Coyne, & Smith, 1985) books, she has presented, both nationally and internationally, many papers and speeches on a wide variety of subjects related to nursing. In 1987 she was named Christine E. Lynn Eminent Scholar in Nursing at Florida Atlantic University. Dr. Parse has many years of experience in theory development, research, administration, and nursing practice and education.

In 1981 Parse presented a unique theory of nursing titled "Man–Living–Health," which synthesized principles and concepts from Rogers (1970, 1984) and concepts and tenets from existential phenomenology. Parse (1981, 1992b) said that man refers to *Homo sapiens,* a generic term for all human beings. She stated that her purpose was to posit an idea of nursing rooted in the human sciences as an alternative to ideas of nursing grounded in the natural sciences. She defined natural science-based nursing as having to do with the quantification of man and illness rather than the qualification of man's total experience with health.

In 1987 Parse refined this discussion by presenting two paradigms, or worldviews, of nursing. The first discussed is the totality paradigm in which man is posited as a total summative being whose nature is a combination of bio-psycho-social-spiritual aspects. The environment is viewed as the external and internal stimuli surrounding man. Man interacts and adapts with his environment to maintain equilibrium and to achieve goals. This is a refined definition of the natural, or medical, science approach to nursing. Parse states that the works of Peplau (1952/1988), Henderson (1991), Hall (1965), Orlando (1961), Levine (1989, 1990), Johnson (1980), Roy (1984; Andrews

& Roy, 1986; Roy & Andrews, 1991), Orem (1991), and King (1981, 1989) are representative of the totality paradigm.

The second worldview that Parse (1987) discusses is the simultaneity paradigm, which views man as "a unitary being in continuous mutual interrelationship with the environment, and whose health is a negentropic unfolding . . ." (p. 136). This is a refined definition of the human science approach to nursing. Parse states that her own work and that of Rogers (1992) are representative of the simultaneity paradigm.

In the spring of 1992, Parse (1992b) changed the name of her theory of Man–Living–Health to the theory of Human Becoming. She reworded the assumptions accordingly. No other aspects of the theory were changed. The revision was made as a response to a change in the dictionary definition of the term *man*. The current dictionary definition is gender-based as opposed to the previous use of the word *man* to identify mankind.

SUMMARY OF PARSE'S THEORY

Parse's theory makes assumptions about humans and health and deduces from them the principles, concepts, and theoretical structures of Human Becoming. These assumptions are based on Rogers's principles and concepts and the works of Heidegger (1962, 1972), Sartre (1963, 1964, 1966), and Merleau-Ponty (1973, 1974) on existential-phenomenological thought. Parse uses Rogers's three major principles (helicy, complementarity [now called integrality], and resonancy) and Rogers's four major concepts (energy field, openness, pattern and organization, and four dimensionality [now called pandimensionality]) as part of the theoretical basis for her own assumptions about humans and health. Parse synthesizes these principles and concepts with the following tenets and concepts of existential-phenomenological thought: intentionality, human subjectivity, coconstitution, coexistence, and situated freedom. It is important to remember that the process of synthesis is by definition the combining of elements to create something new and different. Therefore, as will be demonstrated in the discussion of Parse's assumptions, the products of her synthesis are different from the original principles, tenets, and concepts on which they are based.

ASSUMPTIONS

Because the language of this theory has recently changed, it is helpful to look at the assumptions as they were originally stated. In Parse's 1981 book, *Man–Living–Health: A theory of nursing* she posited nine assumptions, each of which was based on 3 of the 12 previously identified principles, tenets, and concepts from Rogers's theory and on existential-phenomenological thought. Phillips (1987) points out that for 6 of the 9 assumptions, 2 of the 3 concepts used as the basis for each assumption come from Rogers; leaving 3 assumptions for which 2 of the 3 concepts come from existential-phenomenology. Quantitatively, Phillips implies a greater grounding of the assumptions in Rogers' theory than in existential-phenomenology. In contrast, Winkler (1983) states that Parse's assumptions come primarily from philosophical sources and secondarily from Rogers' theory.

Parse's (1981) original nine assumptions are the following:

1. Man is coexisting while coconstituting rhythmical patterns with the environment (based on *pattern and organization, coconstitution,* and *coexistence*).
2. Man is an open being, freely choosing meaning in situation, bearing responsibility for decisions (based on *energy field, openness,* and *situated freedom*).
3. Man is a living unity continuously coconstituting patterns of relating (based on *energy field, pattern and organization,* and *coconstitution*).
4. Man is transcending multidimensionally with the possibles (based on *openness, four dimensionality,* and *situated freedom*).
5. Health is an open process of becoming, experienced by man (based on *openness, coconstitution,* and *situated freedom*).
6. Health is a rhythmically coconstituting process of the man–environment interrelationship (based on *pattern and organization, four dimensionality,* and *coconstitution*).
7. Health is man's pattern of relating value priorities (based on *openness, pattern and organization,* and *situated freedom*).
8. Health is an intersubjective process of transcending with the possibles (based on *openness, coexistence,* and *situated freedom*).
9. Health is unitary man's negentropic unfolding (based on *energy field, four dimensionality,* and *coexistence*).

Using Parse's 1992 language revision, the original nine assumptions now read as four assumptions concerning humans and five assumptions concerning becoming. They are

HUMAN

1. The human is coexisting while coconstituting rhythmical patterns with the universe.
2. The human is an open being, freely choosing meaning in situation, bearing responsibility for decisions.
3. The human is a living unity continuously coconstituting patterns of relating.
4. The human is transcending multi-dimensionally with the possibles.

BECOMING

5. Becoming is an open process, experienced by the human.
6. Becoming is a rhythmically coconstituting process of the human–universe interrelationship.
7. Becoming is the human's pattern of relating value priorities.
8. Becoming is an intersubjective process of transcending with the possibles.
9. Becoming is human unfolding.

In 1985, Parse set forth three assumptions about Man–Living–Health (Parse, Coyne, & Smith, 1985). These three assumptions have also been revised to reflect Human Becoming, as follows:

1. Human Becoming is freely choosing personal meaning in situations in the intersubjective process of relating value priorities.
2. Human Becoming is cocreating rhythmical patterns of relating in open interchange with the universe.
3. Human Becoming is cotranscending multidimensionally with the unfolding possibilities.

The first assumption states that Human Becoming is a subject-to-subject, subject-to-universe interchange where the meaning assigned to the experience reflects one's personal values. This assumption appears to be a synthesis of numbers two, five, and seven of her original nine, which are based on the concepts of energy field, openness, situated freedom, coconstitution, and pattern and organization.

The second assumption states that Human Becoming is an open interchange with the universe and that *together* the human being and the environment create rhythmical patterns. This assumption appears to be a synthesis of original assumptions one, three, and six, which are based on the concepts of energy fields, openness, situated freedom, pattern and organization, and coconstitution.

The third assumption states that Human Becoming is moving beyond the self at all levels of the universe as dreams become realities. Parse (1992b) defines cotranscending as a moving beyond with others and the universe multidimensionally. Multidimensionally refers to the various levels of the universe that humans experience "all at once" and choose possibles from in various situations. This assumption appears to be a synthesis of original assumptions four, eight, and nine, which are based on the concepts of openness, four dimensionality, situated freedom, coexistence, and energy field. It is important to note that Parse is viewing humans as being multidimensional, not four dimensional, which is congruent with Rogers's current terminology of pandimensionality.

Parse (1987) cites the following distinctives of her theory:

1. That humans are more and different than the sum of their parts.
2. That human beings evolve mutually with the environment.
3. That human beings cocreate personal health by choosing meaning in situations.
4. That human beings convey meanings that are personal value which reflect their dreams and hopes.

PRINCIPLES

Three main themes can be identified in Parse's (1987) assumptions: meaning, rhythmicity, and cotranscendence. Each leads to a principle of Human Becoming (see Fig. 19–1):

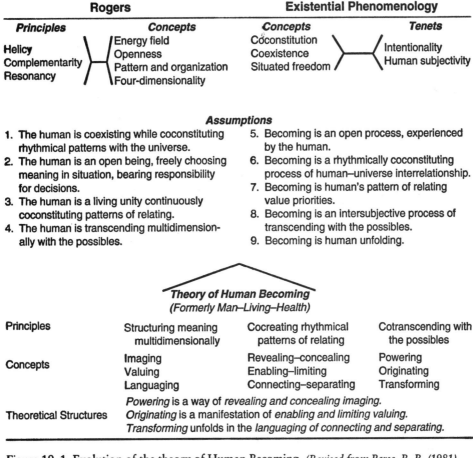

Rogers		Existential Phenomenology	
Principles	*Concepts*	*Concepts*	*Tenets*
Helicy Complementarity Resonancy	Energy field Openness Pattern and organization Four-dimensionality	Coconstitution Coexistence Situated freedom	Intentionality Human subjectivity

Assumptions

1. The human is coexisting while coconstituting rhythmical patterns with the universe.
2. The human is an open being, freely choosing meaning in situation, bearing responsibility for decisions.
3. The human is a living unity continuously coconstituting patterns of relating.
4. The human is transcending multidimensionally with the possibles.

5. Becoming is an open process, experienced by the human.
6. Becoming is a rhythmically coconstituting process of human–universe interrelationship.
7. Becoming is human's pattern of relating value priorities.
8. Becoming is an intersubjective process of transcending with the possibles.
9. Becoming is human unfolding.

Theory of Human Becoming
(Formerly Man–Living–Health)

Principles	Structuring meaning multidimensionally	Cocreating rhythmical patterns of relating	Cotranscending with the possibles
Concepts	Imaging Valuing Languaging	Revealing–concealing Enabling–limiting Connecting–separating	Powering Originating Transforming
Theoretical Structures	*Powering* is a way of *revealing and concealing imaging.* *Originating* is a manifestation of *enabling and limiting valuing.* *Transforming* unfolds in the *languaging of connecting and separating.*		

Figure 19–1. Evolution of the theory of Human Becoming. *(Revised from Parse, R. R. (1981). Man–Living–Health: A theory of nursing (pp. 70–71). New York: Wiley. Used with permission.)*

I. *Structuring meaning multidimensionally is cocreating reality through the languaging of valuing and imaging.*

Parse's (1992b) first principle interrelates the concepts of *imaging, valuing,* and *languaging,* showing that human beings structure meaning to reality that is based on lived experiences. The meaning changes or is stretched to different possibilities, depending on lived experiences. Cocreating in this principle refers to the human–environment mutual participation in the creation of the pattern of each. Languaging reflects images and values through speaking and movements. Valuing is the process of living cherished beliefs while adding to one's personal worldview. Imaging refers to knowing and includes both explicit and tacit knowledge.

From this principle, Parse has identified a nursing practice dimension and a process (see Fig. 19–2). The practice dimension is illuminating

DIMENSIONS

Illuminating meaning is shedding light through uncovering the what was, is, and will be, as it is appearing now; it happens in *explicating* what is.

Synchronizing rhythms happens in *dwelling with* the pitch, yaw, and roll of the interhuman cadence.

Mobilizing transcendence happens in *moving beyond* the meaning moment to what is not yet.

PROCESSES

Explicating is making clear what is appearing now through languaging.

Dwelling with is giving self over to the flow of the struggle in connecting–separating.

Moving beyond is propeling toward the possibles in transforming.

Figure 19–2. Human Becoming Practice Methodology. *(From Parse, R. R. (1987). Nursing science: Major paradigms, theories, and critiques (p. 167). Philadelphia: Saunders. Used with permission.)*

meaning by "shedding light through uncovering the what was, is, and will be, as it is appearing now" (Parse, 1987, p. 167). This happens by explicating or making clear what is appearing now through languaging (the process). Nurses guide individuals and families to relate the meaning of a situation by making the meaning more explicit.

II. *Cocreating rhythmical patterns of relating is living the paradoxical unity of revealing–concealing, enabling–limiting, while connecting–separating.*

The second principle of the theory of Human Becoming interrelates the concepts of *revealing–concealing, enabling–limiting,* and *connecting–separating.* This principle speaks to human beings cocreating a multidimensional universe in rhythmical patterns of relating while living a paradox. The paradoxes identified are revealing–concealing, enabling–limiting, and connecting–separating. Parse (1981) states that these rhythmical patterns are not opposites; they are two sides of the same rhythm and are simultaneous. In interpersonal relationships, one reveals part of the self but also conceals other parts. Making choices or decisions enables an individual in some ways but limits in others. Connecting–separating is a rhythmical process of moving together and moving apart.

The practice dimension Parse (1987) describes for this principle is the synchronizing of rhythms, which happens in dwelling with the pitch, yaw, and roll of interhuman cadence. She likens dwelling with as moving with the flow of the individual/family leading them to recognize the harmony that exists within its own lived context. The nurse does not try to calm or balance rhythms or attempt to help the family adapt.

III. *Cotranscending with the possibles is powering unique ways of originating in the process of transforming.*

The third principle of the theory of Human Becoming interrelates the concepts of *powering, originating,* and *transforming.* Powering is an energizing force the rhythm of which is the pushing–resisting of inter-human encounters. Transforming is defined as the changing of change and is recognized by increasing diversity (Parse, 1981).

The practice dimension identified by Parse (1987) for this principle is mobilizing transcendence, which happens in moving beyond the meaning of the moment to what is not yet. The process she identifies is moving beyond or "propelling toward the possibles in transforming" (p. 167). In this the nurse guides individuals and/or families to plan for the changing of lived health patterns.

THEORETICAL STRUCTURES

The theoretical structures of the theory of Human Becoming are noncausal in nature and consistent with the assumptions and principles. They are designed to guide research and practice (see Fig. 19-3). To operationalize the structures for research and practice, practice propositions must be derived. The three theoretical structures identified are: (1) powering is a way of revealing–concealing imaging, (2) originating is a manifestation of enabling–limiting valuing, and (3) transforming unfolds in the languaging of connecting–separating (Parse, 1981).

In her 1987 book, Parse restates her theoretical structures at a less abstract level in order for them to be used to guide nursing practice. She explains that *"powering is a way of revealing–concealing imaging,* can be stated as *struggling to live goals discloses the significance of the situation"* (p. 170). The nursing practice focus "is on illuminating the process of revealing–concealing unique ways a person or family can mobilize transcendence in considering new dreams, to image new possibles" (p. 170). Parse describes a nurse–family situation in which members share their thoughts and feelings about a situation, which both reveals and conceals all they know about their struggle to meet personal goals. In disclosing the significance of the situation, the meaning of the situation changes for the family members and therefore the meaning changes for the family.

According to Parse (1987), "the second theoretical structure, *originating is a manifestation of enabling–limiting valuing,* can be [restated] as *creating anew shows one's cherished beliefs and leads in a directional movement"* (p. 170). The nursing practice focus with a person or family would be on illuminating ways of being alike and different from others in changing values. By synchronizing rhythms, the members discover opportunities and limitations created by the decisions made in choosing ways to be together. Parse states that the choices of new ways of being together mobilize transcendence.

As a restatement of the third theoretical structure, *"transforming unfolds in the language of connecting–separating,"* Parse (1987) suggests *"changing views emerge in speaking and moving with others"* (p. 170). The nursing practice focus would be "on illuminating the meaning of relating ways of being together as various changing perspectives shed different light on the

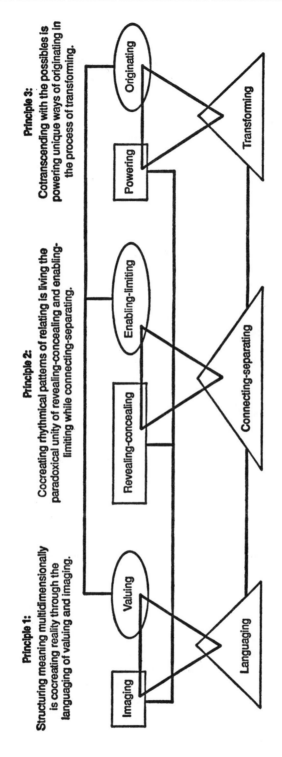

Principle 1:
Structuring meaning multidimensionally is cocreating reality through the languaging of valuing and imaging.

Principle 2:
Cocreating rhythmical patterns of relating is living the paradoxical unity of revealing-concealing and enabling-limiting while connecting-separating.

Principle 3:
Cotranscending with the possibles is powering unique ways of originating in the process of transforming.

Relationship of the concepts in the *squares*: *Powering* is a way of *revealing and concealing imaging.*
Relationship of the concepts in the *ovals*: *Originating* is a manifestation of *enabling and limiting values.*
Relationship of the concepts in the *triangles*: *Transforming* unfolds in the *languaging of connecting and separating.*

Figure 19–3. Relationship of principles, concepts, and theoretical structures of human becoming. *(From Parse, R. R. (1981). Man–Living–Health: A theory of nursing (p. 69). New York: Wiley. Used with permission.)*

familiar, which gives rise to new possibles" (p. 170). Parse suggests that in synchronizing rhythms in a nurse–family situation, members relate their values through speech and movement. In so doing, their views change and, through mobilizing transcendence, the ways of relating change.

PARSE'S THEORY AND NURSING'S METAPARADIGM

The theory of Human Becoming is discussed here in terms of Parse's beliefs about human beings, the universe, health, and nursing. Parse (1987) identifies her theory and that of Rogers as being representative of the simultaneity paradigm. Hence, her assumptions about the four concepts of nursing's metaparadigm are congruent with those of this paradigm.

Human Beings/Universe

Parse's (1992b) first four assumptions specify the human being as an open being in mutual process with the universe, cocreating patterns of relating with others. She states that the human being "lives at multidimensional realms of the universe all at once, freely choosing ways of becoming as meaning is given to situations" (p. 37).

Human beings are central to Parse's theory of Human Becoming. Her views about human beings are evident in all elements of her theory–assumptions, principles, theoretical structures, and practice dimensions. Parse views human beings and universe as inseparable, each coparticipating in the creation of the experience of living. It is not possible or appropriate to define human beings or universe alone, for together they create a lived experience greater than and different from each seen separately.

The concept of relationships (society) is assumed under the larger view of human beings–universe. In her discussion of the concept of cotranscending, Parse (1987) speaks to "moving beyond with others and the environment multidimensionally" (p. 162). She also states that what humans choose from the multiple possibles unfolds and surfaces in relationships with others and the universe. Although human beings are described as having unique rhythmical patterns, it is difficult to interpret if Parse makes a difference in actual pattern between individuals and the human–universe interchange. If one assumes that "others" are a part of the human's universe, the interpretation becomes clearer.

Parse's view of human–universe is consistent with that of Rogers's (1984) presentation of the person–environment as inseparable, complementary, and evolving together. Parse's language revisions, however, delete general system terminology that is still evident in Rogers's work. Parse's view of human–universe is also consistent with the existentialist view of a person being in the world all-at-once and together, and the phenomenological belief that the universe is made up of everything shown to the person in the lived experience (Husserl, 1931/1962; Idie, 1967).

Winkler (1983) notes that although Parse states that all lived experiences are relevant, the omission of any references to biological manifestations of the person in his or her being and becoming limits Parse's theory. Phillips (1987) rejects this criticism and states that the lived experience deals with the wholeness of the person. Cody and Mitchell (1992) also reject this criticism, stating that Parse does not ignore "biological manifestations" but subsumes them within the experience of the person, which is the focus of the inquiry and practice guided by her theory.

Health

Parse (1992b) describes health as a process of becoming that is experienced by the person, coconstituted through the human–universe experience, and incarnated as patterns of relating value priorities. Parse proposes that health is a personal commitment and that individuals are the creative authors of their own unfolding (health). She emphasizes that this unfolding cannot be prescribed or described by societal norms; it can only be lived by the person. Health is viewed by Parse as a process of changing life's meanings, a personal power emerging from the individual's collective relationships with others and the universe (Parse, 1990a).

The concept of situated freedom is evident in Parse's perspective of health. Individuals choose various ways of unfolding and have personal responsibility for their choices. Phillips (1987) describes Parse's theory as a way of dealing with experience, a coming to know rather than a product orientation. He states that the fundamental tenet of Parse's theory is that man participates in health.

Parse's theory speaks to health as man's lived experience as it unfolds negentropically. This is a very different conceptualization of health from that of the totality paradigm theorists. From the totality world view, health is a state of balance or well-being to which man can aspire. The totality world-view infers a norm or standard of health to which individuals and their health care providers aspire. These two different worldviews have very different nursing practice methodologies that are presented in the next section.

Nursing

Parse (1992a) defines nursing as a scientific discipline, the practice of which is a performing art. She places nursing in the company of drama, music, and dance, in each of which the artist creates something unique. The knowledge base of the discipline is the science of the art, and the performance is the art creatively lived. Parse states:

> So too, the nurse, an artist like the dancer, unfolds the meaning of the moment with a person or family consistent with personal knowledge and cherished beliefs. The nurse artist creatively lives knowledge about the human–universe–health connectedness (nursing's phenomenon of concern), which incarnates personal cherished beliefs. The knowledge and beliefs are there in the way the nurse approaches the person, the way the nurse talks and listens to

the person, what the nurse is most concerned about and how the nurse moves with the flow of the person. When the nurse artist is guided by a particular nursing theory or framework, the art form reflects that theory or framework, which represents a school of thought in nursing (p. 147).

Parse (1981) states that nursing's responsibility to society is in the guiding of individuals and families in choosing possibilities in changing the health process, which is accomplished by intersubjective participation with people. She further states that nursing practice involves innovation and creativity, which are not encumbered by prescriptive rules.

This theorist contends that the goals of nursing focus on the quality of life from the person's perspective. Nursing is practiced with all individuals and families, regardless of societal designations of health/illness status. Parse's (1987) theory guides practice that focuses on illuminating meaning and moving beyond with the person/family relative to changing health patterns. An important aspect in regard to Parse's view of nursing is that the client, not the nurse, is the authority figure and prime decision maker in the relationship. The client, in presence with the nurse, determines the activities for changing health patterns. According to this theory, nursing is "a loving, true presence with the other to promote health and the quality of life" (p. 169). The practice of nursing is not a prescriptive approach based on medical or nursing diagnoses, nor is it the offering of professional advice and opinions that stem from the personal value system of the nurse.

Parse (1987) has presented a practice methodology for her theory of Human Becoming that includes dimensions and processes (see Fig. 19–3). The dimensions are *illuminating meaning, synchronizing rhythms,* and *mobilizing transcendence.* The processes are the empirical activities of *explicating, dwelling with,* and *moving beyond.* There is a clear flow of these dimensions and processes from her assumptions and principles.

In Parse's theory the nurse is an interpersonal guide who acts in true presence, an active, energetic way of being with. Authority, responsibility, and the consequences of decisions are accorded to the client. The traditional nursing roles of caregiver, advocate, counselor, and leader do not appear to be congruent with Parse's view of nursing. Teaching, however, is reflected in the dimension of illuminating meaning by explicating, and acting as a change agent is reflected in the dimension of mobilizing transcendence by moving beyond the meaning to what is not yet.

In an editorial in *Nursing Science Quarterly,* Parse (1989) proposes a set of fundamentals essential for fully practicing the art of nursing, which include the following:

- Know and use nursing frameworks and theories.
- Be available to others.
- Value the other as a human presence.
- Respect differences in view.

- Own what you believe and be accountable for your actions.
- Move on to the new and untested.
- Connect with others.
- Take pride in what you do.
- Like what you do.
- Recognize the moments of joy in the struggles of living.
- Appreciate the mystery and be open to new discoveries.
- Be competent in your chosen area.
- Rest and begin anew.

Parse (1987) defines the contextual situations of nursing practice as being nurse–person or nurse–group participation. She does not define specific practice settings as being more or less appropriate for practice application of the theory of Human Becoming. She does, however, advise the nurse to approach the person/family as a nurturing gardener, not as a fix-it mechanic.

PARSE'S THEORY AND THE NURSING PROCESS

Parse (1987) states that the nursing process "evolves from the discipline of philosophy and does not flow from an ontological base in the discipline of nursing" (p. 166). She further states that the steps of the nursing process are the steps of the problem-solving method and are not unique to nursing. The assumptions underlying the nursing process, that the nurse is the authority on health and that the person adapts or can be "fixed," are not congruent with the theory of Human Becoming. Parse posits that as practice is the empirical life of a theory, the practice of one theory would be different from the practice of another. As Parse's practice dimensions and processes have been previously discussed, two examples of practice applications of the theory of Human Becoming are now presented.

Martin, Forchuk, Santopinto, and Butcher (1992) describe how the nurse, guided by the theory of Human Becoming, relates to Mrs. W., a terminally ill cancer client:

Emergent Patterns of Health for Mrs. W.

1. Mrs. W. says she does not want to discuss her situation with her family, yet she makes plans to broach the subject with them.
2. Mrs. W. says that this is the worst time of her life, yet she says that she has never enjoyed the natural world so much as now.

Mrs. W.–Nurse Activities

1. Be truly present with Mrs. W. as she imagines familiar and unfamiliar ways of engaging with and withdrawing from

family during the coming days and weeks. Through presence, seek deeper levels of meaning as she describes her hopes and dreams for the days ahead. Be with her as she shares how she intends to make these hopes come to pass and what meaning these hopes hold for her. Be present with Mrs. W. as she imagines new ways of being close to her family. Invite her to describe how her relationships are changing for her.

2. Be with Mrs. W. while she imagines aspects of nature which have special meaning for her. Invite her to describe how she can come to enjoy these aspects in her current situation. Be with her as she creates words, images and movements which bring her in touch with nature (p. 84).

Mitchell (1986) describes the application of the theory of Human Becoming to Mrs. M., an elderly woman in a long-term-care facility. In true presence with Mrs. M., Mitchell is able to tease out the multiple and complex realities the client experiences. The client transcends time and space to be all-at-once a child, a mother, and a lonely elder. All the realities lived and valued by Mrs. M. continue to be lived despite the passage of time. (Illuminating meaning.)

To understand the meaning of Mrs. M.'s languaging, the nurse dwells with her. The nurse does not try to bring Mrs. M. back to reality or to control or alter Mrs. M.'s experience. The nurse goes with the flow to assist the client in finding meaning. In doing so, the nurse has the opportunity to validate feelings with the client. Mrs. M. states that she felt joy when her mother met her after school. The nurse then states, "You feel good when your mother is waiting for you." Mrs. M. responded by saying, "Yes, she's waiting for me now too. I'm waiting to go home." (Synchronizing rhythms.)

This statement helps the nurse to understand that Mrs. M. perceives her present environment to be a temporary waiting area, that the client's detached behavior has occurred because she attaches little meaning to her current surroundings. Two nursing interventions are selected to guide Mrs. M.'s care. First, the nurse continues to facilitate the expression of Mrs. M.'s meaning in the present situation. Second, the nurse provides Mrs. M. with information and the freedom to make choices such as participation or detachment from unit activities. (Mobilizing transcendence.)

Parse's approach to practice is clearly one of nurses *in presence with* people rather than doing for people. Articles detailing Parse's practice applications are presented as case studies, which, by virtue of the format, tend to be lengthy. Practice-related articles are listed in the bibliography at the end of the chapter.

PARSE'S WORK AND THE CHARACTERISTICS OF A THEORY

1. Theories can interrelate concepts in such a way as to create a different way of looking at a particular phenomenon. Parse's (1992) theory of Human Becoming creates a new way of looking at human beings, health, environment, and nursing. Parse has synthesized Rogers's principles of helicy, complementarity (now called integrality), and resonancy, and her four concepts of openness, energy field, pattern and organization, and four dimensionality (now called pandimensionality) with the tenets of existential-phenomenological thought. This synthesis created the nine assumptions upon which the theory is based.

Parse's (1987) synthesis creates a theory in which humans are open beings who, with their universe, cocreate health. She views nursing as being rooted in the human sciences and having the goal of quality of life from the perspective of the person. In this worldview, the health–illness continuum is irrelevant as are care plans based on health problems. The authority, responsibility, and consequences of decision making reside with the person, not with the nurse. The nurse is presented as a guide who focuses on illuminating meaning, synchronizing rhythms, and mobilizing transcendence with the person or family relative to changing health patterns.

2. Theories must be logical in nature. Parse's theory of Human Becoming describes a logical sequence of events. Parse (1981) presents Rogers's principles and concepts as well as tenets and concepts from existential-phenomenological thought. She then synthesizes these tenets, principles, and concepts to create her nine assumptions. Each assumption is based on three concepts. Six of the assumptions are based on two concepts from Rogers and one concept from existential-phenomenology; the other three assumptions are based on two concepts from existential-phenomenology and one concept from Rogers (Phillips, 1987).

Parse presented three assumptions about Human Becoming (formerly Man–Living–Health) (Parse, Coyne, & Smith, 1985) that are derived from the nine assumptions of the theory and flow from them with logical precision. The principles of the theory of Human Becoming are derived from the assumptions, with each principle relating three concepts to each other (see Fig. 19–3).

Parse then derived three theoretical structures, each of which uses three concepts, one from each principle (see Fig. 19–3). She defines theoretical structure as a statement that interrelates concepts in a way that can be verified (Parse, 1992b). Phillips (1987) points out that the stem of each theoretical structure is taken from the third principle. He speculates that greater importance might be attached to this principle but qualifies this thought by saying that Parse makes it clear that other theoretical structures may be generated from her principles.

Levine (1988), Phillips (1987), and Winkler (1983) speak to the difficulty of Parse's terminology for those unfamiliar with existential-phenomenology. They concur, however, that there is consistency in meaning at each level of discourse.

3. Theories should be relatively simple yet generalizable. Although Parse's theory can be generalized to any lived experience, it is far from simple. Bringing the theory from an abstract level to a practical level is complicated. Terminology that is difficult and unfamiliar to nurses is used and may be a cause of confusion. The range of possibilities that exists in the lived experiences of open, interrelating beings makes this theory inherently complex.

4. Theories can be bases for hypotheses that can be tested or for theory to be expanded. Because Parse's theory is rooted in the human sciences rather than the natural sciences, qualitative rather than quantitative research methodologies are used to expand it. Qualitative research methodologies do not pose hypotheses in the cause–effect or associative relationship tradition of quantitative research methods. Instead, qualitative research methods focus on entities for study that are lived experiences (Parse, 1987).

Parse (1987) describes the theory of Human Becoming research methodology that includes the identification of major entities for study, the scientific processes of investigation, and the details of the processes appropriate for inquiry. She states that the two aspects of lived experience to consider in selecting an entity for study are nature and structure. The aspect of nature refers to common lived experiences that surface in the human–universe interrelationship and are health related; examples include "being–becoming, value priorities, negentropic unfolding, and quality of life" (p. 174). Parse cites the example of "waiting" as being consistent with her definition of a common lived experience.

The second aspect of lived experience to consider in selecting an entity for study is structure. Parse (1987) defines structure as "the paradoxical living of the remembered, the now moment, and the not-yet all at once" (p. 175). Thus, the research question could be: "What is the structure of the lived experience of waiting?" (p. 175). The researcher would then proceed to uncover the structure of this lived experience.

Whereas quantitative research methods test hypotheses or tentative assumptions about phenomena, the theory of Human Becoming research methodology explores questions about the lived experience.

5. Theories contribute to and assist in increasing the general body of knowledge within the discipline through the research implemented to validate them. The book *Nursing research: Qualitative methods* by Parse, Coyne, and Smith (1985) reports support of the theory of Human Becoming as a theory, through phenomenological, descriptive, and ethnographic methods. Five major qualitative studies are reported in this book. They focus on such topics as the phenomenology of health, persisting in change, the lived experience of being exposed to toxic chemicals, aging, and retirement. Parse states that these five studies demonstrate similar findings that are supportive of Human Becoming. She reports that meaning, rhythmicity, and transcendence, the major themes in her theory, can be seen in varying ways in all the studies.

Published research studies guided by this theory have generated descriptive and theoretical structures about the lived experience of hope (Parse, 1990b), the meaning of living with AIDS (Nokes & Carver, 1991), the lived experience of aging and health in the oldest old (Wondolowski & Davis, 1991), the drive to be ever thinner (Santopinto, 1989b), recovering from addiction (Banonis, 1989), and living through unemployment (Smith, 1990).

6. Theories can be used by practitioners to guide and improve their practice. As previously discussed, the theory of Human Becoming is not congruent with the traditional use of the nursing process. The theory of Human Becoming guides practice through its own practice methodology, which is composed of dimensions and processes. The dimensions are *illuminating meaning, synchronizing rhythms,* and *mobilizing transcendence,* and the processes are *explicating, dwelling with,* and *moving beyond* (Parse, 1987). A cardinal rule of this practice methodology is that the authority and responsibility for decision making lies with the person (client), not with the nurse.

There is little doubt that use of Parse's theory would individualize nursing care. Critical care situations and situations where the client is unconscious require that the nurse have a deep understanding of the concept of true presence.

Frik and Polluck (1993) report use of Parse's theory by graduate students practicing in chronic illness settings, a community mental health setting, and an emergency department. The theory was used in promoting compliance in adults with diabetes, implementing hypertensive screening in the emergency room, promoting effective coping skills related to drug abuse, and improving the nutrition of neurologically impaired adults.

Mitchell (1991) reports successful use of Parse's theory on an acute medical–surgical unit. Cody and Mitchell (1992) report successful use of this theory by Jonas (1989) in an outpatient setting, and by Santopinto (1989a) in a long-term care setting. Cody and Mitchell report that nurses in all these studies reported initial difficulties in changing their approach to being with persons and giving up the urge to apply the nursing process in the traditional manner. However, increased professional satisfaction convinced them of the validity of the new approach.

7. Theories must be consistent with other validated theories, laws, and principles but will leave open unanswered questions that need to be investigated. Parse's theory of Human Becoming is consistent with Rogers's principles and concepts and with the tenets and concepts of existential-phenomenological thought. However, as Phillips (1987) points out, Parse has synthesized these concepts and created a new product, which does not speak the same language as that of her sources.

Consistent with other nurse theorists, Parse addresses the phenomena of human beings, health, environment, and nursing. Although Parse's (1981) definition of human beings as an open being who cocreates health multidimensionally is unique, it is similar to that of other nurse theorists. Fitzpatrick (1989), Newman (1986), and Rogers (1992) speak to man and environment interacting to manifest health. Parse's view of the importance of the lived experience and quality of life is congruent with Paterson and Zderad (1976/1988), and Newman. As the theory of Human Becoming focuses on lived experiences, innumerable research questions can be posed for further investigation.

STRENGTHS AND WEAKNESSES

A strength of Parse's theory is the logical flow from construction of her assumptions to the deductive derivation of principles, theoretical structures, practice dimensions, and processes. Another strength of the theory of Human Becoming is that it focuses on all individuals, not only those defined by societal norms as being ill. The individual in the nurse–person relationship discovers the meaning of his or her lived experience. The nurse is in true presence with the client, and together, they discover by illuminating meaning, synchronizing rhythms, and mobilizing transcendence. This occurs as individuals and families interrelate with the nurse multidimensionally.

Phillips believes that Parse's theory of Human Becoming will speed the transformation from a mechanistic approach to health care to one that has a unitary perspective of the health care of humans. This is a laudable goal, but there is a need for research studies to expand the knowledge base about human beings' lived experiences. The uniqueness of lived experiences increases the complexity of this task. However, Parse does report that common elements and themes are surfacing in the current research findings. As these common elements and themes are validated further, they should give direction to a unitary perspective of the health care of humans.

A strength of this theory is the assumption about humans freely choosing personal meaning in the process of relating value priorities. Coupled with this assumption is the thinking that the authority and responsibility of choices resides with the person or client, not the nurse. This is an opposing stance to the tradition of paternalistic health care, in which physicians make decisions and nurses and patients accept them without question. It is a very contemporary stance. Consumers do in fact question health care professionals, seek other opinions and alternative treatment modalities, and resort to the legal system for redress of their perceived damages.

A limitation of the theory of human becoming is its lack of articulation with the body of knowledge and psychomotor skills that most nurses and society generally attribute to the practice of professional nursing. It is an entirely new conceptualization of nursing practice, and it is not congruent with the "assess, diagnose, and treat" language of current nurse practice acts.

A question posed to this author by graduate students in nursing is whether you have to be a nurse to practice the theory of Human Becoming. Many students felt that true presence could be achieved by physicians, social workers, therapists, and members of the clergy. Parse (personal communication, 1994) responded to this idea by noting that as the knowledge base is different in each discipline, what occurs in true presence with the client will be different. She also noted that other disciplines have different goals. Different goals affect and direct a professional's ability to be in true presence with the client.

Parse's theory has been criticized in the past for its exclusion of the discussion of the role of natural sciences in nursing practice. Parse does not address this specifically in relation to her theory, but she does advocate a preprofessional core curriculum that would be appropriate for the professions of law, medicine, theology, and nursing. This undergraduate preprofessional core assumes professional education to occur at the graduate level. Parse's proposed preprofessional core contains a strong natural science and liberal arts base.

Parse has clearly been successful in creating a new paradigm or worldview. Because of its incongruence with traditionally accepted definitions, roles, and nursing process, this new paradigm raises many questions and may be unacceptable as a theory of nursing to some. The strong philosophical base of Human Becoming and the use of philosophical terminology makes this theory difficult for many nurses to understand, and understanding is necessary before individuals will consider a change in their worldview. However, competing paradigms do exist in the discipline of nursing. This competition is seen by scholars as a hallmark of scientific growth (Meleis, 1991).

REFERENCES

Andrews, H. A., & Roy, C. (1986). *Essentials of the Roy Adaptation Model.* Norwalk, CT: Appleton & Lange.

Banonis, B. C. (1989). The lived experience of recovering from addiction: A phenomenological study. *Nursing Science Quarterly, 2,* 37–43.

Cody, W. K., & Mitchell, G. J. (1992). Parse's theory as a model for practice: The cutting edge. *Advances in Nursing Science, 15*(1), 52–65.

Fitzpatrick, J. J. (1989). A Life Perspective Rhythm Model. In J. J. Fitzpatrick, & A. L. Whall (Eds.), *Conceptual models of nursing* (2nd ed.) (pp. 401–407). Norwalk, CT: Appleton & Lange.

Frik, S. M., & Pollock, S. E. (1993). Preparation for advanced nursing practice. *Nursing and Health Care, 14,* 190–195.

Hall, L. (1965). *Another view of nursing care and quality.* Address given at Catholic University Workshop, Washington, DC.

Heidegger, M. (1962). *Being and time.* New York: Harper & Row.

Heidegger, M. (1972). *On time and being.* New York: Harper & Row.

Henderson, V. (1991). *The nature of nursing—Reflections after 25 years.* New York: National League for Nursing.

Husserl, E. (1962). *Ideas: General introduction to pure phenomenology.* New York: Collier-Macmillan. (Originally published, 1931).

Idie, J. M. (1967). Transcendental phenomenology and existentialism. In J. J. Kockelmans (Ed.), *Phenomenology.* New York: Doubleday.

Johnson, D. E. (1980). The Behavioral System Model for Nursing. In J. P. Riehl, & C. Roy (Eds.), *Conceptual models for nursing practice* (2nd ed.) (pp. 207–216). New York: Appleton-Century-Crofts. [out of print]

Jonas, C. M. (1989). *Practicing Parse's theory with groups of individuals in the community.* Paper presented at The Queen Elizabeth Hospital, Toronto, Ontario.

King, I. M. (1981). *A theory for nursing: Systems, concepts, process.* New York: Wiley. [out of print]

King, I. M. (1989). King's general systems framework and theory. In J. Riehl-Sisca (Ed.), *Conceptual models for nursing practice* (3rd ed.) (pp. 149–158). Norwalk, CT: Appleton & Lange.

Levine, M. E. (1989). The conservation principles of nursing: Twenty years later. In J. Riehl-Sisca (Ed.), *Conceptual models for nursing practice* (3rd ed.) (pp. 325–337). Norwalk, CT: Appleton & Lange.

Levine, M. E. (1988). Book Review: Nursing Science by R. R. Parse. *Nursing Science Quarterly, 1,* 184–185.

Levine, M. E. (1990). Conservation and integrity. In M. E. Parker (Ed.), *Nursing theories in practice.* New York: National League for Nursing.

Martin, M. L., Forchuk, C., Santopinto, M., & Butcher, H. K. (1992). Alternative approaches to nursing practice: Application of Peplau, Rogers, and Parse. *Nursing Science Quarterly, 5,* 80–85.

Meleis, A. I. (1991). *Theoretical nursing: Development and progress* (2nd ed.). Philadelphia: Lippincott.

Merleau-Ponty, M. (1963). *The structure of behavior.* Boston: Beacon Press.

Merleau-Ponty, M. (1973). *The prose of the world.* Evanston, Ill: Northwestern University Press.

Merleau-Ponty, M. (1974) *Phenomenology of perception.* C. Smith (Trans.). New York: Humanities Press.

Mitchell, G. (1986). Utilizing Parse's Theory of Man–Living–Health in Mrs. M's neighborhood. *Perspectives, 10*(4), 5–7.

Mitchell, G. J. (1991). Distinguishing practice with Parse's Theory. In I. E. Goertzen (Ed.), *Differentiating nursing practice: Into the 21st century.* Kansas City: American Academy of Nursing.

Newman, M. (1986). *Health as expanding consciousness.* St. Louis: Mosby.

Nokes, K. M., & Carver, K. (1991). The meaning of living with AIDS: A study using Parse's theory of Man–Living–Health. *Nursing Science Quarterly, 4,* 175–180.

Orem, D. E. (1991). Nursing: Concepts of practice (4th ed.). St. Louis: Mosby.

Orlando, I. J. (1961). *The dynamic nurse–patient relationship: Function, process and principles.* New York: Putnam's.

Parse, R. R. (1981). *Man–living–health: A theory of nursing.* New York: Wiley.

Parse, R. R. (1987). *Nursing science—Major paradigms, theories, and critiques.* Philadelphia: Saunders.

Parse, R. R. (1989). Editorial: Essentials for practicing the art of nursing. *Nursing Science Quarterly, 2,* 111.

Parse, R. R. (1990a). Health: A personal commitment. *Nursing Science Quarterly, 3,* 136–140.

Parse, R. R. (1990b). Parse's research methodology with an illustration of the lived experience of hope. *Nursing Science Quarterly, 3,* 9–17.

Parse, R. R. (1992a). Editorial: The performing art of nursing. *Nursing Science Quarterly, 5,* 147.

Parse, R. R. (1992b). Human Becoming: Parse's theory of nursing. *Nursing Science Quarterly, 5,* 35–42.

Parse, R. R., Coyne, A. B., & Smith, M. J. (1985). *Nursing research: Qualitative methods.* Bowie, Md.: Brady Communications.

Paterson, J. E., & Zderad, L. T. (1988). *Humanistic nursing.* New York: National League for Nursing. (Originally published 1976, Wiley).

Peplau, H. E. (1988). *Interpersonal relations in nursing.* NY: Springer. (Original work published 1952, New York: Putnam's).

Phillips, J. R. (1987). A critique of Parse's Man–Living–Health Theory. In R. R. Parse (Ed.), *Nursing science: Major paradigms, theories, and critiques* (pp. 181–204). Philadelphia: Saunders.

Rogers, M. E. (1970). *The theoretical basis of nursing.* Philadelphia: Davis. [out of print]

Rogers, M. E. (1984). *Science of Unitary Human Beings: A paradigm for nursing.* Paper presented at International Nurse Theorist Conference, Edmonton, Alberta.

Rogers, M. E. (1992). Nursing science and the space age. *Nursing Science Quarterly, 5*(1), 27–34.

Roy, C. (1984). *Introduction to nursing: An adaptation model* (2nd ed.). Englewood Cliffs, NJ: Prentice–Hall.

Roy, C., & Andrews, H. A. (1991). *The Roy Adaptation Model: The definitive statement.* Norwalk, CT: Appleton & Lange.

Santopinto, M. D. A. (1989a). *An evaluation of Parse's practice methodology in a chronic care setting.* Paper presented at the 19th Quadrennial Congress of the International Council of Nurses, Seoul, Korea.

Santopinto, M. D. A. (1989b). The relentless drive to be ever thinner: A study using the phenomenological method. *Nursing Science Quarterly, 2,* 29–36.

Sartre, J. P. (1963). *Search for a method.* New York: Alfred A. Knopf.

Sartre, J. P. (1964). *Nausea.* New York: New Dimensions.

Sartre, J. P. (1966). *Being and nothingness.* New York: Washington Square Press.

Smith, M. C. (1990). Struggling through a difficult time for unemployed persons. *Nursing Science Quarterly, 3,* 18–28.

Winkler, S. J. (1983). Parse's theory of nursing. In J. J. Fitzpatrick, & A. L. Whall (Eds.), *Conceptual models of nursing—Analysis and application* (pp. 275–294). Bowie, MD: Brady.

Wondolowski, C., & Davis, D. K. (1991). The lived experience of health in the oldest old: A phenomenological study. *Nursing Science Quarterly, 4,* 113–122.

HELEN C. ERICKSON, EVELYN M. TOMLIN, AND MARY ANN P. SWAIN

Noreen Cavan Frisch
Susan Stanwyck Bowman

■ ■ ■

Helen Erickson completed her initial nursing education in 1957 with a diploma from Saginaw General Hospital in Saginaw, Michigan. She went on to earn a bachelor of science in nursing, a masters in nursing, and a doctorate in educational psychology at the University of Michigan. Erickson is accomplished in all three areas of nursing. She is a clinician, a teacher, and a scholar. As a clinician, she has practiced in many different areas of nursing in both direct care and supervisory roles. She has practiced in both the United States and Puerto Rico. She continues with an independent nursing practice while fulfilling her present faculty commitments.

As a teacher, Erickson has held both instructional and administrative positions and taught in both undergraduate and graduate curricula. She has been on the faculty of the University of Michigan and the University of South Carolina and currently holds the position of professor at the University of Texas at Austin. She has received several awards for excellence in teaching, including recognition as one of only two nursing faculty in the 100-year history of the University of Michigan to receive the Amoco Good Teaching Award.

As a scholar, Erickson has worked on articulating the theory of Modeling and Role-Modeling since her return to graduate school. She published the book on the theory in 1983 in collaboration with Evelyn Tomlin and Mary Ann Swain. She is continually involved in research and publications relating to the theory of Modeling and Role-Modeling. She received the Sigma Theta Tau Rho chapter award for excellence in nursing in 1980. Erickson was also the first president of the Society for the Advancement of Modeling and Role-Modeling from 1986 to 1990. She has presented the theory at many nursing meetings nationally and internationally.

Evelyn Tomlin received a baccalaureate degree in nursing from the University of Southern California and a masters in psychiatric nursing from the University of Michigan. She has extensive clinical practice experience both in the United States and in Afghanistan. She has been involved in staff nursing, critical care, home health, and independent practice as well as many areas of nursing education. She presently enjoys maintaining her independent nursing practice in Illinois. She has published an article relating Modeling and Role-Modeling with spiritual concerns in nursing in the first monograph published by the Society for the Advancement of Modeling and Role-Modeling.

Mary Ann Swain's educational background is in psychology with a bachelor of arts degree from DePauw University in Greencastle, Indiana, and both a masters of science and a doctoral degree from the University of Michigan. Although not a nurse, much of Swain's career has been involved with nursing. She has taught research methods and statistics as well as psychology to nurses at DePauw University and the University of Michigan. Swain has held the positions of director of the doctoral program in nursing, chairperson of nursing research, professor of nursing research and associate vice president for academic affairs at the University of Michigan. She is presently provost and vice president for academic affairs at the State University of New York, Binghampton. She has received many awards for academic excellence and is an honorary member of Sigma Theta Tau. She is active in the Society for the Advancement of Modeling and Role-Modeling and is the immediate past president of the Society.

The book describing the theory of Modeling and Role-Modeling presents the theory in a very informal and readable style (Erickson, Tomlin, & Swain, 1983). It includes many case studies and clinical examples of the use of this theory in nursing. The basis of the theory is always to focus on the person receiving nursing care—not on the nurse, not on the care, and not on the disease. The concept of modeling a person's world is credited to Milton H. Erickson, MD, who was the father-in-law of the principal author of this theory, Helen Erickson. Erickson credits her father-in-law with a great deal of influence on this theory. His initial beliefs in the mind–body connection in health, healing, and disease as well as his belief that the most important thing a nurse can do to help a client is modeling that person's world provided the underlying themes for this theory.

Erickson returned to graduate school after many years of clinical practice to "label and articulate" practice-based knowledge that she knew was important to and consistent in nursing care. She believed this knowledge needed to be shared with other nurses. Both her master's thesis and doctoral dissertation were instrumental in developing the theory of Modeling and Role-Modeling (Erickson, 1976, 1984). Other early research that contributed to this theory was supported by two federal grants: "Influencing compliance among hypertensives" from the National Heart, Lung, and Blood Institute (HL–17045) (Erickson & Swain, 1977; Swain & Stickel, 1981) and "Health promotion among diabetics: Comparing nursing systems" from the Division of Nursing (NU–00658). At the present time, Erickson and Dr. Carolyn Kinney are conducting a federally funded study at the University of Texas to relate Modeling to people with Alzheimer's disease.

The combination of talents of the three authors who collaborated at the University of Michigan in the mid-1970's was advantageous for the development of a nursing theory that was useful and related to practice, education, and research. All three authors have been involved in nursing education. Two are expert nursing clinicians and remain actively involved in clinical practice, and two remain active in research and scholarly pursuits.

THE THEORY OF MODELING AND ROLE-MODELING

Modeling and Role-Modeling is an interpersonal and interactive theory of nursing that requires the nurse to assess (*Model*), plan (*Role-Model*), and intervene (*Five aims of intervention*) on the basis of the client's perspective of the world. The nurse always acknowledges the uniqueness and individuality of the client and appreciates that individuals, at some level, know what makes them ill and what makes them well (*Self-care knowledge*). Two additional concepts important in this theory are (1) *affiliated-individuation,* and (2) *adaptive potential.*

Modeling

Modeling is the process used by the nurse to develop an understanding of the client's world as the client perceives it. The way an individual perceives life and all of its aspects and components; the way an individual thinks, communicates, feels, believes, and behaves; and the underlying motivation and rationale for beliefs and behaviors—all these comprise the individual's model of the world. This concept is based on the works of Milton Erickson, who believed that an appreciation for a client's model of the world was a prerequisite for providing holistic care (Erickson, Tomlin, & Swain, 1983). Modeling is both an art and a science. The art of modeling is the empathetic development of an understanding of the present situation within the client's context of the world—that is, the development of a "model" of the situation from the client's perspective. The science of modeling is the analysis of the information collected about the client's world. To truly understand the client's model of the world, the nurse must have a strong theoretical base in the physical and social sciences. The client's perspective is analyzed on the basis of knowledge and theory regarding human behavior, development, cultural diversity, interaction, pathophysiology, human needs, and so forth (Erickson, Tomlin, & Swain, 1983).

Role-Modeling

Role-Modeling is the facilitation of health. It is also both an art and a science. The art of Role-Modeling involves the individualization of care based on the client's model of the world; the science of role-modeling is the use of theoretical bases when planning and implementing nursing care. Role-Modeling is the facilitation of the individual in attaining, maintaining, or promoting health through purposeful interventions based on the individual's personal perceptions as well as the theoretical base for the practice of nursing (Erickson, Tomlin, & Swain, 1983).

Five Aims of Intervention

The aims of intervention are based on five principles pertaining to similarities among humans (see Table 20–1). Because each individual is unique and has his or her own model of the world, it is not possible to formulate standardized interventions. However, because all human beings have some similarities, the aims of intervention can be standardized. Individualized interventions are based on the client's model of the world and guided by the five aims of intervention defined as follows.

Build Trust. Nursing requires a trusting relationship. This relationship involves honesty, acceptance, respect, empathy, and a belief in the client's model of the world. Therapeutic communication skills are essential in building trust. Trust is basic to any interpersonal relationship and is easily threatened if clients perceive that nurses lack respect for their view of the world or feel that nurses consider the clients' concerns or beliefs to be invalid, unwarranted, erroneous, or inappropriate.

Promote Positive Orientation. Nursing interventions need to promote clients' self-worth as well as hope for the future. Reframing can be used to assist clients in changing their perception of a situation from one of threat to one of challenge, from one of hopelessness to one of hope, and from something negative to something positive.

TABLE 20–1. RELATIONSHIP OF HUMAN SIMILARITY PRINCIPLES AND AIMS FOR INTERVENTION

Principle	Aim
1. The nursing process requires that a trusting and functional relationship exist between nurse and client.	Build trust.
2. Affiliated-individuation is dependent on the individual's perceiving that he or she is an acceptable, respectable, and worthwhile human being.	Promote client's positive orientation.
3. Human development is dependent on the individual's perceiving that he or she has some control over his or her life, while concurrently sensing a state of affiliation.	Promote client's control.
4. There is an innate drive toward holistic health that is facilitated by consistent and systematic nurturance.	Affirm and promote client's strengths.
5. Human growth is dependent on satisfaction of basic needs and facilitated by growth–need satisfaction.	Set mutual goals that are health-directed.

(From Erickson, H. C., Tomlin, E. M., & Swain, M. A. P. (1983). Modeling and role-modeling: A theory and paradigm for nursing (p. 170). Lexington, SC: Pine Press. Used with permission.)

Promote Perceived Control. Human development depends on individuals' perceiving that they have some control over their lives. Nurses may understand that clients have control over what happens to them and may understand that clients are required to give informed consent for any procedure done to them. However, many clients do not perceive that they have any control. It is not enough for the nurse to promote client control; the nurse must promote the client's *perception* of control.

Promote Strengths. Identification and promotion of strengths is a means of assisting clients to mobilize resources. In the face of stressors, individuals may become overwhelmed with their perceived weaknesses and not be able to identify or use strengths.

Set Mutual Goals That Are Health Directed. Nurses must use the individual's innate drive to be as healthy as he or she can be. The nurse's and client's goals are the same—to meet the client's basic needs. When the nurse's and client's goals appear to differ, the nurse has most likely not fully modeled the client's world. Incomplete modeling can be the result of inadequate data gathering and empathy or a lack of knowledge for analysis and interpretation of the data collected.

Self-Care

There are three aspects of self-care in the theory of Modeling and Role-Modeling: *self-care knowledge, self-care resources,* and *self-care action.*

Self-care Knowledge. In most situations, individuals can describe what they perceive to be their health problem; they can also identify what they think will make them feel better. According to Erickson, Tomlin, and Swain, self-care knowledge is knowledge one has about "what has made him or her sick, lessened his or her effectiveness, or interfered with his or her growth. The person also knows what will make him or her well, optimize his or her effectiveness or fulfillment (given circumstances), or promote his or her growth" (Erickson, Tomlin, & Swain, 1983, p. 48). In an analysis of case studies reported by Erickson (1990), the following four themes were found that relate to the nature of self-care knowledge:

1. An individual's perception of factors associated with his [or her] personal health problems are rarely obvious to the health care provider.
2. The individual's perceptions of what is needed to help him or her can best be defined by that person.
3. A nurse's role is to facilitate clients to articulate what they perceive to be associated with their problem and what can be done to help them feel better.
4. Another nursing role is to assist the clients to resolve their problems in ways that meet personal needs and are health and growth directed.

Self-care Resources. All individuals have internal and external resources (strengths and support) that will help gain, maintain, and promote an optimum level of holistic health. It is important for the nurse to assess these resources to assist the client in self-care action.

Self-care Action. Self-care action is the development and use of self-care knowledge and self-care resources. The basis of nursing is assisting clients in self-care actions related to health.

The concept of self-care is used differently in the theory of Modeling and Role-Modeling than in Orem's (1991) Self-Care Deficit Theory. Orem's theory focuses on delineating *when* nursing is needed. Self-care is a universal need met through the ability to care for one's self; nurses assist clients in meeting self-care needs when there is a deficit in the clients' ability to meet their own needs. Self-care in Modeling and Role-Modeling focuses on the individual's personal knowledge about what makes him or her well or ill. All clients have self-care knowledge, and the nurse facilitates the client's identification and use of that knowledge. Self-care, then, in Modeling and Role-Modeling is used in planning implementations rather than being used for determining the *need* for nursing implementations, as is the situation in Orem's self-care theory.

Affiliated-Individuation

All individuals are seen as having simultaneous needs to be attached to other individuals and to be separate from them. This concept is described in Modeling and Role-Modeling as "affiliated-individuation" and considered to be a motivation for human behavior. "Affiliated-individuation occurs when a person perceives himself or herself as simultaneously close to and separate from a significant other" (Erickson, Tomlin, & Swain, 1983, p. 68). Affiliated-individuation is different from interdependence in that it is an intrapsychic phenomenon and can occur without being reciprocated.

Adaptive Potential

Adaptive potential refers to the individual's ability to mobilize resources to cope with stressors. The Adaptive Potential Assessment Model (APAM) has the three categories of *equilibrium, arousal,* and *impoverishment.* Equilibrium has two possibilities: *adaptive equilibrium* and *maladaptive equilibrium.* Arousal and impoverishment are both stress states. They differ in that those in impoverishment must seek to deal with the stress with diminished, if not depleted, resources (Erickson, Tomlin, & Swain, 1983). Adaptive potential is dynamic, and individuals can move from any of the three states to any other of the states, as shown in Figure 20–1. Movement among the states is influenced by the individual's ability to cope. The APAM identifies states (not traits) of coping that can assist the nurse in planning interventions for the client. Assessment of adaptive potential has been well documented (Barnfather, Swain, & Erickson, 1989a, 1989b; Campbell,

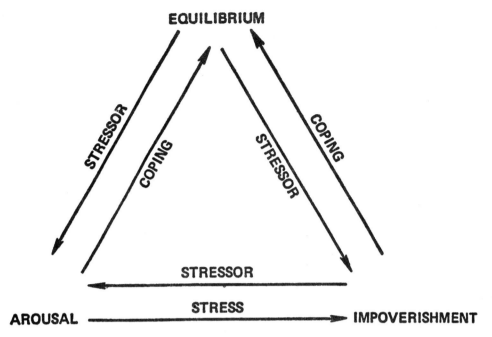

Figure 20–1. An illustration of the dynamic relationship among the states of the Adaptive Potential Assessment Model. *(From Erickson, H., Tomlin, E., & Swain, M. A. (1983).* Modeling and Role-Modeling: A theory and paradigm for nursing *(p. 82). Lexington, SC: Pine Press. Used with permission.)*

Finch, Erickson, & Swain, 1985; Erickson & Swain, 1982). Figure 20–2 identifies how interventions can be guided by the individual's ability to mobilize his or her own resources. A person who is impoverished is not in a situation to be an autonomous, independent person eager to learn and to perform self-care. An impoverished person requires that affiliation needs be met, internal strengths be promoted, and external resources be provided. A client in arousal is in a stress state and has difficulty mobilizing resources. This client has stronger individuation needs and responds to guidance, directions, assistance, and teaching that are all aimed at self-care. The client in equilibrium is in a nonstress state. Adaptive equilibrium is different from maladaptive equilibrium in that the adaptive client has all subsystems in harmony, whereas the maladaptive client places one or more subsystems in jeopardy to maintain equilibrium. The importance of equilibrium, whether adaptive or maladaptive, is that the client sees no reason to change because equilibrium already exists. Interventions for the client in maladaptive equilibrium need to focus on motivation strategies to develop a desire for change.

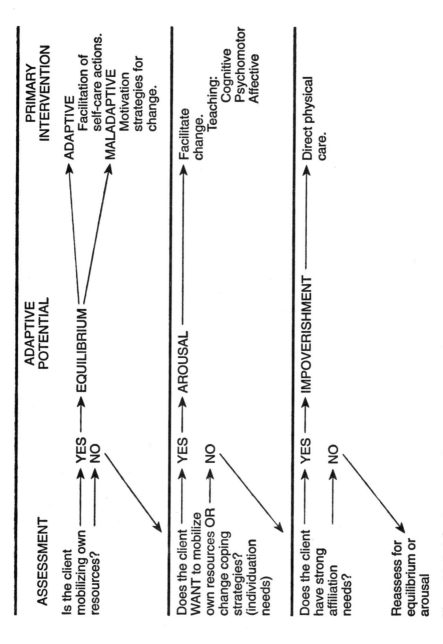

Figure 20–2. Adaptive potential as a guide to planning nursing interventions. *(Bowman, S. S. (1992). Adaptive potential as a guide to planning nursing interventions. Presented at the Fourth National Modeling and Role-Modeling Conference, Boston, MA. Used with permission.)*

MODELING AND ROLE-MODELING AND NURSING'S METAPARADIGM

Human beings are holistic persons with interacting subsystems (biophysical, psychological, social, and cognitive) and inherent genetic bases and spiritual drive (see Fig. 20–3).

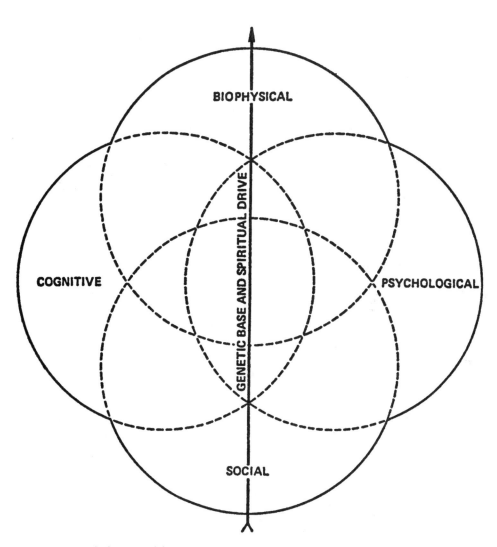

Figure 20–3. A holistic model. *(From Erickson, H., Tomlin, E., & Swain, M. A. (1983). Modeling and Role-Modeling: A theory and paradigm for nursing (p. 45). Lexington, SC: Pine Press. Used with permission.)*

"Holism" implies that the whole is greater than the sum of the parts and is differentiated from "wholism," which implies that a person is an aggregate of parts and the whole is equal to the sum of the parts (Erickson, Tomlin, & Swain, 1983). Modeling and Role-Modeling describes individuals as being born with an inherent desire to fulfill their self-potential. The developmental theories of Erik Erikson, Abraham Maslow, Jean Piaget, and George Engel are basic to describing how people are alike. People are seen as alike in that they are all holistic beings who want to develop their potential. All individuals have basic needs that motivate behavior, including a drive called *affiliated-individuation* (Erickson, Tomlin, & Swain, 1983). Although human beings share these commonalities, each individual is unique. People differ from one another as a result of their individual inherited endowment, their situational ability to mobilize their resources to respond to life's stressors, and their models of the world.

Environment is seen as internal and external and includes both stressors and resources for adapting to stressors. Stressors exist in life at all times and are necessary for overall growth and life enhancement. All individuals have both internal and external resources for dealing with stressors. Potential resources exist and individuals may need assistance in becoming aware of and constructively mobilizing them.

The definition of *health* is consistent with that of the World Health Organization in that Erickson, Tomlin, and Swain (1983) write that health is a state of physical, mental, and social well-being, not merely the absence of disease or infirmity. These authors also write that health connotes a state of dynamic equilibrium among the various subsystems. This dynamic equilibrium implies an adaptive equilibrium whereby the individual learns to cope constructively with life's stressors by mobilizing internal and external coping resources and leaving no subsystem in jeopardy when adaptation occurs.

Nursing is a process between the nurse and the client and requires an interpersonal and interactive nurse–client relationship. Three characteristics of the nurse in this theory are facilitation, nurturance, and unconditional acceptance. Facilitation implies that the nurse aids the individual to identify, mobilize, and develop his or her own strengths. Nurturance is the fusing and integrating of cognitive, psychological, and affective processes with the aim of assisting a client toward holistic health. Unconditional acceptance is the acceptance of each individual as unique, worthwhile, and important with no strings attached. The Modeling and Role-Modeling definition of nursing as given by Erickson, Tomlin, and Swain (1983) is as follows:

> Nursing is the holistic helping of persons with their self-care activities in relation to their health. This is an interactive, interpersonal process that nurtures strengths to enable development, release, and channeling of resources for coping with one's circumstances and environment. The goal is to achieve a state of perceived optimum health and contentment (p. 49).

Additional statements by Erickson, Tomlin and Swain (1983) to define nursing are the following:

> Nursing is the nurturance of holistic self-care.
> Nursing is assisting persons holistically to use their adaptive strengths to attain and maintain optimum bio-psycho-socio-spiritual functioning.
> Nursing is helping with self-care to gain optimum health.
> Nursing is an integrated and integrative helping of persons to take better care of themselves (p. 50).

MODELING AND ROLE-MODELING AND THE NURSING PROCESS/NURSING PRACTICE

The authors of the Modeling and Role-Modeling theory acknowledge two distinct meanings of the nursing process. The first is the formalized, step-by-step problem-solving process that includes gathering and analyzing data, planning and implementing interventions, and evaluating outcomes. The second is a more basic use of the term and refers to an interactive process—the exchange between nurse and patient in which the nurse has a purpose of nurturing and supporting the client's self-care.

There has been much emphasis in schools and in practice areas on the formalized steps of the nursing process. The Modeling and Role-Modeling theory, however, emphasizes the primacy of the interactive, interpersonal definition. Nursing involves an ongoing exchange of information, feelings, and behaviors; the nursing process describes this exchange. Thus, the nursing process begins with the first interaction between nurse and patient. The Modeling and Role-Modeling theory accepts the view, expressed by Lucille Kinlein (1977) in the 1970s, that nursing care begins with the first patient encounter because the nurse's immediate contributions to care include the nurse himself or herself—the presence, the unconditional acceptance, and the support and comfort that are offered from one human being to another.

Because the theory directs the nurse to begin where the client is in modeling the client's world, a comprehensive assessment is rarely done to initiate nursing care. The client will always be asked to express his or her questions, concerns, and needs. Client concerns have utmost priority because a person whose immediate needs are unattended will not progress in other ways. Thus, the theory directs the nurse's priorities of care quite simply, beginning where the client requests care to begin, knowing that as one need is met, other unmet needs will emerge to direct care. At any point, assessment is dictated by client needs, and the nurse will gather whatever information is required to understand and care for the client's expressed concerns.

The interactive nursing process includes formal, logical thinking; Erickson, Tomlin, and Swain (1983) make it clear that they value scientific thinking. However, when using Modeling and Role-Modeling, there are no preset steps in applying the nursing process. Nurses provide care at the first moment of contact, they *assess* while they *implement,* they *analyze* while *evaluating.* They write, "When we view the nursing process predominantly as an ongoing, interactive, interpersonal relationship that includes use of the formal scientific mode of thought, we can regard documentation of the nursing process primarily as a valuable way to communicate with others and keep records" (p. 105).

In providing care, client data are gathered to model the client's world. An evaluation of the client's stress and adaptation is essential, as well as information on self-care knowledge, resources, and actions. Diagnoses include adaptive potential, that is, the client's potential for mobilizing resources needed to contend with stressors.

Erickson, Tomlin, and Swain do not address the use of the nursing diagnoses taxonomy developed by the North American Nursing Diagnoses Association (NANDA) with Modeling and Role-Modeling. For many nurses in practice and in education, however, Modeling and Role-Modeling has been incorporated with the NANDA taxonomy. The Brigham and Women's Hospital in Boston was the first institution in the country to adopt Modeling and Role-Modeling as the base for practice house-wide. Nurses there who were already using NANDA diagnoses to articulate nursing concerns readily adapted by continuing to use them to document nursing concerns while using Modeling and Role-Modeling to understand the etiology of the diagnoses. For example, the nurses may write a NANDA diagnosis of "Fatigue r/t continued state of impoverishment secondary to stressors of hospitalization and isolation." In this way, the NANDA taxonomy is used as an atheoretical labeling of a nursing concern; Modeling and Role-Modeling provides the theoretical base for understanding and intervening with that concern. A similar meshing of Modeling and Role-Modeling with NANDA has occurred at Humboldt State University, where Modeling and Role-Modeling is being used as the conceptual basis for nursing care in an undergraduate nursing curriculum. The case study "Harold" presented in Table 20–2 provides an illustration of how nursing care and diagnoses differ when using nursing diagnoses atheoretically and when using nursing diagnoses with Modeling and Role-Modeling as the theoretical base.

In carrying out nursing care, the nurse must "role-model," that is, help the client in attaining, maintaining, or promoting health through purposeful interventions. Care is based on the five aims of interventions and is consistent with the client's adaptive potential (see Figure 20–2). The nurse's role is to facilitate, nurture, and provide unconditional acceptance while assisting the client to achieve health. Evaluation of nursing care is directed toward goals mutually determined between patient and client.

TABLE 20–2. "HAROLD" A CASE STUDY DEMONSTRATING THE DIFFERENCE BETWEEN THE ATHEORETICAL USE OF NURSING DIAGNOSES AND THE USE OF NURSING DIAGNOSES WITH MODELING AND ROLE-MODELING AS THE THEORETICAL BASE

CASE STUDY—	Nursing Care Based on Admission Data:	Revised Nursing Care Based on Modeling and Role Modeling:
Harold is a 72-year-old unemployed truck driver who was admitted to the hospital with severe COPD, unstable angina, and severe skin lesions on his legs. He is a homeless man who lives in a nonfunctioning car on the beach. He has been admitted 7 times in the past 6 months with exacerbations of COPD, R/O sepsis, and cellulitis. He presented at this admission with a TPR of 101, 138, and 44. Laboratory results demonstrated high WBCs, abnormal blood gases, and subtherapeutic digoxin and aminophylline serum levels. Harold was dirty, odorous, and had open, draining sores on this legs. The medical regimen was aminophylline, anti-inflammatory agents, antibiotics, and his routine medications, which consisted of digoxin, brethine, etc. He was receiving oxygen but was really uncomfortable. He was also very quiet.	**INITIAL DIAGNOSES**	**REVISED DIAGNOSES**
	Ineffective breathing pattern	Impaired mobility
		Fatigue
	Altered gas exchange	Powerlessness
	Self-care deficit: bathing and hygiene	
Harold was seen as "difficult" by the nurses. The nurses were frustrated by his repeated admissions. Harold was frustrated because he thought people had "judged" him and that they wanted him to "change his whole life."	Altered health maintenance	
	Fear	
	INITIAL INTERVENTIONS	**REVISED INTERVENTIONS**
Additional data were gathered to model Harold's world. Harold said that he came to the hospital because he was sick and didn't want to burden his friends. He said that he believed people at the hospital didn't like him because they wanted him to change things he didn't want to change—like where he lived. Harold said that he had always had skin problems with his legs, but the new problem was that his dog had sand fleas and that he couldn't seem to manage. He ran out of medication because his car didn't work and didn't take his theophylline because he thought it altered his sexual functioning. When asked what he saw as his major problem, he said: "I can't get to the shower because I'm so tired—then my legs get worse!"	Positioning	Increasing Harold's role in his care
	Maintaining oxygenation	Increasing Harold's perceived control
	Administering the appropriate medications	Clustering nursing care activities because of fatigue
	Skin care: bathing & hygiene	
	Reassuring Harold	Discussing Harold's specific discharge planning (dog baths; medication delivery, etc.)

How did Modeling and Role Modeling-based practice change Harold's nursing care?
- Harold got holistic, individualized care.
- Harold's attitude and self-esteem improved.
- Harold participated more in self-care activities.
- There was less frustration with the nurses.
- Harold increased his adherence to treatment.
- Ten months after discharge, he had still not been readmitted.

Adapted from a presentation at the Fourth National Modeling and Role-Modeling Conference, 1992, developed by Wendy Woodward, Humboldt State University. Used with permission.

COMPARISON OF MODELING AND ROLE-MODELING AND CHARACTERISTICS OF A THEORY

1. Theories can interrelate concepts in such a way as to create a different way of looking at a particular phenomenon. Modeling and Role-Modeling provides a unique way of understanding nursing. The client is seen in a truly holistic manner, as a person with an understandable and individual worldview. Nursing's task becomes that of knowing the client, discovering the client's needs and concerns, affirming that the client is directing all health-related actions, and facilitating the client's striving toward health. Theories long studied by nursing students—Maslow, Erikson, Piaget, Selye, and Engel—emerge in a new perspective as these psychosocial and developmental theories become useful and immediate in understanding the client's world. Modeling and Role-Modeling provides a sense of the true meaning of client-directed care, for the client is trusted as knowing what he or she needs from the nurse to achieve health.

2. Theories must be logical in nature. Modeling and Role-Modeling provides a logical framework from which to understand nursing and from which to plan and provide care. Major concepts of the definition of the person, the meaning of health, and the client's responsibility for self-care are clear. The five aims of intervention emphasize the importance of the nurse–client relationship. The view of the nursing process as an interpersonal process is readily accepted by nurses who understand the interactive nature of what they are doing.

3. Theories should be relatively simple but generalizable. The simplicity of Modeling and Role-Modeling is its beauty. Trusting that the client knows what he or she needs, and planning nursing care around what the client wants is a simple, yet profound, idea. The basic concepts can be readily understood by beginning students in their first nursing course, while still being useful to advanced practitioners. Modeling and Role-Modeling has been applied to clients who are individuals, families, and communities, and it has been applied to clients in all nursing specialty areas of practice.

4. Theories can be the basis for hypotheses that can be tested or for theory to be expanded. Several areas of scholarly inquiry have emerged from the Modeling and Role-Modeling theory. Investigations have been reported involving assessing and understanding adaptive potential as well as use of the theory as a basis to nursing assessment in general (Barnfather, Swain, & Erickson, 1989a, 1989b; Erickson & Swain, 1982; Finch, 1990) . Other studies have involved evaluating the concept of self-care knowledge (Erickson, 1990). Further studies are being done to document outcomes of theory-based practice, including cost-effectiveness. The Society for the Advancement of Modeling and Role-Modeling meets biannually for the purpose of disseminating knowledge relating to the theory acquired through research, practice, and teaching. In providing a new way of understanding nursing, it stimulates evaluation and the study of nursing's effect on a client's health.

5. Theories contribute to and assist in increasing the general body of knowledge within the discipline through the research implemented to validate them. Modeling and Role-Modeling has contributed to the general body of knowledge within nursing, for the theory has both stimulated research and promoted theory-based practice in acute care settings. Modeling and Role-Modeling provides nurses with a language to describe the essence of holistic practice and to empower their clients to direct their own care.

6. Theories can be used by practitioners to guide and improve their practice. There are numerous examples of how Modeling and Role-Modeling has assisted nurses to improve patient care. The case study in Table 20–2 provides an example of how Modeling and Role-Modeling has positively directed patient care.

7. Theories must be consistent with other validated theories, laws, and principles but will leave open unanswered questions that need to be investigated. Modeling and Role-Modeling is built upon a strong base of theory from the social sciences. It is consistent with a view of individuals as developing beings who are moving through various life stages as they encounter challenges of living and growing. Stress is understood as part of living; a person's ability to adapt to stress depends on prior experiences. The person is viewed holistically, with the recognition that health is achieved when the subsystems are supporting the whole. Unanswered questions emerge that are related to the ability of the self to know and direct health care and to the essence of nursing as facilitating and nurturing.

STRENGTHS AND LIMITATIONS

The theory has many strengths including a strong holistic approach and emphasis on the nurse–client interaction and client–centeredness, as has been described. Its major limitation may be that it is relatively unknown and appears simplistic. Nurses coming to learn about the theory have felt that it merely describes what they have always done intuitively, and that it is too simple merely to put the client in charge of his or her health care. A limitation in practice, particularly for inexperienced nurses, has been that the mandate to "model the client's world" leads to role confusion between being a caring professional and a caring friend.

Nurses at any level can quickly learn how to develop a model of the client's world and gain rewards from this practice. In practice, the development of empathetic assessment is so enticing that nurses may fail to develop the science of modeling. The science of modeling requires professional education. The scientific base for the analysis of data relating to the client's model of the world includes a broad understanding of both the physical and social sciences. To be complete in modeling the client's world, the nurse must draw on many theories in other disciplines, such as psychology, sociology, cultural anthropology, physiology, and pathophysiology.

SUMMARY

The Modeling and Role-Modeling theory suggests an interactive, interpersonal role for nursing. Modeling is the process used to develop an understanding of the client's world; role-modeling is the process of facilitating health-promoting behaviors. Nursing care is based on clients' adaptive potential and directed toward the five aims of intervention: building trust, promoting positive orientation, promoting perceived control, promoting strengths, and setting mutual, health-directed goals. From within this theory, the client is empowered to direct care, based on self-care knowledge, self-care resources, and self-care actions, as the client's perceived needs are addressed. The theory has been applied to work with clients who are individuals, families, and communities. Currently, the theory is being used in both practice and education, and research is being conducted to document and evaluate components of the theory.

REFERENCES

Barnfather, J. S., Swain, M. A. P., & Erickson, H. C. (1989a). Evaluation of two assessment techniques for adaptation to stress. *Nursing Science Quarterly, 2,* 172–182.

Barnfather, J. S., Swain, M. A. P., & Erickson, H. C. (1989b). Construct validity of an aspect of the coping process: Potential adaptation to stress. *Issues in Mental Health Nursing, 10,* 23–40.

Campbell, J., Finch, D., Erickson, H., & Swain, M. A. P. (1985). A theoretical approach to nursing assessment. *Journal of Advanced Nursing, 10,* 111–115.

Erickson, H. (1976). *Identification of states of coping utilizing physiological and psychological data.* Unpublished master's thesis, University of Michigan.

Erickson, H. (1984). *Self-care knowledge: Relations among the concepts support, hope, control, satisfaction with daily life, and physical health status.* Doctoral dissertation, University of Michigan. *Dissertation Abstracts International, 45,* 1731, University Microfilms No. 84-12136.

Erickson, H. (1990). Self-care knowledge: An exploratory study. *Modeling and role-modeling: Theory, practice and research,* monograph, *1*(1), The Society for Advancement of Modeling and Role-Modeling.

Erickson, H., & Swain, M. A. (1977). The utilization of a nursing care model for the treatment of essential hypertension. *Circulation* (abstract).

Erickson, H., & Swain, M. A. (1982). A model for assessing potential adaptation to stress. *Research in Nursing and Health, 5,* 93–101.

Erickson, H. C., Tomlin, E. M., & Swain, M. A. P. (1983). *Modeling and role modeling: A theory and paradigm for nursing.* Lexington, SC: Pine Press.

Finch, D. (1990). Testing a theoretically based nursing assessment. In H. Erickson, & E. Kinney (Eds.), *Modeling and role-modeling: Theory, research and practice.* monograph, *1*(1), (pp. 203–213). Austin, TX: The Society for Advancement of Modeling and Role-Modeling.

Kinlein, L. (1977). *Independent nursing practice with clients.* Philadelphia: Lippincott.

Orem, D. E. (1991). *Nursing: Concepts and practice* (4th ed.). St. Louis: Mosby.

Swain, M. A., & Stickel, S. B. (1981). Influencing adherence among hypertensives. *Research in Nursing and Health, 4,* 213–222.

Tomlin, E. M. (1990). Spiritual concerns in nursing: The interface of Modeling and Role-modeling with professional nursing's Christian roots and values. In H. Erickson, & C. Kinney (Eds.), *Modeling and role-modeling: Theory, practice and research.* monograph, *1*(1), (pp. 40–66). Austin, TX: The Society for the Advancement of Modeling and Role-Modeling.

BIBLIOGRAPHY

Erickson, H. (1983). Coping with new systems. *Journal of Nursing Education, 22,* 132–135.

Erickson, H. (1988). Modeling and role-modeling: Ericksonian techniques applied to physiological problems. In J. Zeig, & S. Lankton (Eds.), *Developing Ericksonian therapy: State of the art.* New York: Brunner/Mazel.

Erickson, H. (1990). Modeling and role-modeling with psycho-physiological problems. In J. Zeig (Ed.), *Brief therapy: Myths and methods.* New York: Brunner/Mazel.

Kinney, C., & Erickson, H. (1990). Modeling the client's world: A way to holistic care. *Issues in Mental Health Nursing, 11,* 93–108.

C H A P T E R   2 1

MADELEINE M. LEININGER

Julia B. George

■ ■ ■

Madeleine M. Leininger received her basic nursing education at St. Anthony's School of Nursing, Denver, CO, and graduated in 1948. In 1950 she earned a bachelor of science from Benedictine College, Atchison, KS; in 1953 a master of science in nursing from Catholic University, Washington, DC; and in 1965 a PhD in anthropology from the University of Washington, Seattle. She is a Fellow in the American Academy of Nursing and holds an LhD from Benedictine College.

Dr. Leininger is the founder of the transcultural subfield of nursing. She is Professor of Nursing and Anthropology and Human Care Research, Colleges of Nursing and Liberal Arts, Wayne State University. She has held both faculty and administrative appointments in nursing education and has published extensively.

In the 1940s Leininger (1991) recognized the importance of caring to nursing. Statements of appreciation for nursing care made by patients alerted her to caring values and led to her longstanding focus on care as the dominant ethos of nursing. During the mid-1950s, she experienced what she describes as cultural shock while she was working in a child guidance home in the midwestern United States. While working as a clinical nurse specialist with disturbed children and their parents, she observed recurrent behavioral differences among the children and concluded that these differences had a cultural base. She identified a lack of knowledge of the children's cultures as the missing link in nursing to understand the variations in care of clients. This experience led her to become the first professional nurse in the world to earn a doctorate in anthropology, and led to the development of the new field of transcultural nursing as a subfield of nursing.

Leininger first used the terms "transcultural nursing," "ethnonursing," and "cross-cultural nursing" in the 1960s. In 1966, at the University of Colorado, she offered the first transcultural nursing course with field experiences and has been instrumental in the development of similar courses at a number of other institutions (Leininger, 1979). In 1979, Leininger defined transcultural nursing as:

> a learned subfield or branch of nursing which focuses upon the comparative study and analysis of cultures with respect to nursing and health–illness caring practices, beliefs, and values with the

goal to provide meaningful and efficacious nursing care services to people according to their cultural values and health–illness context (p. 15).

At the same time she defined ethnonursing as:

the study of nursing care beliefs, values, and practices as cognitively perceived and known by a designated culture through their direct experience, beliefs, and value system (p. 15).

The term "transcultural nursing" (rather than "cross-cultural") is used today to refer to the evolving knowledge and practices related to this new field of study and practice. Leininger (1991) stresses the importance of knowledge gained from direct experience or directly from those who have experienced and labels such knowledge as *emic*, or people-centered. This is contrasted with *etic* knowledge, which describes the professional perspective. She contends that *emically* derived care knowledge is essential to establish nursing's epistemological and ontological base for practice.

Leininger built her theory of transcultural nursing on the premise that the peoples of each culture not only can know and define the ways in which they experience and perceive their nursing care world but also can relate these experiences and perceptions to their general health beliefs and practices. Based upon this premise, nursing care is derived and developed from the cultural context in which it is to be provided.

Leininger (1991) asserts that human care is central to nursing as a discipline and as a profession. She, and others, have studied the phenomena of care for over four decades. They recognize and are proponents of the preservation of care as the essence of nursing. With this increasing recognition of care as essential to nursing knowledge and practice, Leininger labeled her theory Culture Care. She drew upon anthropology for the culture component and upon nursing for the care component. Her belief that cultures have both health practices that are specific to one culture and prevailing patterns that are common across cultures led to the addition of the terms "diversity" and "universality" to the title of her theory. Thus, the most current title of Leininger's theory is Culture Care or Culture Care Diversity and Universality.

LEININGER'S THEORY

In 1985, Leininger published her first presentation of her work as a theory, and in 1988 and 1991 she presented further explication of her ideas. In the 1991 presentation, she provided orientational definitions for the concepts of culture, cultural care, cultural care diversity, cultural care universality, nursing, worldview, cultural and social structure dimensions, environmental context, ethnohistory, generic (folk or lay) care system, professional care system, cultural congruent nursing care, health, care/caring, cultural care preservation, cultural care accommodation, and cultural care repatterning. Some of these definitions were from earlier works and some were original to the 1991 work. Leininger points out that these definitions are provisional guides that may be altered as a culture is studied.

In addition to the definitions, she presented assumptions which support her prediction that "different cultures perceive, know, and practice care in different ways, yet there are some commonalities about care among all cultures of the world" (Leininger, 1985, p. 210). She refers to the commonalities as universality and to the differences as diversity.

Culture is the "learned, shared and transmitted values, beliefs, norms, and lifeways of a particular group that guides their thinking, decisions, and actions in patterned ways" (Leininger, 1991, p. 47). A related assumption is that the values, beliefs, and practices for culturally related care are shaped by, and often embedded in, "the worldview, language, religious (or spiritual), kinship (social), political (or legal), educational, economic, technological, ethnohistorical, and environmental context" of the culture (p. 45).

Cultural care diversity indicates "the variabilities and/or differences in meanings, patterns, values, lifeways, or symbols of care within or between collectives that are related to assistive, supportive, or enabling human care expressions" (Leininger, 1991, p. 47). In contrast, cultural care universality indicates the "common, similar, or dominant uniform care meanings, patterns, values, lifeways or symbols that are manifest among many cultures and reflect assistive, supportive, facilitative, or enabling ways to help people" (p. 47). It is assumed that, while human care is universal across cultures, caring may be demonstrated through diverse expressions, actions, patterns, lifestyles, and meanings. *Cultural care* is defined as "the subjectively and objectively learned and transmitted values, beliefs, and patterned lifeways that assist, support, facilitate, or enable another individual or group to maintain their well-being, health, improve their human condition and lifeway, or to deal with illness, handicaps or death" (p. 47). A related assumption is that cultural care is "the broadest holistic means to know, explain, interpret, and predict nursing care phenomena to guide nursing care practices" (p. 44).

Worldview is the way in which people look at the world, or at the universe, and form a "picture or value stance" about the world and their lives (Leininger, 1991, p. 47). *Cultural and social structure dimensions* are defined as involving "the dynamic patterns and features of interrelated structural and organizational factors of a particular culture (subculture or society) which includes religious, kinship (social), political (and legal), economic, educational, technologic and cultural values, ethnohistorical factors, and how these factors may be interrelated and function to influence human behavior in different environmental contexts" (p. 47). *Environmental context* is "the totality of an event, situation, or particular experience that gives meaning to human expressions, interpretations, and social interactions in particular physical, ecological, sociopolitical and/or cultural settings" (p. 48). *Ethnohistory* includes "those past facts, events, instances, experiences of individuals, groups, cultures, and institutions that are primarily people-centered (ethno) and which describe, explain, and interpret human lifeways within particular cultural contexts and over short or long periods of time" (p. 48). "Knowledge of meanings and practices derived from world views, social structure factors, cultural values, environmental context, and language uses are essential to guide nursing decisions and actions in providing cultural congruent care" (Leininger, 1988, p. 155).

Generic (folk or lay) care systems are "culturally learned and transmitted, indigenous (or traditional), folk (home-based) knowledge and skills used to provide assistive, supportive, enabling, or facilitative acts toward or for another individual, group, or institution with evident or anticipated needs to ameliorate or improve a human lifeway, health condition (or well-being), or to deal with handicaps and death situations" (Leininger, 1991, p. 48). Generic or folk knowledge is emic. *Professional care system(s)* are defined as "formally taught, learned, and transmitted professional care, health, illness, wellness, and related knowledge and practice skills that prevail in professional institutions usually with multidisciplinary personnel to serve consumers" (p. 48). Professional care knowledge is etic. *Health* is "a state of well-being that is culturally defined, valued, and practiced, and which reflects the ability of individuals (or groups) to perform their daily role activities in culturally expressed, beneficial, and patterned lifeways" (p. 48). The related assumptions are that all cultures have generic or folk health care practices, that professional practices usually vary across cultures, and that in any culture there will be cultural similarities and differences between the care-receivers (generic) and the professional care-givers.

Care as a noun is defined as those "abstract and concrete phenomena related to assisting, supporting, or enabling experiences or behaviors toward or for others with evident or anticipated needs to ameliorate or improve a human condition or lifeway" (Leininger, 1991, p. 46). Care is assumed to be a distinct, dominant, unifying and central focus of nursing, and, while curing and healing cannot occur effectively without care, care may occur without cure. *Care* as a verb is defined as "actions and activities directed toward assisting, supporting, or enabling another individual or group with evident or anticipated needs to ameliorate or improve a human condition or lifeway or to face death" (p. 46). Assumptions related to care and caring include that they are essential for the survival of humans, as well as for their growth, health, well-being, healing, and ability to deal with handicaps and death. The expressions, patterns, and lifeways of care have different meanings in different cultural contexts. The phenomenon of care can be discovered or identified by examining the cultural group's view of the world, social structure, and language.

Along with the universal nature of human beings as caring beings, the cultural care values, beliefs, and practices that are specific to a given culture provide a basis for the patterns, conditions, and actions associated with human care. Knowledge of these provides the base for three modes of nursing care decisions and actions, all of which require the coparticipation of the nurse and clients. *Cultural care preservation* is also known as maintenance and includes those "assistive, supporting, facilitative, or enabling professional actions and decisions that help people of a particular culture to retain and/or preserve relevant care values so that they can maintain their well-being, recover from illness, or face handicaps and/or death" (Leininger, 1991, p. 48). *Cultural care accommodation,* also known as negotiation, includes those "assistive, supporting, facilitative, or enabling creative professional actions and decisions that help people of a designated culture to adapt to or negotiate with others for a beneficial or satisfying health outcome with professional care providers" (p. 48). *Cultural care repatterning,* or restructuring, includes "those assistive, supporting, facilitative, or enabling professional actions and decisions that help a client(s) reorder, change, or greatly modify their lifeways for new, different, and beneficial health care pattern [sic] while respecting the client(s) cultural values and beliefs and still providing a beneficial or healthier lifeway than before the changes were coestablished with the client(s)" (p. 49). Repatterning requires the creative use of an extensive knowledge of the client's culture base and must be done in a way that is sensitive to the client's lifeways while using both generic and professional knowledge.

Nursing is defined as "a learned humanistic and scientific profession and discipline which is focused on human care phenomena and activities in order to assist, support, facilitate, or enable individuals or groups to maintain or regain their well-being (or health) in culturally meaningful and beneficial ways, or to help people face handicaps or death" (Leininger, 1991, p. 47). *Professional nursing care (caring)* is defined as "formal and cognitively learned professional care knowledge and practice skills obtained through educational institutions that are used to provide assistive, supportive, enabling, or facilitative acts to or for another individual or group in order to improve a human health condition (or well-being), disability, lifeway, or to work with dying clients" (p. 38). *Cultural congruent (nursing) care* is defined as "those cognitively based assistive, supportive, facilitative, or enabling acts or decisions that are tailor-made to fit with individual, group, or institutional cultural values, beliefs, and lifeways in order to provide or support meaningful, beneficial, and satisfying health care, or well-being services" (p. 49). Related assumptions include that nursing, as a transcultural care discipline and profession, has a central purpose to serve human beings in all areas of the world; that when culturally based nursing care is beneficial and healthy it contributes to the well-being of the client(s)—whether individuals, groups, families, communities, or institutions—as they function within the context of their environments. Also, nursing care will be culturally congruent or beneficial only when the clients are known by the nurse and the clients' patterns, expressions, and cultural values are used in appropriate and meaningful ways by the nurse with the clients. Finally, it is assumed that if clients receive nursing care that is not at least reasonably culturally congruent (that is, compatible with and respectful of the clients' lifeways, beliefs, and values), the client will demonstrate signs of stress, noncompliance, cultural conflicts, and/or ethical or moral concerns.

Leininger named her theory Culture Care Diversity and Universality and depicts it in the Sunrise Model (see Figure 21–1). This model may be viewed

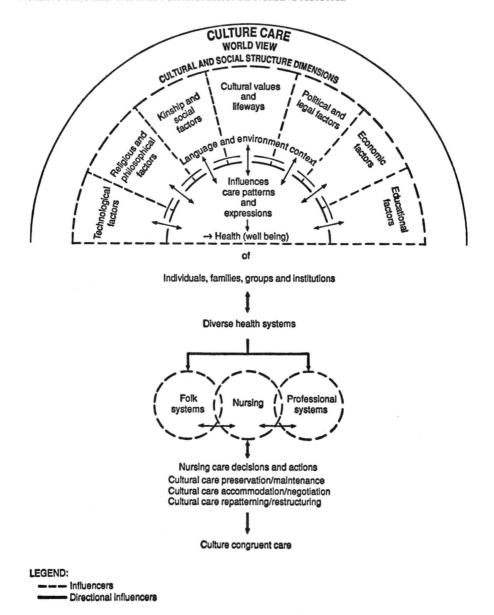

Figure 21–1. Leininger's Sunrise Model depicts dimensions of Cultural Care Diversity and Universality. *(From Leininger, M. (1991). Culture Care Diversity & Universality: A theory of nursing (p. 43). New York: National League for Nursing. Used with permission.)*

as a cognitive map that moves from the most abstract to the least **abstract.** The top of the model is the worldview and social system level, which **directs** the study of perceptions of the world outside of the culture—the suprasystem in general system terms. Leininger (1985) states this level leads to the study of the nature, meaning, and attributes of care from three perspectives. Values and social structure could be a part of each of the perspectives. The microperspective studies individuals within a culture; these studies typically would be on a small scale. The middle perspective focuses on more complex factors in one specific culture; these studies are on a larger scale than micro-studies. The macro-studies investigate phenomena across several cultures and are large in scale.

The cultural care worldview flows into knowledge about individuals, families, groups, communities, and institutions in diverse health care systems. This knowledge provides culturally specific meanings and expressions in relation to care and health. The next focus is on the generic or folk system, professional care system(s), and nursing care. Information about these systems includes the characteristics and the specific care features of each. This information allows for the identification of similarities and differences or cultural care universality and cultural care diversity.

Next are nursing care decisions and actions which involve cultural care preservation/maintenance, cultural care accommodation/negotiation and cultural care repatterning/restructuring. It is here that nursing care is delivered. Within the Sunrise Model, culture congruent care is developed. This care is both congruent with and valued by the members of the culture.

Leininger (1991) points out that the model is not the theory but a depiction of the components of the theory of Culture Care Diversity and Universality. The purpose of the model is to aid the study of how the components of the theory influence the health status of, and care provided to, individuals, families, groups, communities, and institutions within a culture. She presents cogent arguments for the use of the model to guide discovery research that uses qualitative and ethnographic methods of study. She speaks strongly against the use of operational definitions and preconceived notions, and the use of causal or linear perspectives in studying cultural care diversity and universality. She supports the importance of finding out what *is*, of exploring and discovering the essence and meanings of care.

LEININGER'S THEORY AND NURSING'S METAPARADIGM

Leininger defines health but does not specifically define the major concepts of human being, society/environment, and nursing. However, her view of these concepts can be derived from her conceptual definitions and assumptions. She also presents an argument for care as the central concept in nursing's metaparadigm (Leininger, 1991).

Human beings are best represented in her assumptions. Humans are believed to be caring and to be capable of being concerned about the needs, well-being, and survival of others. Human care is universal, that is, seen in all cultures. Humans have survived within cultures and through place and time because they have been able to care for infants, children, and the elderly in a variety of ways and in many different environments. Thus, humans are universally caring beings who survive in a diversity of cultures through their ability to provide the universality of care in a variety of ways according to differing cultures, needs, and settings. Leininger (1991) also indicates that nursing as a caring science should focus beyond traditional nurse–patient interactions and dyads to include "families, groups, communities, total cultures, and institutions" (p. 22) as well as worldwide health institutions and ways to develop international nursing care policies and practices. She points out that in many non-Western cultures family and institutions dominate. In these cultures, person is not an important concept. Indeed, there may be no term in the language for person.

Leininger defines *health;* this definition appears earlier in this chapter. She speaks of health systems, health care practices, changing health patterns, health promotion, and health maintenance. Health is an important concept in transcultural nursing. Because of the emphasis on the need for nurses to have knowledge that is specific to the culture in which nursing is being practiced, it is presumed that health is viewed as being universal across cultures but defined within each culture in a manner that reflects the beliefs, values, and practices of that particular culture. Thus, health is both universal and diverse.

Society/environment are not terms that are defined by Leininger; she speaks instead of worldview, social structure, and environmental context. However, society/environment, if viewed as being represented in culture, are a major theme of Leininger's theory. Environmental context is defined as being the totality of an event, situation, or experience. Leininger's (1991) definition of culture focuses on a particular group (society) and the patterning of actions, thoughts, and decisions that occurs as the result of "learned, shared, and transmitted values, beliefs, norms, and lifeways" (p. 47). This learning, sharing, transmitting, and patterning occur within a group of people who function in an identifiable setting or environment. Therefore, although Leininger does not use the specific terms of society or environment, the concept of culture is closely related to society/environment, and is a central theme of her theory.

Nursing is defined by Leininger; this definition appears earlier in this chapter. She expresses concern that nurses do not have adequate preparation for a transcultural perspective and that they neither value nor practice from such a perspective to the fullest extent possible. She presents three types of nursing actions that are culturally based and thus congruent with the needs and values of the clients. These are cultural care preservation/maintenance, cultural care accommodation/negotiation, and cultural care repatterning/restructuring and have been defined earlier in this chapter. These three modes of action can lead to the delivery of nursing care that best fits with the client's culture and thus decreases cultural stress and potential for conflict between client and caregiver.

CULTURE CARE DIVERSITY AND UNIVERSALITY AND THE NURSING PROCESS

After careful review of the Sunrise Model, it becomes apparent that there are parallels between the model and the nursing process. This is true, in part, because both represent a problem solving process. The focus of the nursing process is the client who is the recipient of nursing care. The client is also a focus of the Sunrise Model, but the importance of knowledge and understanding of the client's culture is a major shaping force in the Model.

Gaining knowledge and understanding of another's culture may be very time consuming for the nurse who is not familiar with that culture. Leininger (1978) speaks with concern about the possibility of the nurse being involved in culture shock or cultural imposition. *Culture shock* may result when an outsider attempts to comprehend or adapt effectively to a different cultural group. The outsider is likely to experience feelings of discomfort and helplessness and some degree of disorientation because of the differences in cultural values, beliefs, and practices. Culture shock may lead to anger and can be reduced by seeking knowledge of the culture before encountering that culture. *Cultural imposition* refers to efforts of the outsider, both subtle and not so subtle, to impose his or her own cultural values, beliefs, behaviors upon an individual, family, or group from another culture. Cultural imposition has been particularly prevalent in efforts to impose Western health care practices upon other cultures.

The upper portions of the Sunrise Model involve the development of knowledge about cultures, people, and care systems. When appropriately used, they could help prevent culture shock and cultural imposition. These levels are similar to the *assessment* and *diagnosis* phases of the nursing process. However, in the Sunrise Model, knowledge of the culture could be gained before identifying a specific client who would be the focus of the nursing process. First, one is assessing or gathering knowledge and information about the social structure and worldview of the client's culture. Other information that is needed includes the language and environmental context of the client as well as the factors of technology, religion, philosophy, kinship, social structure, cultural values and beliefs, politics, legal system, economics, and education. Much of this knowledge could be gathered before the identification of a particular client and would be useful in preventing both culture shock and cultural imposition.

Worldview and social structure knowledge needs to be applied to the situation of the client, whether that client is an individual, a family, a group, a community, or a sociocultural institution. Next, it is recognized that the client exists within a health system and the values, beliefs, and behaviors of the generic (folk), professional, and nursing care portions of that health system need to be identified. Throughout this assessment process, it is important to recognize and identify those characteristics which are universal or common across cultures and those which are diverse or specific to the culture being assessed. After identifying the cultural care diversities and universalities for the culture, a nursing diagnosis can be developed based upon those areas in which the client is not meeting a cultural expectation of the client's culture.

Once the diagnosis has been established, *planning* and *implementation* occur within Nursing Care Decisions and Actions. Again, the nursing care decisions and actions need to be culturally based to best meet the needs of the client and provide culture congruent care. The three modes of action are cultural care preservation/maintenance, cultural care accommodation/negotiation, and cultural care repatterning/restructuring. In cultural care preservation/maintenance, the professional actions focus on supporting, assisting, facilitating, or enabling clients to preserve or retain favorable health, to recover from illness or to face handicaps or death. An example would be facilitating an elderly person's access to grocery shopping so that the individual can continue to prepare healthy meals—or encouraging the sharing of those meals with another in a manner which is culturally acceptable.

Cultural care accommodation/negotiation create professional efforts to facilitate, enable, assist, or support actions which represent ways to negotiate with or adapt or adjust to the client's health and care patterns for a beneficial or satisfying health outcome. For example, in planning for prenatal classes for multigravidas in a Hispanic community, provision for child care needs to be included as Hispanic mothers place very high value on caring for their children and do not use babysitters as freely as do many mothers in American society. The Hispanic mother's care pattern is to provide care for her child and to have the child near her. She will choose to not attend the class rather than leave her child at home with a babysitter. Those who do not understand this may become involved in cultural imposition and label the mother as not caring when she does not attend meetings at which child care is not available.

Cultural care repatterning/restructuring refers to professional actions that seek to help clients change meaningful health or life patterns to patterns that will be healthier for them while respecting the client's cultural values. For example, Charles Sanders, whose dietary pattern has been to eat fried and salted foods at every meal, is found to have hypertension and elevated blood cholesterol levels. Fried chicken with a salty batter is an important element in Mr. Sanders' diet—it is a food which appears on the menu at family celebrations and one which is frequently packed in the brown bag meal he carries to work. Fortunately, the chicken itself is one of the forms of protein which is recommended in low cholesterol diets. The repatterning which can occur relates to the way in which the chicken is prepared. The food preparer in the Sanders family could be taught to skin the chicken (helps lower the cholesterol), use a coating of herbs (rather than salt to help with the hypertension), and bake in the microwave oven with no added fat rather than fry with a salty batter (helps with both cholesterol and hypertension). Such change would repattern the preparation of a favorite food into a way that could provide for the continued inclusion of this food in the diet on a regular basis. At the same time, important changes in the way in which Mr. Sanders eats would be supported. Similar repatterning could occur with other foods, for example, instead of cooking green beans with salt pork, the beans could be cooked with herbs and a little polyunsaturated or monosaturated oil.

The Sunrise Model does not include an area identified as *evaluation*. However, in Leininger's (1991) discussion of transcultural nursing, she places a great deal of importance upon the need for nursing care to provide ways in which care will benefit the client and on the need to systematically study nursing care behaviors to determine which care behaviors are appropriate to the lifeways and behavioral patterns of the culture for healing, health, or well-being. Such study certainly is the equivalent of evaluation. Without evaluation of the outcomes of a particular plan of care that used the nursing process, or a series of such plans, the systematic study that Leininger advises cannot be completed.

CULTURE CARE DIVERSITY AND UNIVERSALITY AND THE CHARACTERISTICS OF A THEORY

Beginning with the identification of a need to understand the culture of clients, through the introduction of the terms transcultural nursing and ethnonursing care, to the presentation of the Sunrise Model, Madeleine Leininger has developed the theory she calls Culture Care Diversity and Universality. This theory will be discussed in relation to the characteristics of a theory presented in Chapter 1.

1. **Theories can interrelate concepts in such a way as to create a different way of looking at a particular phenomenon.** Leininger has developed the Sunrise Model to demonstrate the interrelationships of the concepts in her theory of Culture Care Diversity and Universality. The worldview and social structure portion of the model does not differ significantly from any other view of culture and its interaction with human beings, with the possible exception of the inclusion of care and health patterns. The Model focuses on individuals, families, groups, communities, and sociocultural institutions which is similar to other theories of nursing. The inclusion of the term "cultural" does provide a distinguishing feature since no other nursing theory has this emphasis on culture. Health systems include generic, professional, and nursing care systems. The inclusion of the generic system is unique to the cultural care theory. Nursing care decisions and actions are identified as supporting, accommodating to, or repatterning current health and care practices. The focus of nursing care decisions and actions is shared with many other theories. The division of actions into supporting, accommodating, or repatterning is specific to this theory. The Sunrise Model of Culture Care Diversity and Universality in itself supports the concepts of diversity and universality. The worldview, social structure, and description of individuals, families, groups, communities, and institutions are essentially universal as they have much in common with many other theories. The identified care systems and types of nursing care actions are diverse, or more specific and unique to this particular theory. Overall, the theory of Culture Care was the first to focus specifically on human care from a transcultural perspective (Leininger, 1991). It provides a holistic rather than a fragmented view of people. This view includes "worldview; biophysical state; religious (or spiritual) orientation; kinship patterns; material (and nonmaterial) cultural phenomena; the political, economic, legal, educational, technological, and physical environment; language; and folk and professional care practices" (p. 23). Thus, Leininger

has interrelated concepts in a way which provides a different way of looking at the phenomenon of nursing care.

2. Theories must be logical in nature. There is an inherent logic in the thought that as more is known about a client, the opportunity to provide care that meets that client's needs increases. Leininger has focused on a particular area of knowledge as being important—that area is the culture of the client with culture having a broad definition. The Sunrise Model has a logical order to it. This order is reflected in the movement from a worldview through language and environmental context, care patterns and expressions of individuals, families, groups, communities, and institutions into diverse health systems to nursing care decisions and actions to culture congruent nursing care (see Figure 21–1).

3. Theories should be relatively simple yet generalizable. Leininger's theory is essentially parsimonious in that the necessary concepts are incorporated in such a manner that the theory and its model can be applied in many different settings. The theory and model are not simple in terms of being easily understood upon first contact. However, Leininger's presentations of the theory and model support the need for each of the concepts and demonstrate how the concepts are interrelated. Once the interrelationships are grasped, simplicity is more apparent. The theory and model are excellent examples of being generalizable. The concepts and relationships that are presented are at a level of abstraction which allows them to be applied in many different situations. They provide a guide for knowledge that moves from initial generation of knowledge through affirmation of substantive knowledge to application of that knowledge in a caring process. While the knowledge is to be specific to the situation in which the nursing care is to occur, the process of generating and applying the knowledge is universal.

4. Theories can be the bases for hypotheses that can be tested or for theory to be expanded. During the development of the Culture Care Diversity and Universality theory many studies have been conducted that demonstrate the theory can be the basis for research. A number of these studies were presented during four national transcultural nursing conferences held from 1975 to 1978 at the College of Nursing, University of Utah. The proceedings of these conferences are presented in *Transcultural Nursing* (Leininger, 1979). These proceedings reflect the importance of ethnographic research in the development of this theory. Leininger (1985) presented a number of relational statements that provide a foundation for further study (see Table 21–1). In addition, Leininger (1991) developed a method of study which she labelled ethnonursing research method. She includes examples of ethnonursing research studies of Filipino and Anglo-American nurses, old order Amish, urban Mexican–Americans, Ukrainian pregnancy and childbearing, the Gadsup Akuna, dying patients, and Greek Canadian widows.

It is important to note that the theory of Culture Care Diversity and Universality is based upon, and calls for, qualitative rather than quantitative research. The development of hypotheses is characteristic of positivistic, quantitative research. The development of research questions, and of relational

TABLE 21–1. HYPOTHESES DERIVED FROM LEININGER'S THEORY

- There is an identifiable, positive relationship between the way people of different cultures define, interpret, and know care with their recurrent patterns of thinking and living.
- The *emic* (inside views) of cultural care values, beliefs, and practices of cultures will show a close relationship to their daily life care patterns.
- The meaning and use of cultural care concepts varies cross-culturally and influences nursing care-giver and care-receiver practices.
- There is a meaningful relationship between social structure factors and worldview with generic (folk) and professional care practices.
- Nursing care subsystems are closely related to professional health care systems but differ markedly from generic health care systems.
- Nursing care decisions or actions that reflect the use of the client's cultural care values, beliefs, and practices will be positively related to client's satisfactions with nursing care.
- Nursing care actions or decisions that are based upon the use of cultural care preservation, accommodation, and/or repatterning in client care will be positively related to beneficial nursing care.
- Signs of intercultural care conflicts and stresses will be evident if caregivers fail to use cultural care values and beliefs of clients.
- Marked differences between the meanings and expressions of care givers and care recipients lead to dissatisfactions for both.
- High dependency of the clients upon technological nursing care activities will be closely related to cultural care that reflects decreased personalized care actions.
- Religion and kinship care factors will be more resilient to change than technological factors.
- Western views of cultural care values will be markedly different from non-Western care values.
- Self-care practices will be evident in cultures that value individualism and independence; other care practices will be evident in cultures that support human interdependence.
- Anglo-American nurse-client teaching methods will be dysfunctional with clients of non-Western cultural value orientations.

(Adapted from Leininger, M. M. (1985). Transcultural Care Diversity and Universality: A theory of nursing. Nursing and Health Care, 6, 210, 212.)

statements, is characteristic of qualitative research. Leininger (1991) states that nursing science should be defined "as the creative study of nursing phenomena which reflects the systematization of knowledge using rigorous and explicit research methods within either the qualitative or quantitative paradigm in order to establish a new or to advance nursing's discipline knowledge" (p. 30). Therefore, from the viewpoint of qualitative research, this criterion is met.

5. **Theories contribute to and assist in increasing the general body of knowledge within the discipline through the research implemented to validate them.** The research that has been conducted on transcultural nursing has contributed to the general body of knowledge within the discipline of nursing. One of the outcomes of this research is the identification of major cultural care constructs. Leininger indicates that, as of 1991, ethnonursing research identified 172 care constructs from 54 cultures. These constructs have more diversity than universality of meaning. Included in these constructs

are anticipation of, attentiveness to, comfort, compassion, coping, empathy, engrossment, helping, nurturance, protection, restoration, support, stimulation, stress alleviation, succorance, surveillance, tenderness, touch, and trust (Leininger, 1979, 1985).

Leininger (1991) has directed her research for the last three decades in the epistemological search to establish care as the essence of, and a distinct construct of, nursing. She has sought to explicate the illusive and embedded diverse culture specific and cultural universals of care. The goal of her theory is to provide *culturally congruent care* for the health or well-being of individuals, families, communities, and institutional environments. She views transcultural nursing as the arching framework for all nursing education, theory, research, and practice as nurses are expected to *care* for all people of diverse cultures worldwide. Her ideas have moved nursing beyond unicultural reference to a multicultural perspective.

6. Theories can be utilized by the practitioners to guide and improve their practice. In her presentation of the theory, Leininger presents examples of research findings which can guide and improve the practice of nursing. One example presents the differences in the interpretations of care by American nurses in several general hospitals, Canadian nurses, and Polynesian nurses in Hawaii. The American nurses interpreted care as first dealing with stress alleviation and then comfort. Canadian nurses reported care as being primarily support. Polynesian nurses in Hawaii first identified care as sharing with others in personalized cultural ways and then added being generous to others to achieve signs of harmony among people and their environment. Knowing the diversity in nurses' interpretation of care supports the diversity which will be present in clients and reinforces the need to be knowledgeable about this diversity. Care is universal, the meaning of care is diverse. Leininger (1991) also presents the use of the theory in nursing administration. She states that "the goal of the theory is to improve and to provide culturally congruent care to people that is beneficial, will fit with, and be useful to the client, family, or culture group healthy lifeways" (p. 39).

7. Theories must be consistent with other validated theories, laws, principles but will leave open unanswered questions that need to be investigated. Leininger's theory is certainly consistent with all theories that include the concept of the importance of knowing the client as a person rather than as a problem. Leininger's discussion of the seriousness of unintentional cultural imposition practices by nurses, and of the nurse's need to be aware of his or her own culture and its implications for the nurse–client situation, is very similar to King's (1981) emphasis on the importance of perceptions and the need for the nurse to be alert to both client and personal perceptions. This is but one example of areas of agreement with other theories. It is important to note that while Leininger, Watson (1988), and Boykin and Schoenhofer (1993) all speak of the importance of caring, they approach caring differently.

The unanswered questions that remain to be investigated are greater in number than those that have been answered. Since cultures are diverse not only among cultures but within them, and individuals, even within the same culture, respond differently to the same stimuli, each nurse–client situation provides new questions to be explored.

STRENGTHS AND LIMITATIONS

A major strength of Leininger's theory is the recognition of the importance of culture and its influence on everything that involves the recipients and providers of nursing care. The development of this theory over a number of years has allowed its concepts and constructs to be tested by a number of people in a variety of settings and cultures. The Sunrise Model provides guidance for the areas in which information needs to be collected.

Some limitations, as identified by Leininger (1991), include the limited number of graduate nurses who are academically prepared to conduct the investigations needed to provide transcultural nursing care. While there has been some increase in the number of nurses prepared in transcultural nursing, it is important to note the danger of cultural biases and cultural imposition occurring with nurses' personal cultural values. An associated concern is that too few nursing programs include courses and planned learning experiences that provide a knowledge base for transcultural nursing practice. There is also a need for research funds to support continued study of caring practices—both those that are universal and those that are particular to a culture.

In some of her writings, Leininger is not consistent in her terminology. For example, in *Transcultural Nursing* (1979), she refers to ethnocultural care constructs and then to ethnonursing care constructs. In her theory presentation she refers to these same constructs as major cultural care constructs (Leininger, 1988). Since the constructs are listed it is relatively easy to be aware that these terms all refer to the same constructs. However, the reader's mental energy could be conserved for understanding the theory and model if the terminology were more consistent.

The complexity of the Sunrise Model can be viewed as both a strength and a limitation. The complexity is a strength in that it emphasizes the importance of the inclusion of anthropological and cultural concepts in nursing education and practice. On the other hand, the complexity can lead to misinterpretation or rejection, both of which are limitations.

SUMMARY

Madeleine Leininger has been working since the 1950s on the development of her theory of Culture Care Diversity and Universality. In the 1960s, she first began to use the terms transcultural nursing and ethnonursing. While she has slightly different definitions of these terms, she often uses them interchangeably, an action that can be confusing to the reader.

The major concepts of her theory are culture, cultural care diversity and universality, cultural care, nursing, worldview, cultural and social structure dimensions, environmental context, ethnohistory, generic (folk) care system, professional care system, health, care, caring, cultural care preservation, cultural care accommodation, cultural care repatterning, and cultural congruent nursing care. She defines each of these concepts and presents assumptions that are related to them. The concepts and their interrelationships provide the basis for the Sunrise Model of this theory.

The Sunrise Model presents a cognitive model which, when viewed from the top down, moves from the cultural and social structure through individuals, families, groups, communities, and institutions in generic, professional, and nursing care systems to nursing care decisions and actions that are cultural care preserving, accommodating, and repatterning. The Model also indicates the need to move from knowledge generation through substantive knowledge to application of the knowledge. In discussing the Model, Leininger (1991) presents the idea that care patterns and processes may be universal or diverse. Universal care indicates care patterns, values, and behaviors that are common across cultures. Care diversities represent those patterns and processes that are unique or specific to an individual, family, or cultural group. Leininger believes, and research has supported, that care diversities are greater in number than are universal care patterns.

The theory of Culture Care Diversity and Universality is of significance in a society that is becoming more and more aware of the cultural diversity within its boundaries. While this theory does not provide specific directions for nursing care, it does provide guidelines for the gathering of knowledge and a framework for the making of decisions about what care is needed or would be of the greatest benefit to the client. Leininger has clearly identified what has been a major deficit in our provision of nursing care and provided a road map to begin to fill the gaps created by that deficit.

REFERENCES

Boykin, A., & Schoenhofer, S. (1993). *Nursing as caring: A model for transforming practice*. New York: National League for Nursing.

Leininger, M. (1978). *Transcultural nursing: Concepts, theories, and practices*. New York: Wiley. [out of print]

Leininger, M. (1979). *Transcultural nursing*. New York: Masson. [out of print]

Leininger, M. M. (1985). Transcultural Care Diversity and Universality: A theory of nursing. *Nursing and Health Care, 6*, 209–212.

Leininger, M. M. (1988). Leininger's theory of nursing: Cultural Care Diversity and Universality. *Nursing Science Quarterly, 1*, 152–160.

Leininger, M. M. (1991). *Culture Care Diversity and Universality: A theory of nursing*. New York: National League for Nursing.

King, I. (1981). *A theory for nursing: Systems, concepts, process*. New York: Wiley. [out of print]

Watson, J. (1988). *Nursing: Human science and human care*. New York: National League for Nursing.

BIBLIOGRAPHY

Gaut, D., & Leininger, M. M. (1991). *Care: The compassionate healer.* New York: National League for Nursing.

Leininger, M. M. (1970). *Nursing and anthropology: Two worlds to blend.* New York: Wiley.

Leininger, M. M. (1973). *Contemporary issues in mental health nursing.* Boston: Little, Brown.

Leininger, M. M. (Ed.) (1976). *Transcultural health care issues and conditions.* Philadelphia: Davis.

Leininger, M. M. (1980). Caring: A central focus of nursing and health care services. *Nursing & Health Care, 1,* 135–143, 176.

Leininger, M. M. (Ed.) (1980). *Transcultural nursing: Teaching, practice and research.* Salt Lake City: University of Utah College of Nursing.

Leininger, M. M. (Ed.) (1981). *Care: An essential human need.* Thorofare, NJ: Slack.

Leininger, M. M. (1981). Transcultural nursing: Its progress and its future. *Nursing & Health Care, 2,* 365–371.

Leininger, M. M. (Ed.) (1984). *Care: The essence of nursing and health.* Thorofare, NJ: Slack.

Leininger, M. M. (1984). *Reference sources for transcultural health and nursing.* Thorofare, NJ: Slack.

Leininger, M. M. (1984). Transcultural nursing: An overview. *Nursing Outlook, 32,* 72–73.

Leininger, M. M. (Ed.) (1985). *Qualitative research methods in nursing.* Orlando, FL: Grune & Stratton.

Leininger, M. M., & Watson, J. (1990). *The caring imperative in nursing education.* New York: National League for Nursing.

MARGARET NEWMAN

Julia B. George

■ ■ ■

Margaret Newman (b. 1933) received a BSHE in home economics and English from Baylor University in Texas in 1954; a BS in nursing from the University of Tennessee, Memphis, in 1962; an MS in nursing from the University of California, San Francisco, in 1964; and the PhD in nursing science and rehabilitation nursing from New York University in 1971. She relates that she resisted the feeling that she should become a nurse as she completed her first bachelor's degree and during the next eight years while she served as the primary caregiver during her mother's struggle with amyotrophic lateral sclerosis. Her mother died just as Newman had prayed that she was willing to become a nurse. Within two weeks of her mother's death, Newman was a nursing major at the University of Tennessee and quickly decided that nursing was right for her.

Newman has held faculty positions at the University of Tennessee, New York University, and The Pennsylvania State University. She is currently professor in the School of Nursing at the University of Minnesota. In addition to these faculty positions, she has served as director of nursing for the University of Tennessee Clinical Research Center, acting director of nursing for the PhD program in nursing science at New York University, and professor-in-charge of the graduate program in research at The Pennsylvania State University.

She is an active scholar and the recipient of many honors. She has served, or is serving, on the editorial boards of many scholarly nursing journals, including Advances in Nursing Science, Journal of Professional Nursing, Nursing and Health Care, Nursing Research, Nursing Science Quarterly, *and* Western Journal of Nursing Research. *She is a Fellow in the American Academy of Nursing, listed in* Who's Who in American Women, *and the recipient of the Outstanding Alumnus Award from the University of Tennessee College of Nursing and the Distinguished Alumnus Award from the New York University Division of Nursing. She has been a Latin American Teaching Fellow and an* American Journal of Nursing *Scholar. She has conducted workshops and conferences and served as a consultant around the world, including Australia, Brazil, Canada, Czechoslovakia, France, Finland, Germany, Japan, New Zealand, Poland, and the United Kingdom, in addition to the United States.*

Margaret Newman has stated that during her doctoral study she was interested in theory in nursing (Wallace & Coberg, 1990). More specifically, as a result of her experiences during her mother's illness, she was interested in the relationships between movement, time, and space, for she describes her mother as having been immobilized in time and space. Newman states that she did not intentionally begin to develop a theory but, rather, "slid" into theory development. Her preparations to speak at a conference in 1978 marked the beginning of her defined intention to explicate the temporal and spatial patterns of health. She states that at this time she was moving toward a theory of health. She chose health as a focus because she saw disease as a meaningful aspect of health and believed health needed better definition.

In developing her theory, Newman (1994) was influenced by Martha Rogers (1970), Itzhak Bentov (1978), David Bohm (1980, 1981, 1992), Richard Moss (1981), and Arthur Young (1976a, 1976b). From Rogers she drew upon the concepts of pattern and the unitary nature of human beings with particular emphasis on the importance of the basic assumption of pattern. The unitary human being is open and in interaction with its environment. There are no real boundaries between human and environment; pattern is an identification of the wholeness of the person. Newman identified disease as a manifestation of pattern (Wallace & Coberg, 1990). Bentov's view of consciousness as evolving and being coextensive with the universe supported Newman's concept of health as expanding consciousness. Bohm's discussion of implicate and explicate order supported the idea of health as a pattern of the whole with a normal progression toward higher levels of organization. Moss's presentation of love as the highest level of consciousness was affirming of Newman's views of the nature of health and nursing. Young's discussion of the importance of insight, pattern recognition, and choice provided the impetus for the integration of the concepts of movement, time, and space into a dynamic theory of health.

HEALTH AS EXPANDING CONSCIOUSNESS

Concepts and Assumptions

Newman (1994) states that she began the development of her theory with an effort to follow the demands of logical positivism. Thus, she identified concepts and assumptions for her theory. Her initial assumptions were the following:

1. Health encompasses conditions heretofore described as illness, or in medical terms, pathology.
2. These "pathological" conditions can be considered a manifestation of the total pattern of the individual.
3. The pattern of the individual that eventually manifests itself as pathology is primary and exists prior to structural or functional changes.
4. Removal of the pathology in itself will not change the pattern of the individual.

5. If becoming "ill" is the only way an individual's pattern can manifest itself, then that is health for that person.
6. Health is the expansion of consciousness (Newman, 1979, pp. 56–58).

The initial concepts were movement, time, space, and consciousness (Newman, 1979). Newman discussed *movement* as an essential property of matter and the change that occurs between two states of rest, but she did not define the other concepts initially. She did propose relationships among the concepts as the following:

1. Time and space have a complementary relationship.
2. Movement is a means whereby space and time become a reality.
3. Movement is a reflection of consciousness.
4. Time is a function of movement.
5. Time is a measurement of consciousness (p. 60).

More currently, Marchione (1993) states that Newman's implicit assumptions are that humans have the following characteristics:

- Open energy systems.
- In continual interconnectedness with a universe of open systems (environment).
- Continuously active in evolving their own pattern of the whole (health).
- Intuitive as well as affective and cognitive beings.
- Capable of abstract thinking as well as sensation.
- More than the sum of their parts (p. 6).

The current definition of movement remains the same as Newman's initial definition. *Time and timing* relate the rhythm of living phenomena (Newman, 1994). Examples include the variations in the effectiveness of drug and radiation therapies throughout a 24-hour cycle. Dosages that are therapeutic at one period during the day may be fatal during another period. Individuals who refuse to adhere to the time schedule of a hospital are often identified as uncooperative even though social adherence could be detrimental to the person. For example, a newly diagnosed diabetic women was carefully taught to follow her prescribed diet and insulin plan throughout a standard day of breakfast, lunch, and dinner. It was not until she was readmitted to regain diabetic control that it was discovered she worked nights and was having difficulty following the prescribed meal plan! Time is also seen as a symbol of status. When a person has an appointment with a physician, who is the most likely to have to wait and who is seen as having the greater status? Timing is recognized as important in the provision of nursing care, particularly in home health. A description supporting the importance of timing follows:

When . . . [the client was] ready to express her feelings of confine-
ment and explore options for opening her world, I made weekly
home visits. When she returned to insulin use, I made weekly
home visits plus three or four telephone calls per week for about
one and a half months. During times when she let me know in her
ways that it [was] not her time for change, I allowed the interval
between visits to increase to a month and relied on her to call me
if needed (Newman, Lamb, & Michaels, 1992, p. 406).

Space is discussed in conjunction with time and movement and not defined
separately.

Newer concepts include consciousness and expanding consciousness, pattern, pattern recognition, and transformation. *Consciousness* is "the *information* of the system; the capacity of the system to interact with the environment" (Newman, 1994, p. 33). In humans this "informational capacity
includes not only all the things we normally associate with consciousness, such
as thinking and feeling, but also all the information embedded in the nervous
system, the endocrine system, the immune system, the genetic code and so on"
(p. 33). As human beings develop, consciousness grows, or expands. As consciousness expands, the more it coexists with the universe. Consciousness is
the essence of all matter; persons do not possess consciousness, they *are* consciousness. The direction of life is ever toward higher levels of consciousness.

Pattern depicts the whole and is characterized by movement, diversity, and
rhythm. Movement is constant and rhythmic, and the parts are diverse.
Pattern is relatedness; the process of patterning occurs as human energy fields
penetrate one another and transformation occurs. *Transformation* is change
that occurs all-at-once rather than in a gradual and linear fashion. As more
information is obtained, pattern evolves unidirectionally and becomes more
highly organized.

Pattern recognition occurs within the observer. Although we may predict
the next event in a sequence, on the basis of knowledge of the sequence to
date, we cannot make such predictions *with certainty* because additional
information that indicates a change in the sequence has not happened
(Bateson, 1979). Thus, if given a sequence of 3, 6, 9, 12 we are likely to predict that the next number would be 15 when in reality the sequence is 3, 6, 9,
12, 16, 20, 24, 28, 33, 38, and so on. It may not be possible to see the pattern all at once. We need to remind ourselves that the piece of reality that is
known to us is only a portion of the total reality. Newman (1994) suggests
that more of the pattern is revealed as the time frame is expanded. We follow
this concept of increased knowledge of pattern with increased time when
we need three elevated blood pressure readings taken at different times
to identify an individual as hypertensive. It is also important to note that each
pattern is embedded in another pattern. The pattern in the individual
is embedded in the pattern of the family and of the family in the pattern of
the community and so on. The more we comprehend the whole, the more
knowledge of the parts becomes meaningful. Paradoxically, the whole may be

seen in the parts. A change in the way an individual walks may communicate an overall mood of sadness or glee.

Health and Disease

Newman (1994) believes that a new view of *health* is needed. The old view that health is the absence of disease has been associated with a tendency to view those without health as inferior. She proposes that Hegel's dialectical fusion of opposites to form a synthesized new could fuse disease and nondisease to form a new concept of health. She adds Jantsch's (1980) idea that such fusion may transcend synthesis and, indeed, opposites come to include each other. Bohm (1981) states that when such synthesis is followed to its logical conclusion the opposites pass into each other, reflect each other, and are recognized as identical to each other. From these viewpoints, disease becomes "a meaningful reflection of the whole [of health]" (Newman, 1994, p. 7). Newman states that Rogers (1970) eliminated the view of health and disease as dichotomies when she proposed persons as unitary human beings. Within such a view, health and disease are not separate entities but *"are each reflections of the larger whole"* (Newman, 1994, p. 9). Again drawing upon Bohm, Newman uses the example of the two views of the same scene provided by cameras that photograph that scene from different angles. Just as the pictures from each camera provide different pictures of the same whole, disease and nondisease provide different views of health.

Newman states that health, disease, and the pattern of the whole are consistent with Bohm's (1980) theory of implicate and explicate order. Implicate order is that "unseen, multidimensional pattern that is the ground, or basis, for all things" (Newman, 1994, p. 10). Explicate order arises out of the implicate order and includes the tangibles—those things we can identify with our senses—of the world. Because we can see, touch, hear, feel the tangibles we tend to identify them as primary, which is contrary to Bohm's statement that implicate order is primary. In this sense, *"manifest health, encompassing disease and non-disease, can be regarded as the explication of the underlying pattern of person-environment"* (Newman, 1994, p. 11).

Newman proposes that those fluctuations in patterns identified as sickness can provide the disturbance needed to reorganize the relationships of a pattern more harmoniously. Illness may achieve what people have wanted but have been unable to acknowledge; it can provide or represent the disequilibrium needed to maintain the vital active exchange with the environment. We grow or evolve through experiencing disequilibrium and learning how to attain a new sense of balance. Thus, disease may be seen as both emergent pattern and expanding consciousness. It is important to remember that although an individual may exhibit the emergent pattern labeled disease, that individual's pattern relates to and affects the patterns of others—family, friends, community. As open energy systems in constant interaction, humans influence one another's patterns and evolve together.

Newman (1994) cites Ferguson's (1980) discussion of the paradigm shift that is occurring in the view of health. She describes it as a shift from an instrumental to a relational view. The shift includes searching for *patterns* instead of treating symptoms; perceiving pain and disease as *information* instead of seeing them as totally negative; viewing the body as a *dynamic field of energy* that is continuous with a larger field instead of as a machine in various states of repair or disrepair; and seeing disease as a *process* rather than an entity. The new paradigm of health, in its embrace of a unitary pattern of changing relationships, is essential to nursing. Within this paradigm the task is not to seek to change the pattern of another but to recognize that pattern as information that represents the whole and to seek to relate to the pattern as it unfolds. The relational paradigm of health incorporates and transforms the old instrumental paradigm. The characteristics of the instrumental paradigm—linear, causal, predictive, rational, controlling, dichotomous—need to be seen as special cases of the new relational paradigm. The characteristics of the new paradigm are pattern, emerging, unpredictable, unitary, intuitive, and innovative.

When health is seen as a pattern of the whole, disease becomes an emergent pattern that can be understood in terms of a pattern of energy (Newman, 1994). Seeing disease as a manifestation of pattern can help people become aware of their pattern of person–environment interaction. The insight that is gained can be transforming, both for the person and the family. Newman draws upon Young's (1976b) discussion of the acceleration of the evolution of consciousness to explain such transformation. Young emphasizes the process of interaction both among individuals and between people and society in reaching the goal of a higher level of development. He describes seven stages in this evolution. The first is potential freedom, which moves into the second stage, or binding. In binding, the collective is primary, the individual is not important, everything is regulated and initiative is not needed. In the third stage, centering, individual identity, self-consciousness and self-determination develop as the person breaks with authority. The fourth stage, choice, is the turning point in which the individual learns the "law." The emphasis in choice is on science and a search for laws with a new awareness of self-limitation. When the law is learned, the fifth stage, or decentering, begins and the emphasis shifts away from self-development to something greater than the individual. Energy is a dominant feature and one's works develop a life of their own; the experience is one of unlimited growth. The sixth stage, unbinding, involves increasing freedom from time, and the seventh stage represents complete freedom and unrestricted choice. Newman (1994) says that most of us do not experience stages six and beyond. She does state that Young's conception of evolution and her own model of health as expanding consciousness are corollaries:

> We come into being from a state of potential consciousness, are bound in time, find our identity in space, and through movement we learn the "law" of the way things work and make choices that ultimately take us beyond space and time to a state of absolute consciousness (p. 46).

It is from Young that Newman derived her emphasis on the importance of a choice point. A choice point occurs when the old ways of doing things no longer work and new answers must be sought. The experience is one of disconnectedness—the familiar does not function in the expected way, things are falling apart. This sense of disorder is a predecessor of a transformation to a higher level of consciousness. Such transformation is characterized by the knowledge that the old rules no longer apply and by the willingness to tolerate some degree of uncertainty and ambiguity until the emerging pattern becomes clearer.

Newman (1994) says that disease is not necessary for evolution to higher levels of consciousness. She cites Bentov (1978) and Moss (1981) in discussing the fact that the degree of flexibility one uses to responding to stress helps to determine how disabling that stress will be. The more open and flexible one is, the more energy can flow through and the less stress has negative effects. Newman recommends that "we accept the experience as *our* experience regardless of how contrary it is to what we might have wished would happen" (p. 29).

In the model of health as expanding consciousness it does not matter where one is in the spectrum. There is no basis for rejecting any experience as irrelevant. The important factor is to be fully present in the moment and know that whatever the experience, it is a manifestation of the process of evolving to higher consciousness (p. 68).

New Paradigm

Newman, Sime, & Corcoran-Perry (1991) have proposed a perspective for nursing that they call the unitary-transformative paradigm. The unitary-transformative paradigm views "the human being as a unitary phenomenon unfolding in an undivided universe" (Newman, 1994, p. 82). Phenomena are identified by pattern and by interaction with the larger whole. Change is unidirectional, unpredictable, and transformative. Change occurs as systems move through periods or stages of organization and disorganization (choice points) to become more complex. Disruptive processes are seen as phases of reorganization. Health is seen as the evolving pattern of the whole, which illustrates the unfolding implicate order. The person is seen as unitary *and* continuous with the undivided wholeness of the universe. As either person or universe transforms, the other transforms and there are no identifiable boundaries.

The appropriate methodology for studying this paradigm is a hermeneutic, dialectic approach (Newman, 1994). Newman supports research as praxis (Newman, 1990a; 1994). She uses Wheeler and Chinn's (1984) definition of praxis as "thoughtful reflection and action that occur in synchrony, in the direction of transforming the world" (p. 2). Newman indicates that both the participants and the researchers experience growth as her interactive research methodology is carried out. She believes that research must focus on practice realities and not be limited to outcomes. It is important that the nursing research help practitioners understand and act in their unique situations. The content of the research is the process of the nursing, seeking pattern recognition. The theory of expanding consciousness is used as *a priori* theory to inform and illuminate the experiences of the participants in the research.

HEALTH AS EXPANDING CONSCIOUSNESS AND NURSING'S METAPARADIGM

Newman (1994) deals with all the concepts in nursing's metaparadigm. *Human beings* are unitary with the *environment*. There are no boundaries. Human beings are identified by their patterns. The patterns of individuals are embedded in those of their family and, in turn, these are embedded in the patterns of the community and society. Humans are moving toward ever-increasing organization and are capable of making their own decisions. Progression to a higher level of organization often occurs after a period of disorganization, or choice point, when the older ways no longer work. Movement is a pivotal choice point in evolving consciousness and is the expression of consciousness. Restriction of movement forces one beyond space–time.

Health is expanding consciousness: "the evolving pattern of the whole, the explication of the unfolding implicate order (Newman, 1994, pp. 82–83). Health is a synthesis of disease and nondisease. Newman's theory is about health; further discussion of health can be found in the presentation of the theory in this chapter.

Newman (1994) discusses *nursing* as a profession, presenting three stages in the growth of the profession. The first stage is formative. In this stage nursing was in the process of becoming, of establishing its identity, and individual practitioners were responsible for their own practice. In the second or normative stage, nursing lost some of its authority and was more competitive and persuasive in relation to the environment. During this stage, nursing moved primarily into the hospital setting and nurses became employees. The third stage is the integrative stage. Newman thinks that nursing is moving into the third stage but has not yet completed the process. In the integrative stage nursing will relate to other health care providers and to clients as partners, in a cooperative, mutual manner. Newman (1990b) suggests that three nursing roles are essential to the integrative model. The professional nursing role is the primary integrative role; Newman refers to this role as nursing clinician/case manager. The other two roles are that of nursing team leader and staff nurse. The nursing clinician/case manager embraces the whole of the nursing paradigm; the staff nurse functions primarily from the medical or disease-oriented paradigm; the nursing team leader serves as a liaison between the two to integrate and coordinate all into individualized care for every client. Notice that these three roles demonstrate the incorporation of the old (disease-oriented paradigm) within the new (nursing paradigm) with the old becoming part of the whole rather than the primary focus of activity.

Newman (1994) defines nursing as *"caring in the human health experience"* (p. 139). She believes that caring is a moral imperative for nursing. On the basis of Moss's (1981) statement on love, she says that caring is something that transforms all of us and all that we do, rather than being something that we do. Caring reflects the whole of the person. Caring requires that we be open. Being open is being vulnerable. Being vulnerable may lead to suffering, which we tend to avoid. Avoiding suffering can impede our efforts to move to higher levels of consciousness. "The need is to let go, embrace our experience, and allow the expansion of consciousness to unfold" (Newman, 1994, p. 142). Without caring, nursing does not occur.

HEALTH AS EXPANDING CONSCIOUSNESS AND THE NURSING PROCESS

> When health is conceptualized as the expansion of consciousness in a universe of undivided wholeness, intervention aimed at producing a particular result becomes a problem. To intervene with a particular solution in mind is to say we know what form the pattern of expanding consciousness will take, and we don't. Moss (1981), who declares himself a *former* general practitioner of medicine, asks where is the world going anyway, except around in circles. Somehow this bigger picture makes it easier to relax and enjoy an authentic involvement/evolvement with another person (Newman, 1994, p. 97).

In the relational paradigm described by Newman (1994), the focus is not on the professional identifying what is wrong (*assessment* and *diagnosis*), or on planning and taking steps to correct the problem (*planning, implementation, evaluation*). Rather, the professional enters into partnership with the client. The situation that brings the client to the attention of the nurse is often one of chaos and, at the minimum, involves circumstances that the client does not know how to handle. The client is at a choice point and is seeking a partner to participate in an authentic relationship. The nurse and client trust that, through the process of the unfolding of the relationship, both will emerge at a higher level of consciousness. The nurse is with the client throughout the process.

The intent of the nurse is to "enter into the process with the client to be present with it, attend to it and live it, even if it appears in the form of disharmony, catastrophe, or disease" (Newman, 1994, p. 99). To accomplish this, the nurse must give up the compulsion to fix things, to shape the world in a previous image of what health is or should be. Newman believes that the joy of nursing is in being present with clients through disorganization and disharmony with "an unconditional acceptance of the unpredictable, paradoxical nature of life" (p. 103). Such acceptance does not mean doing nothing. Action becomes apparent as pattern becomes apparent. In the client situations Newman presents as examples, she identifies the nurse as "doing" many of the things that would be done within the old framework—providing support and information, for example. It is the intent with which these things are done that differs. In the unitary-transformative paradigm, the nurse's actions are part of the process of being with another as both nurse and client seek expanded consciousness. The actions are not oriented toward achieving a preestablished goal determined by the nurse. Newman describes successful outcomes as "a shift from concentration on self to a broader perspective that extends beyond self, a kind of universal perspective . . . manifest in congruence between inner and outer experience and a greater capacity for love and relatedness in the world. The health professional's awareness of being, rather than doing, is the primary mechanism" (p. 103).

Newman describes this nurse–client relationship as similar to the events that occur after two pebbles are thrown into a pool of water. From the entry point of each pebble ripples begin to emanate. These ripples continue to radiate, meet, interact, and develop an interference pattern. The interference pattern spreads and is part of the whole of each of the original patterns. If we substitute two people for the pebbles and the waves of each of their patterns for the ripples in the water, we have an interaction pattern similar to that shown in Figure 22–1. To be in touch with another one needs to be in touch with one's own pattern. The more we know ourselves, the clearer we can be in expressing our patterns to others and in coming to know them. There are no separate parts; the pattern is to be sensed as a whole, as a continuous flow of movement with relationships that continue to merge and move apart. "The nurse–client relationship is a rhythmic coming together and moving apart of the client and the nurse" (Newman, 1994, p. 112).

The five-step nursing process does not apply to Newman's theory. The implication of the five-step process that predictive goals can be set and that outcomes should be measured against these goals is not compatible with

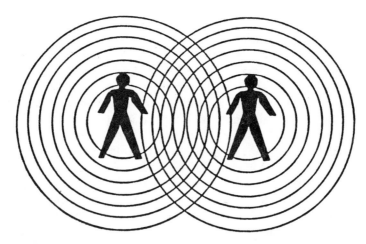

Figure 22–1. Interaction pattern of two persons: A holographic model of intervention. *(Used by permission from Newman, M. (1994). Health as expanding consciousness (2nd ed.). New York: National League for Nursing.)*

Newman's statements that we cannot make predictions with certainty and that we do not know what form expanding consciousness will take. For Newman, the process of nursing is one of coming together as partners during a time of chaos when the client is at a choice point. The nurse is there to be with the client and to accept the unpredictable nature of life. Accepting the circumstances decreases the stress in responding to those circumstances. Although the nurse may share knowledge, provide support, or be an organizing force in the relationship, the primary function for the nurse in this caring relationship is awareness of being. Attending to silence is at least as crucial as attending to utterances and movements. When the client is ready, the nurse and client will again move apart. It is hoped that each will have reached a higher level of consciousness through the experience.

HEALTH AS EXPANDING CONSCIOUSNESS AND THE CHARACTERISTICS OF A THEORY

1. Theories can interrelate concepts in such a way as to create a different way of looking at a particular phenomenon. For nearly three decades, Newman has challenged us to view the phenomenon of health in a different way. Her proposal of health as expanding consciousness, with health and disease parts of the same whole, interrelated space, time, movement, and pattern in a new way. Although concepts are present within her work, they are not primary to understanding the unitary-transformative paradigm. She indicates that she has moved beyond the interrelationship of concepts to the interrelationship of human beings.

2. Theories must be logical in nature. Newman's presentation is logical. She presents the material from which she derived her ideas as needed and discusses with clarity those works that support her theory. There are some contradictions in her work. For example, she describes disease as disequilibrium or disruption and discusses the role played by disequilibrium in growth or the expansion of consciousness. At another point, she states that disease is not necessary and may not occur if human beings can be open to and accepting of the turn of events in their lives. She also describes humans and their environment as an undivided whole and speaks eloquently to the importance of viewing them in this way. Again, in another discussion, she indicates that the whole can be seen in its parts. She does discuss the fact that the smaller the piece being viewed is, the fuzzier the picture of the whole will be.

3. Theories should be relatively simple yet generalizable. Newman's theory of health as expanding consciousness is not limited by person or setting. It is generalizable to anybody, anywhere. Her presentation of nursing within this theory is limited to those situations in which caring occurs. She states that without caring, nursing is not present. Her statement that health is expanding consciousness, seen in the evolving pattern of the whole, is relatively simple. Her ideas represent a paradigm shift in our view of health and of nursing and may be complex to those who do not comprehend the paradigm. This is true for any paradigm shift and should not be seen as a limitation of this theory.

4. Theories can be the bases for hypothesis that can be tested or theory to be exanded. Newman supports the use of the theory of health as expanding consciousness as *a priori* in research. However, she does not support the positivistic view of hypothesis development and testing. In her research methodology, the patterns that are identified through interviews with research participants are tested against the theory. Thus, the theory of health as expanding consciousness can be used in research and in testing. The methodology to be used does not include hypotheses, which represent a view of the world that is incongruent with the theory.

5. Theories contribute to and assist in increasing the general body of knowledge within the discipline through the research implemented to validate them. Research has been conducted by using Newman's theory. Newman has conducted studies on the needs of hospitalized patients (1966), time and movement (1972, 1976), subjective time (1982; Newman & Guadiano, 1984), patterns in persons with coronary artery disease (Newman & Moch, 1991). These studies have both added to the general body of nursing knowledge and served to refine and develop her theory. Fryback's (1993) and Moch's (1990) studies supported Newman's thesis that disease is a part of health and that the emergence of disease allows health to unfold. Schorr, Farnham, and Ervin (1991) also report support for Newman's theory, whereas Mentzer and Schoor (1986) found that perceived duration of time was not related to age. Newman says that Engle's (1984, 1986) conclusion that the faster one moves, the healthier one is, is based on a paradigm other than Newman's even though Engle used the methodology that Newman had identified at that time. It is important to note that in the mid-1980's Newman had not yet explicated a methodology for the unitary-transformative paradigm.

6. Theories can be used by practitioners to guide and improve their practice. Newman's (1994) discussion of research as praxis makes it clear that her intention and belief is that theory must be derived from practice, reflect the realities of practice, and inform practice. She has also proposed a model for practice that is derived from the theory (Newman, 1990b). Bramlett, Gueldner, and Sowell (1990) discussed consumer-centric advocacy as accomplished through the nurse–client interpersonal relationship and supported by Newman's indication of client freedom to be the decision maker. Others have spoken of the utility of Newman's work in guiding and improving practice. Areas of discussion have included parish nursing (Gustafson, 1990); caring for high-risk pregnant women (Kalb, 1990); practicing in a professional manner (Nelson, 1991); and pattern recognition as the essence of practice (Smith, 1990). The use of the theory at Carondelet St. Mary's has also been described (Ethridge, 1991; Michaels, 1992; Newman, Lamb, & Michaels, 1991).

7. Theories must be consistent with other validated theories, laws, and principles but will leave open unanswered questions that need to be investigated. Newman (1994) clearly documents the consistency of her theory with those of Itzhak Bentov (1978), David Bohm (1980, 1992), Richard Moss (1981), Martha Rogers (1970), and Arthur Young (1976a, 1976b). Her statement that nursing does not occur in the absence of caring is consistent with Boykin and Schoenhofer (1993), Leininger (1991), and Watson (1988). Many unanswered questions to be investigated can be derived from this evolving theory. When research is praxis, the questions arise within each nurse–client relationship and within each practice setting.

SUMMARY

Newman developed a theory of health as expanding consciousness in which disease and nondisease are synthesized to form a new view of health. Health is seen as the explication of the underlying pattern of person–environment. Humans are unitary beings moving in space–time and unfolding in an undivided universe toward increasing organization. Humans are ever changing in an unidirectional, unpredictable, and transformative (all-at-once) manner. Change is associated with periods of organization and disorganization. During disorganization, when old ways no longer are effective, humans face choice points. It is during such times that clients and nurses come together.

Nursing is "caring in the human health experience" (Newman, 1994, p. 139). In the unitary-transformative paradigm, caring involves the whole of the nurse and the whole of the client. Nurse and client become partners in living through the period of disharmony and emerging at a higher level of consciousness.

Newman proposes a hermeneutic dialectic approach to research and states that research is praxis. Both the participants and the researchers grow and learn in the interactive process of conducting the research. The experience of the participant and researcher is not unlike that of the client and nurse.

Newman has provided a new view of the world of health in a logical manner. Her theory of health as expanding consciousness can be applied in any setting, and can be used in research and practice. Continued research is needed as this theory evolves.

REFERENCES

Bateson, G. (1979). *Mind and nature: A necessary unity.* Toronto: Bantam.

Bentov, I. (1978). *Stalking the wild pendulum.* New York: E. P. Dutton.

Bohm, D. (1980). *Wholeness and the implicate order.* London: Routledge & Kegan Paul.

Bohm, D. (1981). The physicist and the mystic—is a dialogue between them possible? A conversation with David Bohm conducted by Renee Weber. *Re-Vision, 4*(1), 22–35.

Bohm, D. (1992). On dialogue. *Noetic Sciences Review, 23,* 16–18.

Boykin, A., & Schoenhofer, S. (1993). *Nursing as caring: A model for transforming practice.* New York: National League for Nursing.

Bramlett, M. H., Gueldner, S. H., & Sowell, R. L. (1990). Consumer-centric advocacy: It's connection to nursing frameworks. *Nursing Science Quarterly, 3,* 156–161.

Engle, V. F. (1984). Newman's conceptual framework and the measurement of older adults' health. *Advances in Nursing Science, 7*(1), 24–36.

Engle, V. F. (1986). The relationship of movement and time to older adults' functional health. *Research in Nursing and Health, 9,* 123–129.

Ethridge, P. (1991). A nursing HMO: Carondelet St. Mary's experience. *Nursing Management, 22*(7), 22–27.

Ferguson, M. (1980). *The aquarian conspiracy: Personal and social transformation in the 1980s.* Los Angeles: J. P. Tarcher.

Fryback, P. B. (1993). Health for people with a terminal diagnosis. *Nursing Science Quarterly, 6,* 147–159.

Gustafson, W. (1990). Application of Newman's theory of health: Pattern recognition as nursing practice. In M. E. Parker (Ed.), *Nursing theories in practice* (pp. 141–161). New York: National League for Nursing.

Jantsch, E. (1980). *The self-organizing universe.* New York: Pergamon.

Kalb, K. A. (1990). The gift: Applying Newman's theory of health in nursing practice. In M. E. Parker (Ed.), *Nursing theories in practice* (pp. 163–186). New York: National League for Nursing.

Leininger, M. M. (1991). *Culture Care Diversity and Universality: A theory of nursing.* New York: National League for Nursing.

Marchione, J. (1993). *Margaret Newman: Health as expanding consciousness.* Newbury Park, CA: Sage.

Mentzer, C. A., & Schorr, J. A. (1986). Perceived situational control and perceived duration of time: Expressions of life patterns. *Advances in Nursing Science, 9*(1), 12–20.

Michaels, C. (1992). Carondelet St. Mary's nursing enterprise. *Nursing Clinics of North America, 27,* 77–85.

Moch, S. D. (1990). Health within the experience of breast cancer. *Journal of Advanced Nursing, 15,* 1426–1435.

Moss, R. (1981). *The I that is we.* Millbrae, CA: Celestial Arts.

Nelson, J. I. (1991). A crab or a dolphin: A new paradigm for nursing practice. *Nursing Outlook, 39,* 136–137.

Newman, M. A. (1966). Identifying and meeting patients' needs in short-span nurse–patient relationships. *Nursing Forum, 5*(1), 76–86.

Newman, M. A. (1972). Time estimation in relation to gait tempo. *Perceptual and Motor Skills, 34,* 359–366.

Newman, M. A. (1976). Movement tempo and the experience of time. *Nursing Research, 25,* 273–279.

Newman, M. A. (1979). *Theory development in nursing.* Philadelphia: Davis.

Newman, M. A. (1982). Time as an index of expanding consciousness with age. *Nursing Research, 31,* 290–293.

Newman, M. A. (1990a). Newman's theory of health as praxis. *Nursing Science Quarterly, 3,* 37–41.

Newman, M. A. (1990b). Toward an integrative model of professional practice. *Journal of Professional Nursing, 6,* 167–173.

Newman, M. A. (1994). *Health as expanding consciousness* (2nd ed.). New York: National League for Nursing.

Newman, M. A., & Guadiano, J. K. (1984). Depression as an explanation for decreased subjective time in the elderly. *Nursing Research, 33,* 137–139.

Newman, M. A., Lamb, G. S., & Michaels, C. (1991). Nursing case management: The coming together of theory and practice. *Nursing & Health Care, 12,* 404–408.

Newman, M. A., & Moch, S. D. (1991). Life patterns of persons with coronary artery disease. *Nursing Science Quarterly, 4,* 161–167.

Newman, M. A., Sime, A. M., & Corcoran-Perry, S. A. (1991). The focus of the discipline of nursing. *Advances in Nursing Science, 14*(1), 1–6.

Rogers, M. (1970). *An introduction to the theoretical basis of nursing.* Philadelphia: Davis.

Schorr, J. A., Farnham, R. C., & Ervin, S. M. (1991). Health patterns in aging women as expanding consciousness. *Advances in Nursing Science, 13*(4), 52–63.

Smith, M. C. (1990). Pattern in nursing practice. *Nursing Science Quarterly, 3,* 57–59.

Wallace, D. (Producer), & Coberg, T. (Director). (1990). *Margaret Newman—The nurse theorists: Portraits of excellence* [Video tape]. Oakland, CA· Studio Three Production, Samuel Merritt College of Nursing.

Watson, J. (1988). *Nursing: Human science and human care.* New York: National League for Nursing.

Wheeler, C. E., & Chinn, P. L. (1984). *Peace and power: A handbook of feminist process.* Buffalo: Margaret-daughters.

Young, A. M. (1976a). *The geometry of meaning.* San Francisco: Robert Briggs.

Young, A. M. (1976b). *The reflective universe: Evolution of consciousness.* San Francisco: Robert Briggs.

BIBLIOGRAPHY

Fawcett, J. (1993). *Analysis and evaluation of nursing theories.* Philadelphia: Davis.

Newman, M. A. (1987a). Aging as increasing complexity. *Journal of Gerontological Nursing, 13*(9), 16–18ʼ

Newman, M. A. (1987b). Patterning. In M. Duffy, & N. J Pender (Eds.), *Conceptual issues in health promotion.* A report of proceedings of a Wingspread Conference. Indianapolis: Sigma Theta Tau International.

Newman, M. A. (1989). The spirit of nursing. *Holistic Nursing Practice, 3*(3), 1–6.

Newman, M. A. (1992a). Health conceptualizations. In J. J. Fitzpatrick, R. L. Taunton, & A. K. Jacox (Eds.), *Annual review of nursing research, 9,* 221–243. New York: Springer.

Newman, M. A. (1992b). Prevailing paradigms in nursing. *Nursing Outlook, 40,* 10–13, 32.

Newman, M. A. (1994). Into the 21st Century. *Nursing Science Quarterly, 7,* 44–46.

ANNE BOYKIN AND SAVINA SCHOENHOFER

Julia B. George

■ ■ ■

Anne Boykin (b. 1944) received her bacheors of science in nursing from Alverno College, Milwaukee, WI, her MS in adult nursing from Emory University and the PhD in higher education administration with a nursing emphasis from Vanderbilt University. She has practiced nursing in acute care as well as community settings. She has held faculty positions at Clemson University, Valdosta State College, Marquette University, and Florida Atlantic University. She is dean of the College of Nursing, Florida Atlantic University, Boca Raton, Florida, and president of the International Association for Human Caring. She is active in numerous professional associations including the National League for Nursing, American Association of Colleges of Nursing, and the Southern Council on Collegiate Education. Her publications are in the areas of caring and nursing as a discipline.

Savina Schoenhofer (b. 1940) holds a BA in psychology, a BSN in nursing, an MEd in guidance and counseling, and an MN in nursing from Wichita State University, and the PhD in higher education administration from Kansas State University. She has practiced nursing in community mental health and migrant health care. She has held faculty and administrative positions at Wichita State University and Florida Atlantic University. She is professor of nursing at the University of Mississippi School of Nursing in Jackson, MS. She has published in the areas of nursing home management, nursing values, caring, and touch in nursing in critical care settings.

Boykin and Schoenhofer (1993) propose a grand theory of Nursing as Caring. Major influences in the development of the theory are Mayeroff's (1971) generic discussion of caring and Roach's (1984, 1987, 1992 rev.) discussions of caring person and caring in nursing. Roach's view of caring as process, rather than Mayeroff's view of caring as end, is incorporated in the theory of Nursing as Caring. Parker (1993) describes this theory as one that is personal rather than abstract and advises that one must know oneself as caring person to live the theory. She also points out that the theory of Nursing as Caring focuses on living caring rather than on achieving an end product and may be used alone or with other theories.

Gaut (1993) identifies the process of theory development used by Boykin and Schoenhofer as that of intension as described by Kaplan (1964). She characterizes such knowledge growth as being comparable to the gradual illumination of a room that occurs as people with lights enter a dark room. The first to enter perceive in general what is in the room. As additional people bring more light, details become clearer and clearer. Knowledge developed by intension begins with general awareness of the whole and progresses to more and more indepth identification and awareness of the specifics. Boykin and Schoenhofer (1993) write that work on their theory of Nursing as Caring began in 1983 as they worked together in curriculum development (a general view) and progressed over time to an identification of a level of detail that led them to the label of a general theory of nursing.

SUPPORTING STRUCTURES AND ASSUMPTIONS

Mayeroff's (1971) caring ingredients are drawn upon in the theory of Nursing as Caring. Boykin and Schoenhofer (1993) state that "when we have gone outside the discipline [of nursing] to extend possibilities for understanding, we have made an effort to go beyond application, to think through the nursing relevance of ideas that seemed, on the surface to be useful" (p. xiv). Mayeroff's caring ingredients are summarized by Boykin and Schoenhofer as follows (page numbers within the quotation refer to Mayeroff's work):

- Knowing—Explicitly and implicitly, knowing that and knowing how, knowing directly and knowing indirectly (p. 14).
- Alternating rhythm—Moving back and forth between a narrower and a wider framework, between action and reflection (p. 15).
- Patience—Not a passive waiting but participating with the other, giving fully of ourselves (p. 17).
- Honesty—Positive concept that implies openness, genuineness, and seeing truly (p. 18).
- Trust—Trusting the other to grow in his or her own time and own way (p. 20).
- Humility—Ready and willing to learn more about other and self and what caring involves (p. 23).
- Hope—"An expression of the plenitude of the present, alive with a sense of a possible" (p. 26).
- Courage—Taking risks, going into the unknown, trusting (p. 27). (pp. xiv–xv).

Boykin and Schoenhofer present two major perspectives for the theory of Nursing as Caring. Their perspectives are a perception of persons as caring and a conception of nursing as discipline and profession.

Perception of Persons as Caring

The basic premise of Nursing as Caring is that *all persons are caring* (Boykin & Schoenhofer, 1993, p. 3). Seven major assumptions underlie the theory, as follows:

- Persons are caring by virtue of their humanness
- Persons are caring, moment to moment
- Persons are whole or complete in the moment
- Personhood is a process of living grounded in caring
- Personhood is enhanced through participating in nurturing relationships with caring others
- Nursing is both a discipline and a profession (Boykin & Schoenhofer, 1993, p. 3) and
- Persons are viewed as already complete and continuously growing in completeness, fully caring and unfolding caring possibilities moment-to-moment (p. 21).

The capacity for caring grows throughout one's life. Although the human is innately caring, not every human act is caring. Knowing oneself as caring person leads to a continuing commitment to know self and other as caring. This in turn leads to a moral obligation the quality of which is a "measure of being 'in place' in the world" (Boykin & Schoenhofer, 1993, p. 7). The ways in which one expresses caring are continually developing. The more opportunities one exercises fully to know oneself as caring, the easier it becomes to allow oneself (and others) the space and time to further develop caring. This enhances the awareness of self and consciousness that caring is lived moment to moment and directs one's "oughts." The emerging question becomes "How ought I act as caring person?" (p. 7). The degree of authentic awareness of self as caring person influences how one is with others. It requires the courage to let go of the present to discover new meaning about self and other.

Personhood, a process of living grounded in caring, recognizes the possibilities for caring in every moment and is enhanced through caring relationships with others. Caring is living in the context of relational responsibilities—responsibilities for self and other. The heart of the caring relationship is the importance of person-as-person (Boykin & Schoenhofer, 1993).

Drawing upon Pribram's (1971) discussion of the uniqueness of a hologram as being that any part of a broken hologram is capable of reconstructing the total image, Boykin and Schoenhofer (1993) speak of the necessity to view the person as a whole. The person as a whole is a significant value that communicates respect for all that person is at the moment. Using the holographic perspective, it is recognized that any aspect or dimension of the person reflects the whole. Viewing the person as a whole, as caring and complete, is intentional and does not provide for dividing the other into parts or segments, such as mind, body, or spirit, at any time. The person, both self and other, is at all times whole. Unless the person is encountered as a whole, there is only a failed encounter. The person can be fully known only as a whole.

To understand the person as caring, one needs to focus on valuing, to celebrate the wholeness of humans, to view humans as both living and growing in caring, and to actively seek engagement on a personal level with others. The caring perspective of humans is basic to a view of nursing as an undertaking that focuses on humans, provides service from person to person, exists because of a social need, and is a human science (Boykin & Schoenhofer, 1993).

Conception of Nursing as a Discipline and Profession

The theory of Nursing as Caring is derived from a belief that nursing is both a discipline and a profession. The discipline of nursing originates in the unique social call to which nursing is a response and involves being, knowing, living, and valuing all at once. As a discipline, nursing is a unity of science, art, and ethic. Discipline relates to all aspects of the development of nursing knowledge.

The profession of nursing is based on understanding the social need from which the call for nursing originates and the body of knowledge which is used in creating the response known as nursing. Professions are based in everyday human experiences and responses to one another. Boykin and Schoenhofer (1993) discuss the relationship between the nurse and the nursed as a social contract that involves recognition that a basic need is present in conjunction with the availability of the knowledge and skill required to meet that need. The social call is for a group in society to make a commitment to acquire and use this knowledge and skill for the good of everyone. They also believe that nursing is in transition from social contract relationships to covenantal relationships. In contrast to the impersonal, legalistic emphasis in a social contract, the covenantal relationship emphasizes personal commitment and an always present freedom to choose commitments. The covenantal relationship leads to knowledge that each of us is related to all others as well as to the universe and that caring relationships lead to harmony. While discipline develops knowledge, as a profession nursing uses that knowledge to respond to specific human needs.

GENERAL THEORY OF NURSING AS CARING

The focus of nursing is *"nurturing persons living caring and growing in caring"* (Boykin & Schoenhofer, 1993, p. 21). Nursing is the response to the unique human need to be recognized as, and supported in being, caring person. The nurse must know the person as caring person and take those nursing actions that seek to nurture the person in living and growing in caring.

The focus of nurturing persons living caring and growing in caring is broad in statement but specific to the individual situation in practice. As the nurse seeks to know the nursed who is living and growing in caring, the individual's unique ways of living caring become known. Although it is easy to identify instances of noncaring, it is the nurse's commitment to discover the unique caring individual. For example, the nurse connects with the hope that underlies despair, hopelessness, fear, and anger and recognizes these emotions as personal expressions of the caring value. The nurse enters the world of the nursed with the intention and commitment to know the other as caring person. It is in knowing the other in this way that calls for nursing are heard (Boykin & Schoenhofer, 1993). Knowing *how* the other is living caring and expressing aspirations for growing in caring is as important as knowing the other as caring person. "The call for nursing is a call for acknowledgment and affirmation of the person living caring in specific ways in this immediate situation" (p. 24). The nursing response to this call is a caring nurturance evidenced by specific caring responses to sustain and enhance the nursed in living caring and growing in caring in the immediate situation. Boykin and Schoenhofer liken this being in relationship to a dance of caring persons (see Figure 23–1). The circle represents relating with respect for and valuing of the other in the basic dance to know self and other as caring

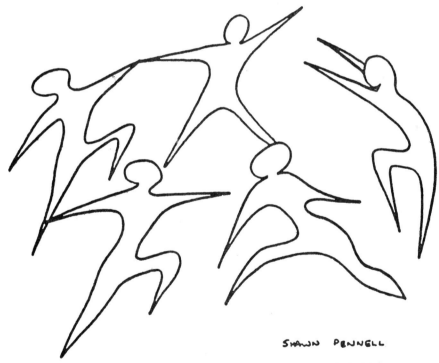

THE DANCE OF CARING PERSONS

Figure 23–1. The Dance of Caring Persons. *(Used with permission from Boykin, A., & Schoenhofer, S. (1993). Nursing as caring: A model for transforming nursing practice. New York: National League for Nursing.)*

person. Each dancer in the circle makes a contribution and moves within the dance as the nursing situation evolves. There is always room for more in the circle and dancers may move in or out as the nursed calls for services. While dancers may or may not connect by holding hands eye-to-eye contact facilitates knowing other as caring.

The *nursing situation* is defined by Boykin and Schoenhofer (1993) as *"a shared lived experience in which the caring between nurse and nursed enhances personhood"* (p. 24). The nursing situation is the context in which nursing exists. It is through the study of the nursing situation that the content and structure of nursing knowledge is known. The nursing situation is composed whenever a nurse engages in a situation from a nursing focus. It is the intention with which the situation is approached and caring is expressed that creates the nursing situation and demonstrates nursing as caring. "As an expression of nursing, *caring is the intentional and authentic presence of the nurse with another who is recognized as person living caring and growing in caring. Here, the nurse endeavors to come to know the other as caring person and seeks to understand how that person might be supported, sustained, and strengthened in their* [sic] *unique process of living caring and growing in caring"* (p. 25).

The call for nursing comes from persons who are living caring and aspiring to grow in caring. The call is for nurturance through personal expressions of caring. The nurse responds to the call of caring person, not to a lack of caring or to noncaring. The nurse brings to this response a deliberately developed, or expert, knowledge of what it means to be human and to be caring; the nurse has made a commitment to recognize and nurture caring in all situations. The nurse risks entering the other's world, comes to know how the other is living caring in the moment, discovers unfolding possibilities for growing in caring, and thus transforms the general knowledge brought to the situation through an understanding of the uniqueness of the specific situation.

Every nursing situation is original and differs from all others because each is a lived experience that involves two individuals who do not have duplicates. The nature of this lived experience is one of reciprocity with personal investment from both the nurse and the nursed. Knowing self and other as caring, which is the crux of the nursing situation, involves a constant and mutual unfolding to discover the living of caring in the moment and the possibilities. For the nurse to enter the world of another, the other must allow such entrance. It is only through openness and willingness from both the nurse and the nursed that true presence in the situation occurs. Boykin and Schoenhofer (1993) identify the phenomenon that develops through the encountering of the nurse and the nursed as *caring between.* When caring between occurs, personhood is nurtured.

It is important that in the theory of Nursing as Caring, the call for nursing is based on neither need nor deficit. In this theory nursing does not seek to right a wrong, solve a problem, meet a need, or alleviate a deficit. Rather, Nursing as Caring is an egalitarian model of helping that celebrates the human in the fullness of being. Nursing responses are as varied as the calls for nursing (Boykin & Schoenhofer, 1993).

THE THEORY OF NURSING AS CARING
AND NURSING'S METAPARADIGM

Of the four concepts in nursing's metaparadigm, human beings, health, environment, and nursing, two are of primary importance in the theory of Nursing as Caring. These are human beings and nursing.

Basic beliefs about *human beings* are reflected in the major assumptions of the theory. Human beings are persons who are caring from moment to moment and are whole and complete in the moment. Humans are enhanced through their participation in nurturing relationships with caring others. All persons are caring, although not all actions are caring.

Nursing involves the nurse knowing self as caring person and coming to know the other as caring. Each expresses unique ways of living and growing in caring. The other expresses a call for caring to which the nurse attends. Nursing includes creating caring responses that nurture personhood and exists when the nurse actualizes personal and professional commitment to the belief that all persons are caring. Not all that a nurse does may express nursing. Any interpersonal experience has potential to become a nursing situation. The nursing situation occurs when the nurse presents self as offering the professional service of nursing and the other presents self as seeking, wanting, and/or accepting such professional service.

The theory of Nursing as Caring is an interpersonal process that can occur wherever nurse and other meet under circumstances that provide for the development of the nursing situation. *Environment* is not an important component of the theory itself. Aspects of the environment would be important only so far as they influence the expression of caring. Similarly, *health* is not defined as part of this theory.

THE THEORY OF NURSING AS CARING
AND THE NURSING PROCESS

The nursing process as a problem-solving approach or mechanism is incompatible with the theory of Nursing as Caring. The problem-solving focus seeks to find something to correct, which Boykin and Schoenhofer (1993) believe distracts nurses from their primary mission of caring and leads to the loss of the context of nursing. In Nursing as Caring, the challenge is to come to know the other as caring person and to nurture that person in ways that are specific to the situation rather than to discover what is missing or needed. Nursing is described as *processual* rather than a process. Boykin and Schoenhofer believe that the telling of stories of nursing situations make evident the service of nursing. One example of such a story is:

Connections

One night as I listened to the change of shift report, I remember the strange feeling in the pit of my stomach when the evening nurse reviewed the lab tests on Tracy P. Tall, strawberry-blonde and freckle-faced, Tracy was struggling with the everyday problems of adolescence and fighting a losing battle against leukemia. Tracy rarely had visitors. As I talked with Tracy this night I felt resentment from her toward her mother, and I experienced a sense of urgency that her mother be with her. With Tracy's permission I called her mother and told her that Tracy needed her that night. I learned she was a single mother with two other small children, and that she lived several hours from the hospital. When she arrived at the hospital, distance and silence prevailed. With encouragement, the mother sat close to Tracy and I sat on the other side, stroking Tracy's arm. I left the room to make rounds and upon return found Mrs. P. still sitting on the edge of the bed fighting to stay awake. I gently asked Tracy if we could lie on the bed with her. She nodded. The three of us lay there for a period of time and I then left the room. Later, when I returned, I found Tracy wrapped in her mother's arm. Her mother's eyes met mine as she whispered "she's gone." And then, "please don't take her yet." I left the room and closed the door quietly behind me. It was just after 6 o'clock when I slipped back into the room just as the early morning light was coming through the window. "Mrs. P," I reached out and touched her arm. She raised her tear-streaked face to look at me. "It's time," I said and waited. When she was ready, I helped her off the bed and held her in my arms for a few moments. We cried together. "Thank you nurse," she said as she looked into my eyes and pressed my hand between hers. Then she turned and walked away. The tears continued down my cheeks as I followed her to the door and watched her disappear down the hall.

Gayle Maxwell (1990)

THE THEORY OF NURSING AS CARING AND THE CHARACTERISTICS OF A THEORY

1. Theories can interrelate concepts in such a way as to create a different way of looking at a particular phenomenon. The theory of Nursing as Caring identifies a focus and nursing situation rather than concepts. Boykin and Schoenhofer (1993) state that they have deliberately not presented the theory in the traditional format of concepts and propositions. Nursing as Caring presents nursing as a living caring that is personal and unique in each nursing situation. The theory does not present new and different definitions of nursing or caring but does provide a different way of looking at the phenomenon of the nursing relationship.

2. Theories must be logical in nature. Boykin and Schoenhofer's (1993) presentation of Nursing as Caring is logical. Their thoughts and beliefs are presented in a manner that connects them clearly and coherently. They anticipate areas in which their presentation differs from a traditional scientific format and explain their rationale for any variations.

3. Theories should be relatively simple yet generalizable. Understanding living and growing in caring may not be viewed as relatively simple by those who prefer to deal with the world in concrete, measurable, and impersonable terms. Those who are comfortable, even excited, by a more cognitive, less measurable and more personal approach will find the theory of Nursing as Caring with its focus on living caring in an interpersonal nursing situation to be relatively simple. The nurse brings general knowledge to the specific situation and uses that knowledge and the unique situation to inform each other. This is not generalizable in the way positivistic research findings are generalizable. However, as a general theory Nursing as Caring applies whenever the nurse approaches a nursing situation from the caring perspective. This *is* generalizable.

4. Theories can be the bases for hypotheses that can be tested or for theory to be expanded. The research methodology that is appropriate for the theory of Nursing as Caring is qualitative, rather than a quantitative, positivistic methodology. Boykin and Schoenhofer (1993) state that the process for coming to know nursing is dialogical rather than dialectical. The purpose of this process is enlightenment rather than control. They write about a research methodology that is totally appropriate for studying Nursing as Caring but that has not yet been developed and suggest that such a method would go beyond hermeneutics, with a phenomenological aspect in an action research orientation. Therefore, the generation of research hypotheses is not appropriate. The generation of research questions is appropriate and possible.

5. Theories contribute to and assist in increasing the general body of knowledge within the discipline through the research implemented to validate them. The general body of knowledge within the discipline and profession of nursing has been increased through the development of the theory of Nursing as Caring. Boykin and Schoenhofer (1993) speak to the need to develop a research methodology that is adequate to study this theory. Throughout the process of theory development, they have validated their work with practitioners of nursing. Beck (1994) reports on three phenomenological studies on the meaning of caring in a nursing program. The results of these studies have implications for nursing education.

6. Theories can be used by practitioners to guide and improve their practice. Boykin and Schoenhofer (1993) describe the theory of Nursing as Caring as a personal theory that requires knowledge of self as caring in order to interact with the other as living caring in the moment. The locus of the theory is the nursing situation. The entire reason for this theory is to guide and improve practice. Kearney and Yeager (1993) provide examples of how Nursing as Caring has guided their practices. They present nursing stories and discuss how the four major themes of Nursing as Caring (seeing the other as caring person, entering the world of the other with the intention of knowing the other, calls for caring nurturance, nursing responses that enhance personhood) have guided them.

7. **Theories must be consistent with other validated theories, laws, and principles but will leave open unanswered questions that need to be investigated.** Boykin and Schoenhofer (1993) state that they have been influenced in the development of the theory of Nursing as Caring by many theoretical works. They list Gaut (1983, 1984, 1985, 1986), Leininger (1978, 1981, 1991), Mayeroff (1971), Paterson and Zderad (1988), Ray (1981, 1984, 1985, 1989), Roach (1984, 1987, 1992 rev.), and Watson (1979, 1988), as major influences in their understanding of caring and caring in nursing. King and Brownell (1976), the Nursing Development Conference Group (1979), and Phenix (1964) are identified as major influences in their understanding of nursing as a discipline. The theory of Nursing as Caring is consistent with these works. As a developing theory, Nursing as Caring leads to many as yet unanswered questions and will create new questions with each nurse–nursed caring encounter.

SUMMARY

Boykin and Schoenhofer (1993) have developed the general theory of Nursing as Caring. Mayeroff's (1971) concepts of knowing, alternating rhythm, patience, honesty, trust, humility, hope, and courage provide a basis for the theory. The two major perspectives of the theory are a perception of persons as caring and a conception of nursing as discipline and profession. All persons are seen as caring. The major assumptions of the theory are that "persons are caring by virtue of their humanness; persons are caring, moment to moment; persons are whole or complete in the moment; personhood is a process of living grounded in caring; personhood is enhanced through participating in nurturing relationships with caring others; nursing is both a discipline and a profession" (Boykin & Schoenhofer, 1993, p. 3), and "persons are viewed as already complete and continuously growing in completeness, fully caring and unfolding caring possibilities moment-to-moment" (p. 21).

The discipline of nursing originates in the unique social call to which nursing is a response, and it relates to all aspects of the development of nursing knowledge. The profession of nursing is based on understanding the social need from which the social call originates and the body of knowledge used to create the response known as nursing.

The general theory of Nursing as Caring has a *focus* and a *locus*. The focus is *"nurturing persons living caring and growing in caring"* (Boykin & Schoenhofer, 1993, p. 21). The locus is the nursing situation defined as *"shared lived experience in which the caring between nursed and nursed enhances personhood"* (p. 24).

The concepts of human being and nursing from nursing's metaparadigm are apparent in the theory of Nursing as Caring. The concepts of society or environment and health are not apparent in this theory. Also, the theory is not congruent with the nursing process.

Boykin and Schoenhofer (1993) have indeed presented a different way of viewing the phenomenon of nursing in their general theory of Nursing as Caring. The relationships which develop when this theory is lived are dynamic and ever changing. They present this theory as one of human science that is not based upon a mathematical structure but upon lived experience.

REFERENCES

Beck, C. T. (1994). Researching experiences of living caring. In A. Boykin (Ed.), *Living a caring-based program* (pp. 93–126). NY: National League for Nursing.

Boykin, A., & Schoenhofer, S. (1993). *Nursing as caring: A model for transforming practice.* New York: National League for Nursing.

Gaut, D. A. (1983). Development of a theoretically adequate description of caring. *Western Journal of Nursing Research, 5,* 312–324.

Gaut, D. A. (1984). A theoretic description of caring as action. In M. Leininger (Ed.), *Care: The essence of nursing and health* (pp. 27–44). Detroit, MI: Wayne State University Press.

Gaut, D. A. (1985). Philosophical analysis as research method. In M. Leininger (Ed.), *Qualitative research methods in nursing* (pp. 73–80). Orlando, FL: Grune & Stratton.

Gaut, D. A. (1986). Evaluating caring competencies in nursing practice. *Topics in Clinical Nursing, 8*(2), 77–83.

Gaut, D. A. (1993). Introduction. In A. Boykin & S. Schoenhofer, *Nursing as caring: A model for transforming practice* (pp. xvii–xxix). New York: National League for Nursing.

Kaplan, A. (1964). *The conduct of inquiry.* San Francisco: Chandler Publishing.

Kearney, C., & Yeager, V. (1993). Practical applications of Nursing as Caring theory. In M. E. Parker (Ed.), *Patterns of nursing theories in practice* (pp. 93–102). New York: National League for Nursing.

King, A., & Brownell, J. (1976). *The curriculum and the disciplines of knowledge.* Huntington, NY: Publishing.

Leininger, M. (1978). *Transcultural nursing: Concepts, theories, and practices.* New York: Wiley.

Leininger, M. (1981). Some philosophical, historical and taxonomic aspects of nursing and caring in American culture. In M. Leininger (Ed.), *Caring: An essential human need* (pp. 133–143). Detroit, MI: Wayne State University Press.

Leininger, M. (1991). *Culture care Diversity and Universality: A theory for nursing.* New York: National League for Nursing.

Maxwell, G. (1990). *Connections. Nightingale Songs, 1*(1). P.O. Box 057563, West Palm Beach, FL 33405–7563.

Mayeroff, M. (1971). *On caring.* New York: Harper & Row.

Nursing Development Conference Group. (1979). *Concept formalization in nursing: Process and product.* Boston: Little, Brown. [out of print]

Parker, M. (1993). Foreword. In A. Boykin, & S. Schoenhofer. *Nursing as caring: A model for transforming practice* (pp. ix–xii). New York: National League for Nursing.

Paterson, J., & Zderad, L. (1988). *Humanistic nursing.* New York: National League for Nursing.

Phenix, P. (1964). *Realms of meaning.* New York: McGraw-Hill.

Pribram, K. H. (1971). *Languages of the brain: Experimental paradoxes and principles in neuropsychology.* Englewood Cliffs, NJ: Prentice-Hall.

Ray, M. (1981). A philosophical analysis of caring within nursing. In M. Leininger (Ed.), *Caring: An essential human need* (pp. 25–36). Detroit, MI: Wayne State University Press.

Ray, M. (1984). The development of a classification system of institutional caring. In M. Leininger (Ed.), *Care: The essence of nursing and health* (pp. 95–112). Detroit, MI: Wayne State University Press.

Ray, M. (1985). A philosophical method to study nursing phenomena. In M. Leininger (Ed.), *Qualitative research methods in nursing* (pp. 81–92). Orlando, FL: Grune & Stratton.

Ray, M. (1989). The theory of bureaucratic caring for nursing practice in the organizational culture. *Nursing Administration Quarterly, 13*(2), 31–42.

Roach, S. (1984). *Caring: The human mode of being, implications for nursing.* Toronto: Faculty of Nursing, University of Toronto.

Roach, S. (1987). *The human act of caring.* Ottawa: Canadian Hospital Association.

Roach, S. (1992 Revised). *The human act of caring.* Ottawa: Canadian Hospital Association.

Watson, J. (1979). *Nursing: The philosophy and science of caring.* Boston: Little, Brown.

Watson, J. (1988). *Nursing: Human science and human care. A theory of nursing.* New York: National League for Nursing. (Originally published 1985, Appleton-Century-Crofts).

C H A P T E R   2 4

NURSING THEORIES AND THE NURSING PROCESS

*Julia B. George**

■ ■ ■

The focus of this chapter is on the professional nurse's use of nursing theories or models as a framework to guide nursing practice. Where appropriate, this applica-tion of theory to practice is discussed through use in the nursing process. As profes-sional nurses, we need to test those theories that we believe can be useful to our practice. When nurses deliberately use the same theories or models in a variety of nursing situations, or a variety of theories and models in similar nursing situations, review and analysis of the results can contribute to the body of nursing knowledge.

A combination of theories or models can be used by the practicing nurse to identify new relationships and new ideas for testing. It is also possible that as nurses consistently use nursing theories or models in practice, we can identify those with which we as professionals feel most confident. We may also find that certain ones work better in selected situations than others. By keeping accurate records and communicating our successes and failures to others, the practice of nursing becomes more capable of responding appropriately in those situations that call for nursing.

A REVIEW OF THE TWENTY-ONE THEORIES

As various nursing theories or models are used as the framework for prac-tice, the focus of nursing practice will differ. Florence Nightingale focused on organizing and manipulating the physical, social, and psychological environ-ment in order to put the person in the best possible conditions for nature to act. She also emphasized that nurses should alleviate and prevent unneces-sary suffering and pain. Nightingale's notions about nursing laid the ground-work for and influenced other nursing theorists (see Chapter 3).

Hildegard Peplau presents nursing as an interpersonal process of thera-peutic interactions between the nurse and patient. The purpose of this interpersonal relationship is to clarify the patient's problems, set mutually

*Gratitude is expressed to Marjorie Stanton for her contributions to this chapter in earlier editions.

acceptable goals, and solve those problems. Conflict may occur if the nurse and patient cannot come to agreement about the goals or the means to achieve them; however, both the patient and nurse should grow from this experience (see Chapter 4). Peplau identifies four phases in the relationship: orientation, identification, exploitation, and resolution. Her influence on the notion of nursing as an interpersonal process is pervasive.

Virginia Henderson views nursing as doing for patients what they cannot do for themselves, and she identifies 14 components of nursing care that need to be considered (see Chapter 5). Her view of nursing seems to foster dependence initially, although her goal is to help the patient return to independence as soon as possible. Henderson's influence is seen in the writings of many of the later nursing theorists.

Lydia Hall's notion of nursing centers around the three components of care, core, and cure. Care represents nurturance and is exclusive to nursing. Core involves the therapeutic use of self and emphasizes the use of reflection. Cure focuses on nursing related to the physician's orders. Core and cure are shared with other health care providers. Hall views the three components as interrelated, with one component taking precedence over the other two at varying points during the patient's course of progress. Hall's focus is primarily on the ill adult who is past the acute stage of illness (see Chapter 6).

Dorothea Orem's theory of nursing (see Chapter 7) consists of the three theories of self-care, self-care deficit, and nursing systems. The theory of self-care includes the human's ability to care for him- or herself (self-care agency), basic conditioning factors, a totality of self-care actions needed (therapeutic self-care demand), and three categories of self-care requisites: universal, developmental, and health deviation. The self-care deficit theory is the core of Orem's general theory of nursing because it identifies when nursing is needed. That is, it identifies that nursing is needed when current or future therapeutic self-care demands exceed self-care agency. The nursing systems theory identifies three nursing systems as wholly compensatory, partly compensatory, and supportive-educative. Orem's theoretical construct of self-care deficit has some similarity to Henderson's general concept of nursing.

Dorothy E. Johnson's behavioral system model for nursing has seven subsystems: attachment or affiliative, dependency, ingestive, eliminative, sexual, aggressive, and achievement. These seven subsystems need nurturance and stimulation for growth, and they also need protection from noxious influences (see Chapter 8). Nursing problems occur when there are insufficiencies in a subsystem's behaviors, discrepancies between the behaviors of a subsystem and those expected of it, incompatibility between two subsystems, or dominance of one subsystem over the others. The goal of nursing is to keep the behavioral system in balance and to maintain stability in the system. Nursing focuses on the behaviors of the person who is ill or is threatened with illness; and medicine, using the biological system model, focuses on the illness itself.

Faye G. Abdellah focuses on problem-solving to move the patient toward health. She provides a means for categorizing overt and covert patient needs under 21 common nursing problems relative to caring for patients (see Chapter 9). There is some similarity to Henderson's 14 components of basic nursing care.

Ida Jean Orlando (Pelletier) advances to some extent Henderson's theory of nursing; she believes that the nurse helps patients meet a perceived need that the patients cannot meet for themselves. Orlando (see Chapter 10) believes that nurses provide direct assistance to meet an immediate need for help in order to avoid or to alleviate distress or helplessness. She emphasizes the importance of validating the need and evaluating care based on observable outcomes. Orlando indicates that nursing actions can be automatic (those chosen for reasons other than the immediate need for help) or deliberative (those resulting from validating the need for help, exploring the meaning of the need, and validating the effectiveness of actions taken to meet the need).

Ernestine Wiedenbach strongly believes that the nurse's individual philosophy or central purpose lends credence to nursing care. She believes that nurses help to meet the individual's need for help through the identification of the needs, ministration of help, and validation that the actions were helpful. This all occurs within the realities of the immediate situation. Wiedenbach also believes nursing to be a deliberative action, as does Orlando (see Chapter 11).

Myra Levine sees nursing as human interaction: the dependency of individuals on one another. Levine identifies four principles of conservation: conservation of energy, conservation of structural integrity, conservation of personal integrity, and conservation of social integrity. She believes this provides a way to view people holistically. Levine views nursing as supporting the process of adaptation to achieve conservation and preserve integrity. Adaptation is based on past experiences (historicity), with task-specific responses (specificity), and the ability of several systems to respond to a demand (redundancy). Conservation is the product of adaptation (see Chapter 12). To Levine, health and disease are patterns of adaptive change, and the purpose of nursing is to take care of others when they need to be taken care of. She is similar to Henderson in her emphasis on the importance of helping the person become independent again as soon as possible.

Imogene King presents a theory of goal attainment from an open systems conceptual framework that integrates personal systems, interpersonal systems, and social systems. The interpersonal systems of nurse and client provide the major emphasis in this theory. Nurse–client interactions are the essential component in goal setting and in identifying the means of goal achievement. King views human beings as the focus of nursing and as open systems interacting with the environment (see Chapter 13).

Martha Rogers developed the principles of homeodynamics, which focus on the wholeness of human beings, the unitary nature of human beings and their environment, and the nature and direction of human and environment change. Humans, as irreducible, indivisible, pandimensional energy fields identified by pattern, benefit from nursing that participates in harmony with their process of change. Rogers believes the science of nursing is the science of unitary human beings (see Chapter 14).

Callista Roy's major emphasis is on the person as an adaptive system. To further describe the client of nursing, the four adaptive modes are identified as physiological, self-concept, role function, and interdependence. The person has two major internal processor subsystems, the regulator and the cognator, which are seen as mechanisms for adapting or coping. The goal of nursing is to promote adaptive responses (see Chapter 15).

Betty Neuman presents the Neuman Systems Model that focuses on the whole person and that person's reaction to stress. Her model can be used in illness or wellness. The model focuses on the human variables, basic structure and energy resources, lines of resistance and defense, stressors and reaction to them, levels of prevention, intra-, inter-, and extrapersonal factors and reconstitution. Nursing's major concern is to help the client system attain, maintain, or regain system stability (see Chapter 16).

Josephine Paterson and Loretta Zderad provide a humanistic nursing practice theory based on their belief that nursing is an existential experience. Nursing is viewed as a lived dialogue that involves the coming together of the nurse and the person to be nursed. The essential characteristic of nursing is nurturance. Humanistic nursing cannot take place without the authentic commitment of the nurse to being with and doing with the client. Humanistic nursing also presupposes responsible choices (see Chapter 17).

Jean Watson's science of caring is built on a framework of seven assumptions and ten carative factors. She emphasizes the interpersonal nature of caring, describes the nurse as a coparticipant with the client, and includes the soul as an important consideration. She includes health promotion and treatment of illness in nursing. The goal of nursing is to help people to achieve a high degree of harmony within themselves (see Chapter 18).

Rosemarie Rizzo Parse's theory of Human Becoming is based on Martha Rogers' principles and concepts and on existential phenomenological thought. She emphasizes free choice of personal meaning in relating value priorities, cocreating of rhythmical patterns in exchange with the environment, and cotranscending in many dimensions as possibilities unfold. She also believes that each choice opens certain opportunities while closing others. Thus, she speaks to revealing–concealing, enabling–limiting, and connecting–separating. Since each individual makes his or her own personal choices, the role of the nurse is that of guide, not decision maker (see Chapter 19).

Helen Erickson, Evelyn Tomlin, and Mary Ann Swain's theory is titled Modeling and Role-Modeling. The focus of this theory is on the person. The nurse models (assesses), role models (plans), and intervenes in this interpersonal and interactive theory. Each individual is unique, has some self-care knowledge, needs simultaneously to be attached to and separate from others, and has adaptive potential. Nurses in this theory facilitate, nurture, and accept the person unconditionally (see Chapter 20).

Madeleine Leininger focuses on the importance of understanding the similarities (universalities) and differences (diversities) of peoples across cultures.

She speaks to the importance of the nurse's awareness of the cultures of the client and of the nurse. She also emphasizes care and caring as the dominant and central domain of nursing (see Chapter 21).

Margaret Newman focuses on health as expanding consciousness (see Chapter 22). Humans are unitary beings in whom disease is a manifestation of the pattern of health. Consciousness is the information capability of the system which is influenced by time, space, and movement and is ever-expanding. Change occurs through transformation. Nursing is involved with human beings who have reached choice points and found that their old ways are no longer effective. Caring is a moral imperative for nursing. As does Parse, Newman eschews the nursing process. The nurse is a partner with the client rather than the goal setter and outcome predictor.

Anne Boykin and Savina Schoenhofer present the grand theory of Nursing as Caring (see Chapter 23). All persons are caring, and nursing is a response to a unique social call. The focus of nursing is on nurturing persons living and growing in caring in a manner that is specific to each nurse–nursed relationship or nursing situation. Each nursing situation is original. As with Newman, Boykin and Schoenhofer identify caring as a moral imperative. They also do not support the nursing process, which they describe as a need-based process. Nursing as Caring is not based on need or deficit but is an egalitarian model of helping.

COMPARISON OF THE THEORIES OR MODELS

A review of the theories presented indicates that there are similarities and differences among them. Many of the theorists were influenced by each other in their advancement of nursing knowledge. This fact is valuable and useful to students of professional nursing practice. The concept of looking specifically at the environment in relation to patients or clients was initiated by Nightingale and considered later by Johnson, King, Neuman, Orem, Roy, Rogers, Leininger, and Newman, but not specifically considered by Henderson, Abdellah, Peplau, and Orlando. The concept of dependency and its role in nursing was identified by Henderson and was also used by Orlando, Orem, and Levine. Independence is a focus in the theories or models of Peplau, Rogers, Hall, King, and Parse. Interdependence is a theme in the works of Erickson, Tomlin, and Swain; Newman; and Boykin and Schoenhofer. Adaptation is considered in the theories or models of Nightingale, King, Levine, Rogers, Roy, and Erickson, Tomlin and Swain; however, where Roy views adaptation as health producing, Roger's concept of adaptation would be viewed as not being conducive to health. Peplau, Levine, Paterson and Zderad, King, Watson, Parse, Leininger, Erickson, Tomlin and Swain, Newman, and Boykin and Schoenhofer emphasize interpersonal or interactive concepts in their writings, although these concepts are not overlooked by other theorists (eg, Hall and Orlando). Systems theory is used specifically by Rogers, King, Roy, Johnson, Neuman, Parse, and

Newman. The theories or models of Henderson, Orlando, and Hall seem primarily useful in the care of the ill, whereas those of Nightingale, Peplau, Wiedenbach, Orem, Levine, King, Rogers, Roy, Watson, Leininger, and Newman are useful for caring for the well and the ill. Abdellah's ideas seem more consistent with the technical aspects of nursing care, whereas the others' ideas do not. Caring is a particular focus of Watson, Leininger, Newman, and Boykin and Schoenhofer.

One way of looking at the differences among the nurse theorists is to explore the variety of ways they characterize nursing behaviors. A quick summary of the theorists presented identifies at least four different forms of nursing behaviors: (1) assuming responsibility for the person until he or she is ready to assume responsibility for self; (2) changing or manipulating the environment to facilitate health; (3) helping the person toward some goal; and (4) being with the person. The reader may be able to identify other similarities and differences.

Practitioners of nursing need to use the theories or models that are most useful in a given situation. As stated earlier, a combination of theories or models can be considered and, if used consistently, should be analyzed by the user as to their effectiveness. By using various nursing theories or models, the focus and consequences of nursing practice may differ, as discussed in the following example.

Consider this situation: Mrs. Mary James is a 68-year-old woman recovering from a stroke that occurred three days ago. She has weakness of the left side of her body. She is left-handed and requires retraining in the following areas: balancing while standing, climbing stairs, self-feeding, bladder control, and personal hygiene activities including dressing. She is in a hospital room with four other patients and is in the bed nearest the door. There is one window in the room. Before her hospitalization for the stroke, Mrs. James maintained her own home, was quite independent, volunteered one day a week at the local hospital, and was active in the local garden club.

Table 24–1 provides a brief overview of the direction a nurse might take using the various nursing theories or models as a framework to guide nursing practice. You will note that although each theorist moves Mrs. James to some point of independence, the methods are different due to different orientations. A fully developed description of care using any one of the theories or models as a framework would provide much more detailed and specific information about Mrs. James than is given in this table. However, the brief overview in Table 24–1 does give the reader an idea of how care might occur if a particular theory were used or differ if another theory were used. It is not intended to be an all-inclusive discussion on nursing care for Mrs. James.

The consistent use of selected nursing theories or models in nursing practice provides a way to validate and test these theories or models. The transmission of such knowledge by practicing nurses and nurse researchers adds to the unique body of knowledge necessary to a profession.

The systematic use of nursing theories or models provides a structure and discipline for nursing practice. It also provides a framework for teaching professional nursing students how to base practice on knowledge.

TABLE 24–1. OVERVIEW OF THEORIES OR MODELS AND NURSING PROCESS

Theorist	Assessment	Nursing Diagnosis	Planning	Implementation	Evaluation
Nightingale	Focus is on environment of patient. What is environment contributing to disability or illness of Mrs. James? What are inhibiting factors, ie, position of bedside table; lack of flowers; too far from window; slippery, cold floor; lack of space (four-bed room); too many people in room; noisy area?	Relates to environment or what is lacking in the environment as a condition to restore health, ie, crowded, restricted environment that inhibits movement toward independence and health.	Focus is on identifying those areas of the environment needing modification or change to provide Mrs. James with the best possible conditions for nature to restore or improve health, ie, remove restrictions, maximize use of right hand, provide sunlight and ventilation, provide for safe environment.	Carries out the actions necessary to change or manipulate the environment to provide optimum conditions for restoration or improvement of health. Move Mrs. James to room with two beds for more space but with companionship; provide chair near the window; place bedside table and things needed by Mrs. James on right side of bed; provide warm, sturdy slippers or shoes; place other patient in room on Mrs. James's right; provide flowers.	Relates to how well changes in or manipulation of the environment worked to effect optimal conditions for restoration or improvement of health, ie, able to move about room with some assistance. Sits by window and talks to patient in room. Uses right hand to feed self and care for other needs. Arranges flowers in room. Taking an interest in what is happening inside and outside the room.
Peplau	Focus is on the orientation phase—Mrs. James has expressed need for help. The nurse, family, and Mrs. James work	Relates to the identification of the health problem or deficit by the nurse and Mrs. James, ie, inability to cope with dependent role caused by	Focus is on the nurse and Mrs. James setting mutual goals for Mrs. James to become more independent through the development of the	Carries out plans mutually agreed upon by nurse and Mrs. James. However, Mrs. James is in control in asking for what she needs, ie, "I don't need to	Relates to how well Mrs. James progressed through orientation, identification, and exploitation phases. Have the needs been

(Continued)

425

TABLE 24-1. (CONTINUED)

Theorist	Assessment	Nursing Diagnosis	Planning	Implementation	Evaluation
Peplau (continued)	together to clarify the problems; Mrs. James's loss of independence, her fear about what has happened to her, how she will cope, how will her family cope.	diminished function of left side of body.	interpersonal relationship. Mrs. James should feel comfortable in discussing how she will become more independent. This is likened to the identification phase.	be fed. Teach me to feed myself. I'm ready." The nurse helps Mrs. James to recognize and explore her feelings when she becomes frustrated in her attempts to feed herself. This can be likened to the exploitation phase.	met? When the answer is yes, terminating the relationship (resolution phase) begins.
Henderson	Focus is on assessing Mrs. James's ability relative to the 14 components of basic nursing care, ie, Mrs. James is left-handed with left-sided weakness (relates to component #2—"eat and drink adequately").	Relates to deficits in the ability of Mrs. James to function in each of the 14 components. Takes into consideration strength, will, and knowledge, ie, inability to feed self due to left-handed weakness (relates to component #2).	Focus is on identifying those areas of the 14 components that Mrs. James cannot do for herself and which therefore the nurse must do or assist in doing, ie, feed Mrs. James until she is able to feed herself with her right hand. This should lead to independence on the part of Mrs. James.	Carries out the plan to initially feed Mrs. James while teaching her to use her right hand to feed herself.	Relates to how soon and how well Mrs. James is able to feed herself with her right hand, ie, for the first three days she needed to be fed; by fourth day, held utensils and fed self with assistance; by seventh day, was able to feed self if food was bite-size.
Hall	Focus is on increasing Mrs. James's self-awareness through observation and reflection. Helps	Statement of Mrs. James's need or problem. Mrs. James is in control, ie, "I need to learn	Focus is on setting goals and priorities with Mrs. James, ie, needs to learn to care for self:	Carries out plans with Mrs. James. Intimate bodily care is given, ie, help her to feed self and begin to	Relates to Mrs. James's progress toward goals, ie, able to feed self with right hand, able to

Mrs. James hear herself, ie, "I'm a sick woman. I can't take care of myself. I can't even dress or feed myself. Everyone is looking at me." Biological data are also being collected, ie, cannot grasp or hold with left hand.	to take care of myself. I need to learn to use my right hand to feed and dress myself. I need to think about myself for awhile and not worry about others."	1. Learn to use right hand to feed and dress self. 2. Walk by self to bathroom. 3. Improve self-concept.	use right hand; assist her to dress until she learns to dress self; support and listen to her.	dress self with assistance, able to walk to bathroom with assistance, states "I think I'll be able to take care of myself."
Orem Focus is on appraising the situation; determining why Mrs. James needs care; considers her life history and life style, the physician's perspective and Mrs. James's perspective, ie, Mrs. James needs help because she has left-sided weakness, is left-handed, and cannot feed herself or walk without assistance.	Relating to therapeutic self-care demand and self-care agency: inability to feed self without assistance, inability to walk without assistance, ability to learn alternate methods of self-care relating to identified deficits.	Focus is on developing nursing system to improve Mrs. James's self-care abilities relative to eating, walking, and other deficits in activities in daily living. Identify Mrs. James's strengths, such as previous independent life style. Reach agreements with Mrs. James and family about role each will play.	Carries out plan to assist Mrs. James in the performance of self-care tasks, ie, learning to feed herself and using walker to assist in walking (supportive-educative nursing system). Help her feed herself until she can do this alone (partly compensatory nursing system).	Relates to monitoring progress of Mrs. James with regard to self-care activities and making adjustments and recommendations as necessary. Is self-care agency equal to or greater than therapeutic self-care demand?
Johnson Focus is on the behavioral subsystems to identify disturbances in structure and	Relates to a description of the behavior that is associated with an actual or	Focus is on identification of short and long term goals in the system or	Carries out the necessary activities to assist Mrs. James in modifying, changing,	Relates to the degree of progress in achieving the goals set during planning.

(Continued)

TABLE 24–1. (CONTINUED)

Theorist	Assessment	Nursing Diagnosis	Planning	Implementation	Evaluation
Johnson (continued)	function of subsystems or a discrepancy in behavioral functioning. *Affiliative and dependency subsystems:* Mrs. James has no family for support and affection. Has relied on her outreach through volunteering and her relationship with garden club members for support and assistance. Limited mobility has curtailed outreach. Came to hospital alone.	potential instability in the subsystem. Diminished ability for social behavior due to immobility. Weakening of affiliative subsystem due to limited access to friends.	subsystem by modifying or changing behavior. *Long range goal:* Diminish the effects of hospitalization and immobilization on Mrs. James. *Short term goals:* Preserve and strengthen Mrs. James's relationships with friends to encourage and enhance her interest in and caring about others.	or regulating behavior so that the goal of each subsystem will be met. Behavioral objectives are used to show progress toward goal. 1. Within two days have Mrs. James contact at least two of her garden club friends. 2. Within four days have Mrs. James, with the use of her walker, visit each client in the room to begin to get to know them.	Mrs. James called her "dearest" friend, Ada Brown, within two days and made plans to call Mrs. Jackson by the next day. Mrs. James also visited each client in the room, using her walker, and decided that she would spend time each day with Mrs. Smith who has no visitors.
Abdellah	Focus is on each of the 21 nursing problems to collect data about Mrs. James, ie, #7—"To facilitate maintenance of elimination." Mrs. James has not had a bowel movement in two days, has difficulty moving about, does not like fruits and vegetables.	Problems with elimination possibly due to insufficient exercise and lack of roughage in diet.	Focus is on facilitating the maintenance of elimination, ie, assisting Mrs. James to walk at least 15 minutes twice daily and move about in bed. Also speak to dietitian regarding diet of grain cereals, sliced fruit or finger fruits, etc. and to increase fluid intake.	Carries out the nursing activities to assist Mrs. James to change position in bed and to walk with walker. Encourages Mrs. James to eat prescribed foods; assists in feeding and praises her for trying foods with fiber.	Relates to the resolution of Mrs. James's elimination problems, is elimination achieved and maintained?

Orlando	Focus is on collecting data relative to the immediate situation and clarifying nurse's reaction to Mrs. James, ie, Mrs. James has left-sided weakness. What does Mrs. James identify as her immediate need—inability to feed self, difficulty in bathing?	Relates to identifying Mrs. James's needs that she cannot meet by herself. Validate these with her, ie, Mrs. James needs to be taught to use her right hand to feed and bathe self.	Focus is on planning with Mrs. James and mutually setting goals, ie, clarifying with Mrs. James that she indeed needs to learn to use her right hand in order to feed and bathe herself.	Carries out the nursing activities necessary to meet Mrs. James's needs, ie, assist Mrs. James to use her right hand to eat—do not feed her; place bedside table on her right; teach her techniques for bathing with her right hand.	Relates to Mrs. James's behavior in terms of feeding and bathing herself using her right hand—has her need to do so been met? Uses right hand to eat but needs encouragement. Able to get out of bed with assistance; can walk to bathroom; able to bathe self except for back and feet.
Wiedenbach	Focus is on the nurse's perception and awareness of the situation, ie, "Mrs. James must feel so helpless since she is unable to feed herself."	Relates to the situation perceived and to identification of person's need, ie, "feeling of helplessness."	Focus is on the nurse and Mrs. James's plan to reduce Mrs. James's feeling of helplessness by teaching her how to eat with her right hand, with food prepared in bite-size pieces.	Ministration of help. "I'll assist you in using your right hand until you can feed yourself. I'll stay with you until you learn how to feed yourself with your right hand."	Relates to validating that Mrs. James feels less helpless when she can use her right hand for feeding herself.
Levine	Focus is on using the four conservation principles as a basis for observing and interviewing Mrs. James to identify adaptation needs. Using the principle	Relates to the stress of illness or altered health reflecting a problem or potential problem with regard to a deficit or threatened deficit, ie, personal integrity	Focus is on planning therapeutic interventions designed to promote adaptation that contributes to healing and restoration of health,	Carries out the actions necessary based on conservation of energy, and structural, personal and social integrity. Mrs. James to sit on side of the bed for 2	Relates to Mrs. James's adaptation to changes in her life style that threaten personal integrity, ie, able to walk with assistance of walker,

(Continued)

429

TABLE 24–1. (CONTINUED)

Theorist	Assessment	Nursing Diagnosis	Planning	Implementation	Evaluation
Levine (continued)	of personal integrity, the nurse questions Mrs. James about her life style before she had the stroke; "What did you usually do each day? How did you get to the garden club?" Analysis of data reflects Mrs. James's balance of strengths and weaknesses in each of the four conservation areas.	threatened due to increased dependency on others in caring for self.	ie, plan to have Mrs. James ambulate to increase her sense of mobility and independence and conserve energy. Start out slowly—10 minutes twice a day, sitting before walking, and using a walker.	minutes, then sit in chair for 10 minutes, walk to bathroom and back using walker; increase time of walking as her strength increases.	manipulate walker very well; out of bed all day.
King	Focus is on the nurse's and Mrs. James's perception of Mrs. James's health status and her ability to adapt to stress and to use resources to achieve potential for daily living. Mrs. James is viewed as a reacting being, a time-oriented being, and a social being, ie, "I hate being dependent on others to feed and	Relates to the nurse's understanding and analysis of the data about Mrs. James's social system, perceptions, interpersonal relations, and health, ie, difficulty coping with feelings of dependency.	Focus is on mutual goal setting and clear communication necessary for setting goals to move Mrs. James toward health. Working with Mrs. James, the nurse and Mrs. James identify ways to increase Mrs. James's independence in the hospital, ie, learn to feed self with right hand; learn to walk	Carries out the activities necessary for Mrs. James to achieve increased independence, ie, teach Mrs. James to eat with right hand. Prepare food so she can do so. Stay with Mrs. James until she feels confident. Assist Mrs. James to use and manipulate walker in walking and using elevator.	Relates to how well the interpersonal process of nursing assisted Mrs. James in meeting the basic activities of daily living and to cope with health and illness, ie, feels less dependent now that she can feed self with right hand; ambulation allows Mrs. James to move out of four-bed room and relate to others; using elevator

	dress me, even to go to the bathroom." Left-handed, no strength in left hand, left sided weakness.	with walker; progress in using cane; learn to manipulate walker for use in elevator.		decreases feelings of dependency. "I feel so much better now that I can go to the bathroom by myself and feed myself."
Rogers	Focus is on collecting data and opinions about the person and the environment relative to principles of integrality, helicy, and resonance, ie, How is Mrs. James interacting with the hospital environment? Mrs. James reports difficulty in sleeping in the hospital. Until she was hospitalized, she slept 6 to 7 hours a night. Was very active, gardened. How has the life process of Mrs. James progressed to date? What patterns characterize Mrs. James?	Relates to rhythms, patterns, and life process and reflects the principles of homeodynamics, ie, alteration in sleep pattern.	Focuses on promoting dynamic repatterning with regard to alteration in Mrs. James's sleeping pattern. Plans are to provide an environment conducive to sleeping; increase activity during the day based on Mrs. James's previous life style; use relaxation techniques to promote readiness for sleep.	Carries out the strategies necessary to strengthen the integrity of the individual—environment relationship. Ask Mrs. James to tend plants on unit, thus increasing walking and providing a purpose. Air and smooth her bed; use appropriate pillows; flex her knees to reduce any pulling on her back muscles; practice relaxation techniques with her.	Relates to optimum state of health, ie, What is Mrs. James's pattern of sleeping by the third day following nursing implementation? How long is she sleeping? How well is she sleeping? Does she wake at night? Does she need sleep medication? How does she feel and look?
Roy	First level: Focus is on collecting data related to each	Relates to the deficits, or excesses of basic needs leading to	Focus is on promoting Mrs. James's adaptation in relation to	Carries out activities necessary to manipulate the	Relates to Mrs. James's goal achievement. After

(Continued)

TABLE 24-1. (CONTINUED)

Theorist	Assessment	Nursing Diagnosis	Planning	Implementation	Evaluation
Roy (continued)	adaptation mode. Physiological mode: Mrs. James's behavior related to rest and sleep. "I'm having trouble sleeping at night. I'm used to 7 hours sleep a night." Nurses during the night note Mrs. James is awake two to three times each night asking for something to sleep. *Second level:* Focal stimuli—Mrs. James is in a new environment. Contextual stimuli—other three people in room snore. Residual stimuli—Mrs. James's internal response to all the recent changes in her life.	Ineffective behavior, ie, inability to sleep throughout the night due to new and noisy environment.	the four modes. Physiologic mode: goal is Mrs. James will sleep if environment conducive to sleep is created.	environment by removing, increasing, decreasing, or altering stimuli. The resulting behavior should be adaptive, ie, provide for fresh air, freshen room at bedtime, reduce light and noise, encourage Mrs. James to fall asleep before others to reduce disturbance from others' snoring, try ear plugs. Introduce Mrs. James to relaxation techniques before sleeping. Consider moving her to another room.	two nights check with Mrs. James about restful sleep. Has sleeping improved? Does she look and feel rested in the morning? Review the night nurses' notes relating to Mrs. James's wakefulness.
Neuman	Focus is on Mrs. James's reaction to known or possible stressors (intra-, inter-, extraper-	Relates to stressors identified in each area—intra-, inter-, extrapersonal, ie, immobility due to	Focus is on setting priorities to facilitate Mrs. James's adaptive behaviors to stress. Teach Mrs.	Carries out the necessary actions to achieve highest level of reconstitution. Focus is on	Relates to the degree of reconstitution achieved. Mrs. James is able to feed self with right

	Assessment	Diagnosis	Goal	Implementation	Evaluation
	sonal). Also looks at lines of defense and resistance. *Intrapersonal:* Mrs. James is left-handed with muscle weakness of left arm, hand, and leg. Incontinent at times. *Interpersonal:* Separated from friends. *Extrapersonal:* Unable to engage in gardening or do volunteer work. Nurse asks Mrs. James, "What are you doing and what can you do to help yourself?" "I'm being fed, but I think I can feed myself. I want to walk to the bathroom."	left-sided weakness; intermittent lack of bladder control; diminished socialization due to immobility.	James to feed herself with right hand. Teach Mrs. James to use walker to become more mobile. Begin exercises for bladder control. Encourage Mrs. James to use walker to get to bathroom.	primary, secondary, and tertiary prevention; ie, primary prevention—reduce the possibility of Mrs. James becoming depressed by increasing independence and assisting her to feed herself immediately. Get Mrs. James out of bed and using walker to go to bathroom. Introduce her to others in the room. Tell her how much she has accomplished. Praise her for her accomplishments.	hand with little assistance. Needs help to cut meat. Able to use walker to get to bathroom. Incontinence occurring less often. Mrs. James tries hard to improve the strength of her right side. She is determined to go home as quickly as possible. She tries to cheer the other people in the room.
Paterson and Zderad	Focus is on describing what is and confirming it with Mrs. James. This begins the interdependent relationship between the nurse and the nursed. Mrs. James is a strong, independent	Based on assessment and relates to comfort–discomfort level. Bruised self-image due to change in body function. Limited support system due to lack of family.	Identification of ways to reduce discomfort and increase comfort to help nursed become all she can be. Assist Mrs. James to become more independent by teaching her how to feed self with	This nurse becomes truly present to Mrs. James and behaves in ways to reduce discomfort and relieve tension. Have Mrs. James call at least two of her garden club friends. Be there for Mrs. James. Feed	The nurse examines how effective her relationship and action with Mrs. James have been in reducing discomfort and alleviating tension. *Increased independence:* Mrs. James

(Continued)

TABLE 24–1. (CONTINUED)

Theorist	Assessment	Nursing Diagnosis	Planning	Implementation	Evaluation
Paterson and Zderad (continued)	woman who has weakness in the left side of her body. She is left-handed, cannot feed or dress herself, cannot walk without help. Depends on garden club friends, has no family. "Mrs. James, I'm Sue Ryan, your nurse. Can you tell me what is happening with you?" "Well, I had a stroke and I can't do anything without help. My friends don't know where I am—I'm a mess."		right hand and how to use walker to become more mobile. This will give her more control over her life and will increase her comfort. Encourage contact with her garden club friends for needed support system.	her when necessary. Share feelings with her. Teach her to use her right hand. Encourage Mrs. James to use walker to increase her mobility and independence. Discuss her plans for the future.	learned to eat with her right hand within two days. Now uses walker with ease. Visits people in room with her. Uses bathroom without assistance. *Decreased discomfort and relieved tension:* Has more control over her situation. Has decided to return home. Sharing her plans for the next few months. Mrs. James and nurse have been truly present with each other. Mrs. James's self-confidence has been bolstered, and she has learned ways to become independent and in control. She has discussed care after discharge. Mrs. James and nurse have planned contact after her discharge.

Watson				
Use the human needs model to guide assessment. *Lower Order Needs:* *Biophysical:* Is she able to obtain adequate food and fluids? Mrs. James needs assistance in this area due to limited use of her dominant left hand. *Elimination needs?* Mrs. James had difficulties with both bowel and bladder control. *Ventilation?* She is in a multibed unit with only one window. *Psychophysical:* *Activity or inactivity?* Mrs. James's left-sided weakness limits her ability to walk alone. She reports difficulty sleeping. *Sexuality?* Mrs. James describes herself as "as mess." *Higher Order Needs:* *Psychosocial— Achievement?* **Mrs.**	Based on assessment and related to human needs. Areas of need include adequacy of food and fluid, bowel and bladder control, ventilation, activity and rest, self-image, and interaction with others.	Plan care around the ten carative factors. Include instilling faith and hope, establishing a helping-trust relationship, acceptance of feelings, interpersonal teaching–learning, a supportive-protective-corrective environment, meeting human needs.	Arrange meeting with therapists to explain what they can do to help Mrs. James regain function. Have a person who has recovered from a stroke visit with Mrs. James. Encourage Mrs. James to discuss her feelings about herself, her stroke, and her current abilities. Arrange environment to maximize use of her right hand—water pitcher to right of her bed, walker available, etc. With Mrs. James, plan a toileting schedule to help her regain bowel and bladder control. Move her to a smaller room so there will be fewer interruptions to her sleep.	Are Mrs. James's human needs being met? Is her food and fluid intake adequate? Is she regaining bowel and bladder control? Is her pattern of sleep nearer to her normal pattern? Is she moving around safely with her walker? How does she describe herself? Is she interacting with other patients, with her friends?

(Continued)

TABLE 24–1. (CONTINUED)

Theorist	Assessment	Nursing Diagnosis	Planning	Implementation	Evaluation
Watson (continued)	James is worried about whether or not she will be able to continue to care for her home and to serve as a hospital volunteer. *Affiliation?* Mrs. James misses her regular contact with her friends in the Garden Club. *Interpersonal?* Mrs. James is concerned about whether others will continue to value her if she can no longer be independent.				
Parse	Assessment and Diagnosis do not fit with this theory as Parse states the nurse–client interaction is not limited by prescriptions.	See Assessment.	Nurse is a guide, not a decision maker. Interaction is evolving.	Nurse serves as a guide to illuminate meaning—guides Mrs. James to identify the personal meaning of the situation to her; to synchronize rhythms—lead Mrs. James to recognize the harmony within her existence; and to mobilize	Because the interaction is not limited by prescription, standards of evaluation cannot be created. Essentially, the nurse can evaluate if Mrs. James has identified personal meaning, recognized harmony, and dreamed of the possibles.

Erickson, Tomlin, and Swain	Begins with first nurse–patient encounter. Nurse asks Mrs. James to express her concerns. Mrs. James says, "I need to learn how to take care of myself all over again I have to learn to use my right hand instead of my left."	Self-care deficit: feeding, bathing/hygiene, dressing/grooming, toileting.	Support Mrs. James in her desire to regain self-care ability. Assist her in learning to use her right hand. Set specific goals and time frames with her, ie, within 2 days can feed self if food is in small bites.	transcendence—guide Mrs. James to move from the present to what is not yet, to dream of the possibles for her. Begins with first nurse–patient encounter. With Mrs. James identify how her things may be arranged to help her use her right hand; what will help her feed herself (tray placement and arrangement, food in small bites); clothing styles she can most easily manage dressing and undressing by herself; use of a walker to get to and from bathroom.	What does Mrs. James say about her progress toward the mutually set goals? What progress is seen by the nurse?
Leininger	Gather data relevant to the Sunrise Model. *Worldview:* She is American, active in a Garden Club and as a hospital volunteer. Her language is American English.	Based on areas of cultural diversity or universality which are not being met. Includes need for independence in mobility, feeding, toileting, sleep, and need for interaction	Based on cultural care preservation, accommodation, repatterning, or any combination of the three.	Include preservation through helping Mrs. James continue contact with member of her Garden Club; accommodation through helping her learn to use a	Are cultural diversities and universalities being met? Does Mrs. James view herself as continuing to be independent?

(Continued)

TABLE 24–1. (CONTINUED)

Theorist	Assessment	Nursing Diagnosis	Planning	Implementation	Evaluation
Leininger (continued)	Until her illness she lived in her own home; she is currently in a multibed ward. Technology—drives a car with a stick shift. Religious preference is unknown. Philosophy— believes independence and service to others are important. Kinship— widow, two children live over 1000 miles away. Social structure—interacts primarily with her own age group. Cultural values and beliefs—values independence, believes children should not have to support parents. Politics—is not politically involved. Legal system—lives in a historic neighborhood that does not allow for	with others of her own age group.		walker for mobility and keeping the walker available for her; repatterning through assisting her in learning to eat with her right hand—arranging her tray to enhance use of her right hand, cutting food into bite size pieces, encouraging her to butter her own bread.	

external modification of dwellings. Economics—Income from a trust fund; has insurance that will cover all costs associated with this illness. Education—college graduate. *Health systems:* Folk—believes use of professional health services is important. Professional—physician is head of the team, various therapists are part of the team. Nursing—part of the team. Identifies needs for care due to limited use of previously dominant side—include eating, toileting, mobility, interaction.

| Newman | Not compatible with nursing process. Nurse is to enter relationship with Mrs. James to be present with her. | See assessment. | Inappropriate to believe outcomes can be predicted. | Nurse in authentic relationship with Mrs. James as a partner during this choice point in which Mrs. James's | Have both nurse and Mrs. James reached higher levels of consciousness? Is Mrs. James ready |

(Continued)

TABLE 24–1. (CONTINUED)

Theorist	Assessment	Nursing Diagnosis	Planning	Implementation	Evaluation
Newman (continued)				old ways no longer work. Partnership includes providing support and information and being an organizing force. Both accept the unpredictable nature of life and work together for Mrs. James to be able to return to her home.	for nurse and client to move apart?
Boykin and Schoenhofer	Incompatible with nursing process; nurse is not seeking something to correct.	See assessment.	See assessment.	Nurse to know Mrs. James as caring person and nurture her in situation specific ways such as cutting up her food, encouraging her efforts to use her right hand.	Nurse tells his or her story of the nursing situation.

GLOSSARY*

■ ■ ■

Abstract concept. An image of something neither observable nor measurable.

Achievement subsystem. (Johnson) The behavioral subsystem relating to behaviors that attempt to control the environment and lead to personal accomplishment.

Adaptation. (Levine) Process of adjusting or modifying behavior or functioning to fit the situation and to achieve conservation; life process by which people maintain wholeness.

Adaptation. (Rogers) Change resulting from the integration of human beings and their environment. The change occurs as an ongoing evolving process that can never return to the original state.

Adaptation. (Roy) Positive response to internal or external stimuli using biopsychosocial mechanisms to promote personal integrity.

Adaptation level. (Roy) Condition of the person, or the individual's range of coping ability.

Adaptive responses. (Roy) Behaviors that positively affect health through promotion of the integrity of the person in terms of survival, growth, reproduction, and mastery.

Agent. (Wiedenbach) The practicing nurse, or the nurse's delegate, who serves as the propelling force in goal-directed behavior.

Aggressive subsystem. (Johnson) The behavioral subsystem that relates to behaviors concerned with protection and self-preservation.

Assumption. Statement or view that is widely accepted as true.

Assumption. (Wiedenbach) The meaning a nurse attaches to an interpretation of a sensory impression.

Attachment or affiliative subsystem. (Johnson) The behavioral subsystem that is the first formed and provides for a strong social bond.

Authority. (King) An active, reciprocal relationship that involves values, experience, and perceptions in defining, validating, and accepting the right of an individual to act within an organization.

---

* When a term relates specifically to a theorist, the name of the theorist appears in parentheses after the term.

Automatic activities. (Orlando) Nursing actions decided on for reasons other than the patient's immediate need.

Basic conditioning factors. (Orem) Aspects that influence the individual's self-care ability; include age, gender, stage of development, state of health, sociocultural orientation, health care system and family system factors, pattern of living, environment, availability and adequacy of resources.

Body image. (King) Individuals' perceptions of their own bodies, influenced by the reactions of others.

Care. (Hall) The exclusive aspect of nursing that provides the patient bodily comfort through "laying on of hands" and provides an opportunity for closeness.

Care. (Leininger) (noun) Phenomena related to assistive, supportive, or enabling behavior toward or for another individual (or group) with evident or anticipated needs to ameliorate or improve a human condition or lifeway.

Caring. (Leininger) (verb) Action directed toward assisting, supporting, or enabling behavior of another individual (or group) with evident or anticipated needs to ameliorate or improve a human condition or lifeway.

Central purpose. (Wiedenbach) The commitment of the individual nurse, based on a personal philosophy, that defines the desired quality of health and specifies the nurse's special responsibility in providing care to assist others in achieving or sustaining that quality.

Clustering of data. The grouping of data pieces that fit together and show relationships.

Cocreating. (Parse) Participation of human and environment in creating the pattern of each.

Cognator mechanism. (Roy) Coping mechanism or control subsystem that relates to the higher brain functions of perception, information processing, learning, judgment, and emotion.

Communication. (King) A direct or indirect process in which one person gives information to another.

Community. (Paterson and Zderad) Two or more persons striving together, living–dying all-at-once.

Concept. An abstract notion; a vehicle of thought that involves images; words that describe objects, properties, or events.

Conceptual framework. Group of interrelated concepts.

Connecting–separating. (Parse) The rhythmical process of distancing and relating.

Consciousness. (Newman) The information of the system; the system's capacity to interact with the environment.

Conservation. (Levine) Defense of the wholeness of a living system; ensures ability to confront change appropriately and retain unique identity.

Conservation of energy. (Levine) Balancing energy output with energy input to avoid excessive fatigue.

Conservation of personal integrity. (Levine) Maintaining or restoring the patient's sense of identity and self-worth.

Conservation of social integrity. (Levine) Acknowledging the patient as a social being.

Conservation of structural integrity. (Levine) Maintaining or restoring the structure of the body.

Contextual stimuli. (Roy) Stimuli of the person's internal or external world, other than those immediately confronting the person, that influence the situation and are observable, measurable, or subjectively reported by the person.

Core. (Hall) The shared aspect with any health professional who therapeutically uses a freely offered closeness to help the patient discover who he or she is.

Covert problem. Hidden or concealed condition of concern.

Cultural Care. (Leininger) The cognitively known values, beliefs, and patterned expressions that assist, support, or enable another individual or group to maintain well-being, improve a human condition or lifeway, or face death and disabilities.

Cultural care accommodation/negotiation. (Leininger) Assistive, supportive, or enabling professional actions and decisions that help clients of a particular culture to adapt to, or negotiate for a beneficial or satisfying health status, or to face death.

Cultural care diversity. (Leininger) The variability of meanings, patterns, values or symbols of care that are culturally derived by humans for their well-being, or to improve a human condition or lifeway, or to face death.

Cultural care preservation/maintenance. (Leininger) Assistive, supportive, or enabling professional actions and decisions that help clients of a particular culture to preserve or maintain a state of health, or to recover from illness, and to face death.

Cultural care repatterning/restructuring. (Leininger) Assistive, supportive, or enabling professional actions or decisions that help clients change their lifeways for new or different patterns that are culturally meaningful and satisfying, or that support beneficial and healthy life patterns.

Cultural care universality. (Leininger) Common, similar or uniform meanings, patterns, values, or symbols of care that are culturally derived by humans for their well-being or to improve a human condition and lifeway or to face death.

Cultural imposition. (Leininger) Efforts of an outsider, subtle and not so subtle, to impose his or her own cultural values, beliefs, or behaviors upon an individual, family, or group from another culture.

Cultural values. (Leininger) Values that are derived from the culture, identify desirable ways of acting or knowing, guide decision making, and are often held over long periods.

Culture. (Leininger) Learned, shared, and transmitted values, beliefs, norms, and lifeway practices of a particular group that guide thinking, decisions, and actions in patterned ways.

Culture. (Rogers) The integrated pattern of human behavior that includes thought, speech, action, and artifacts, and depends on man's capacity for learning and transmitting knowledge to succeeding generations.

Culture shock. (Leininger) Experiencing feelings of discomfort, helplessness, disorientation while attempting to comprehend or adapt effectively to a different cultural group.

Cure. (Hall) An aspect with medical personnel in which the nurse helps the patient and family through medical, surgical, and rehabilitative care.

Decision making in organizations. (King) An active process in which choice, directed by goals, is made and acted upon.

Deliberative actions. (Orlando) Nursing actions that ascertain or meet the patient's immediate need.

Dependency subsystem. (Johnson) The behavioral subsystem in which behaviors evoke nurturing behaviors in others.

Developmental self-care requisites. (Orem) Maintaining conditions to support life and development or to provide preventive care for adverse conditions that affect development.

Dialogue. (Paterson and Zderad) An intersubjective experience in which individuals relate creatively and have a real sharing.

Discrepancy. (Johnson) Action that does not achieve the intended goal.

Dominance. (Johnson) Primary use of one behavioral subsystem to the detriment of the other subsystems and regardless of the situation.

Eliminative subsystem. (Johnson) The behavioral subsystem that relates to socially acceptable behaviors surrounding the excretion of waste products from the body.

Emic. (Leininger) Personal knowledge or explanation of behavior; indigenous, not universal.

Empirical. Measured or observed through the senses.

Enabling–limiting. (Parse) Making choices results in enabling an individual in some ways while limiting in others.

Environment. (Neuman) Those internal and external forces that surround humans at any given point in time.

Environment. (Nightingale) External conditions and influences that affect life and development.

Environment. (Rogers) Four-dimensional, negentropic energy field identified by pattern and encompassing all that is outside any given human field.

Environment. (Roy) All conditions, circumstances, and influences surrounding and affecting the development and behavior of persons or groups.

Environmental context. (Leininger) The totality of an event, situation, or particular experience that gives meaning to human expressions, including physical, ecological, social interactions, emotional, and cultural dimensions.

Equifinality. An open system that may attain a state independent of time or initial conditions and determined only by the system parameters.

Epistemology. The study of the history of knowledge, including the origin, nature, methods, and limitations of knowledge development.

Ethnonursing. (Leininger) The study of nursing care beliefs, values, and practices as cognitively perceived and known by a designated culture through their direct experience, beliefs, and value system.

Existential psychology. The study of human existence using phenomenological analysis.

Exploitation phase. (Peplau) The third phase of Peplau's nurse–patient relationship. The patient takes full advantage of all available services while feeling an integral part of the helping environment. Goals are met through a collaborative effort as the patient becomes independent during convalescence.

Extrapersonal stressors. (Neuman) Forces occurring outside the system that generate a reaction or response from the system.

First-level assessment. (Roy) Behavioral assessment; the gathering of output behaviors of the person in relation to the four adaptive modes.

Flexible line of defense. (Neuman) Variable and constantly changing ability to respond to stressors.

Focal stimuli. (Roy) Stimuli of the person's internal or external world that immediately confront the person.

Folk health system. (Leininger) Traditional or local indigenous health care or cure practices that have special meanings and uses to heal or assist people and are generally offered in familiar home or community environmental contexts with their local practitioners.

Framework. (Wiedenbach) The human, environmental, professional, and organizational facilities that make up the context in which nursing is practiced and that constitute its currently existing limits.

General system theory. A general science of wholeness.

Goal. The end stated in broad terms to identify effective criteria for evaluating nursing action.

Goal. (Wiedenbach) Outcome the nurse seeks to achieve.

Grand theory. Theory that covers broad areas of a discipline; may not be testable.

Growth and development. (King) The process in the lives of individuals that involves changes at the cellular, molecular, and behavioral levels and helps them move from potential to achievement.

Health deviation self-care. (Orem) Care needed by individuals who are ill or injured; may result from medical measures required to correct illness or injury.

Health problem.
Actual. Client need that currently exists.
Potential. Client need that may occur in the future and which may be averted with appropriate action.

Health. (Leininger) A state of well-being that is culturally defined, valued, and practiced and that reflects the ability of individuals (or groups) to perform their daily role activities in a culturally satisfactory way.

Helicy. (Rogers) The nature and direction of human and environmental change; change that is continuously innovative, probabilistic, and characterized by increasing diversity of the human field and environmental field pattern emerging out of the continuous, mutual, simultaneous interaction between the human and environmental fields and manifesting nonrepeating rhythmicities.

Historicity. (Levine) Aspect of adaptation in which responses are based on past experiences.

Holism. A theory that the universe and especially living nature are correctly seen in terms of interacting wholes that are more than the mere sum of the individual parts.

Homeodynamics. (Rogers) A way of viewing man in his wholeness. Changes in the life process of human beings are irreversible, nonrepeatable, rhythmical in nature, and evidence growing complexity of pattern. Change proceeds by continuous repatterning of both human beings and environment by resonating waves, and reflects the mutual simultaneous interaction between the two at any given point in space–time.

Humanism. (Rogers) A doctrine, attitude, or way of life centered on human interests or values. A philosophy that asserts the dignity and worth of human beings and their capacity of becoming through choices.

Identification phase. (Peplau) The second phase of Peplau's nurse–patient relationship. The perceptions and expectations of the patient and nurse become more involved while building a working relationship of further identifying the problem and deciding on appropriate plans for improved health maintenance.

Illness. (Levine) State of altered health.

Illness. (Neuman) State of insufficiency in which needs are yet to be satisfied.

Imaging. (Parse) The picturing or making real of events, ideas, and people.

Incompatibility. (Johnson) Two behavioral subsystems in the same situation being in conflict with each other.

Ineffective response. (Roy) Behaviors that do not promote the integrity of the person in terms of survival, growth, reproduction, and mastery.

Ingestive subsystem. (Johnson) The behavioral subsystem that relates to the meanings and structures of social events surrounding the occasions when food is eaten.

Insufficiency. (Johnson) A behavioral subsystem that is not functioning adequately.

Integrality. (Rogers) The continuous, mutual, simultaneous integration process between human and environmental fields.

Interactions. (King) The observable, goal-directed, behaviors of two or more persons in mutual presence.

Interpersonal stressors. (Neuman) Forces that occur between two or more individuals and evoke a reaction or response.

Intrapersonal stressors. (Neuman) Forces occurring within a person that result in a reaction or response.

Languaging. (Parse) Reflection of images and values through speaking and moving.

Lines of resistance. (Neuman) The internal set of factors that seek to stabilize the person when stressors break through the normal line of defense.

Logical empiricism. Worldview in which truth must be confirmed by sensory experiences.

Means. (Wiedenbach) The activities and devices that enable the nurse to attain the desired goal.

Meeting. (Paterson and Zderad) The coming together of human beings characterized by the expectation that there will be a nurse and a nursed.

Metatheory. Theory about theory development.

Model. Representation of the interactions among and between concepts that shows the patterns of these interactions.

Modeling. (Erickson, Tomlin, and Swain) Process used by the nurse to gain an understanding of the client's world as the client perceives it.

More-being. (Paterson and Zderad) The process of becoming all that is humanly possible.

Movement. (Newman) Change that occurs between two states of rest.

Need for help. (Orlando) A requirement for assistance in decreasing or eliminating immediate distress or in improving the sense of adequacy.

Negentropy. The open system growth process of becoming more complex and efficient.

Normal line of defense. (Neuman) The biological-psychological-sociocultural-developmental-spiritual skills developed over a lifetime to achieve stability and deal with stressors.

Nursing agency. (Orem) The specialized abilities that enable nurses to provide nursing care.

Nursing problem. (Abdellah) A condition faced by the client or client's family with which the nurse can assist through the performance of professional functions.

Nursing process. A deliberate, intellectual activity by which the practice of nursing is approached in an orderly, systematic manner. It includes the following components:
Assessment. The process of data collection that results in a conclusion or nursing diagnosis.
Diagnosis. A behavioral statement that identifies the client's actual or potential health problem, deficit, or concern that can be affected by nursing actions.
Planning. The determination of what can be done to assist the client, including setting goals, judging priorities, and designing methods to resolve problems.
Implementation. Action initiated to accomplish defined goals.
Evaluation. The appraisal of the client's behavioral changes that result from the action of the nurse.
Outcome evaluation. Evaluation based on behavioral changes.
Structure evaluation. Evaluation relating to the availability of appropriate equipment.
Process evaluation. Evaluation that focuses on the activities of the nurse.
Reassessment. The process of collecting additional data during the planning, implementing, and evaluation phases of the nursing process that may lead to immediate changes in those phases, or a change in the nursing diagnosis.

Nursing situation. (Boykin and Schoenhofer) Shared living experience in which personhood is enhanced through caring between nurse and nursed.

Nurturer. (Hall) A fosterer of learning, growing, and healing.

Objective. A specific means by which one proposes to accomplish or attain the goal.

Ontology. A branch of metaphysics that studies the nature of being and of reality.

Organization. (King) An entity made up of individuals who have prescribed roles and positions and who use resources to achieve goals.

Orientation phase. (Peplau) The first phase of Peplau's nurse–patient relationship. Through assessment, the patient's health needs, expectations, and goals are explored and a care plan is devised. Concurrently, the roles of nurse and patient are being identified and clarified.

Originating. (Parse) A continuing process of growing more complex while in mutual energy exchange with the environment.

Overt problem. Apparent or obvious condition of concern.

Paradigm shift. A new way of viewing a phenomenon, or group of phenomena, that attracts a group of adherents and raises many questions to be answered.

Parsimonious theory. Theory that is both simple and generalizable.

Partly compensatory nursing system. (Orem) A situation in which both nurse and patient perform care measures or other actions involving manipulative tasks or ambulation.

Perception. (King) An individual's view of reality that gives meaning to personal experience and involves the organization, interpretation, and transformation of information from sensory data and memory.

Phenomenology. The study of the meaning of phenomena to a particular individual; a way of understanding people from the way things appear to them.

Potential comforter. (Hall) The role of the nurse seen by the patient during the care aspect of nursing.

Potential painer. (Hall) The role of the nurse seen by the patient during the cure aspect of nursing.

Power. (King) A social force and ability to use resources to influence people to achieve goals.

Powering. (Parse) An energizing force the rhythm of which is the pushing–resisting of interhuman encounters.

Prescription. (Wiedenbach) A directive for activity that specifies both the nature of the action and the necessary thought process.

Prescriptive theory. (Wiedenbach) A theory that conceptualizes both the desired situation and the activities to be used to bring about the desired situation.

Presence. (Paterson and Zderad) The quality of being open, receptive, ready, and available to another in a reciprocal manner.

Primary prevention. (Neuman) The application of general knowledge in a client situation to try to identify and protect against the potential effects of stressors before they occur.

Problem-solving process. Identifying the problem, selecting pertinent data, formulating hypotheses, testing hypotheses through the collection of data, and revising hypotheses.

Professional health system. (Leininger) Professional care or cure services offered by diverse health personnel who have been prepared through formal professional programs of study in special educational institutions.

Professional nursing action. (Orlando) What the nurse says or does for the benefit of the patient.

Proposition. A statement explaining relationships among concepts.

Realities in the immediate situation. (Wiedenbach) At any given moment, all factors at play in the situation in which nursing actions occur; realities include the agent, the recipient, the goal, the means, and the framework.

Received view. See Logical empiricism.

Recipient. (Wiedenbach) The vulnerable and dependent patient who is characterized by personal attributes, problems, and capabilities, including the ability to cope.

Reconstitution. (Neuman) The increase in energy that occurs in relation to the degree of reaction to a stressor.

Redundancy. (Levine) Aspect of adaptation related to numerous levels of response available for a given challenge.

Reflective technique. (Hall) The process of helping the patient see who he or she is by mirroring what the person's behavior says, both verbally and nonverbally.

Regulator mechanism. (Roy) Coping mechanism subsystem that includes chemical, neural, and endocrine transmitters and autonomic and psychomotor responses.

Relating. (Paterson and Zderad) The process of nurse–nursed "doing" with each other, being with each other.

Research. Formal, systematic process of gathering data to gain solutions, descriptions, answers and to interpret new ideas, facts or assumptions, and relationships.

Residual stimuli. (Roy) Characteristics of the individual that are relevant to the situation but are difficult to measure objectively.

Resolution phase. (Peplau) The fourth and final phase of Peplau's nurse–patient relationship. This phase evolves from the successful completion of the previous phases. The patient and nurse terminate their therapeutic relationship as the patient's needs are met and movement is made toward new goals.

Resonancy. (Rogers) The identification of the human field and the environmental field by wave pattern manifesting continuous change from lower-frequency longer waves to higher-frequency shorter waves.

Revealing–concealing. (Parse) Actions in interpersonal relationships that reveal one part of oneself and, as a result, conceal other parts.

Role. (King) The set of behaviors and rules that relate to an individual in a position in a social system.

Role Modeling. (Erickson, Tomlin, and Swain) Planning and implementing individualized care based on the client's model of the world.

Secondary prevention. (Neuman) Treatment of symptoms of stress reaction to lead to reconstitution.

Second-level assessment. (Roy) The collection of data about focal, contextual, and residual stimuli impinging on the person.

Self-care. (Orem) Practice of activities that individuals personally initiate and perform on their own behalf to maintain life, health, and well-being.

Self-care action. (Erickson, Tomlin, and Swain) Use of self-care knowledge and self-care resources.

Self-care agency. (Orem) The human ability to engage in self-care.

Self-care deficit. (Orem) The inability of an individual to carry out all necessary self-care activities.

Self-care knowledge. (Erickson, Tomlin, and Swain) Knowledge about what has made one sick, lessened one's effectiveness, or interfered with one's growth; also includes knowledge of what will make one well, fulfilled, or effective.

Self-care resources. (Erickson, Tomlin, and Swain) An individual's strengths and supports that will help gain, maintain, and promote optimal health.

Set. (Johnson) An individual's predisposition to behave in a certain way.

Sexual subsystem. (Johnson) The behavioral subsystem that reflects socially acceptable behaviors related to procreation.

Simultaneity paradigm. (Parse) A view of humans as unitary beings who are in continuous interrelationship with the environment and whose health is a negentropic unfolding.

Social structure. (Leininger) The dynamic nature of interrelated structural and organizational factors of a particular culture (or society) and how those factors function to give meaning and structural order including educational, technological, and cultural factors.

Space. (King) A universal area, known also as territory, that is defined in part by the behavior of those who occupy it.

Specificity. (Levine) Aspect of adaptation in which responses are task specific and particular challenges lead to particular responses.

Status. (King) The relationship of an individual to a group, or a group to other groups, including identified duties, obligations, and privileges.

Stress. (King) A positive or negative energy response to interactions with the environment in an effort to maintain balance in living.

Supportive-educative nursing system. (Orem) A situation in which the patient is able to, or can and should learn to, perform required therapeutic self-care measures but needs assistance to do so.

Supportive intervention. (Levine) Action that maintains the patient's present state of altered health and prevents further health deterioration.

Synergistic wholeness. (Rogers) Cooperative action of discrete agencies such that the total effect is greater than the sum of the effects taken independently.

Tertiary prevention. (Neuman) Activities that seek to strengthen the lines of resistance after reconstitution has occurred.

Theory. A set of interrelated concepts that are testable and provide direction or prediction; systematic way of looking at the world to describe, explain, predict, or control it.

Theory. (Watson) An imaginative grouping of knowledge, ideas, and experience that is represented symbolically and that seeks to illuminate a given phenomenon.

Therapeutic interpersonal relationship. (Peplau) A relationship between patient and nurse in which their collaborative effort is directed toward identifying, exploring, and resolving the patient's need productively. The relationship progresses along a continuum as each experiences growth through an increasing understanding of one another's roles, attitudes, and perceptions.

Therapeutic intervention. (Levine) Action that promotes healing and restoration of health.

Therapeutic self-care demand. (Orem) The sum or total of self-actions needed, during some period, to meet self-care requisites.

Time. (King) The relation of one event to another, uniquely experienced by each individual.

Totality paradigm. (Parse) View of man as a summative being, a combination of bio-psycho-social-spiritual aspects, surrounded by an environment of external and internal stimuli. Man interacts with the environment to maintain equilibrium and achieve goals.

Transactions. (King) Observable behaviors between individuals and their environment that lead to the attainment of valued goals.

Transcultural nursing. (Leininger) A learned subfield or branch of nursing that focuses on the comparative study and analysis of cultures with respect to nursing and health–illness caring practices, beliefs, and values. The goal is to provide meaningful and efficacious nursing care services to people according to their cultural values and health–illness context.

Transformation. (Newman) Change occurring all-at-once.

Unitary humans. (Rogers) Pandimensional, negentropic energy fields identified by pattern and manifesting characteristics and behaviors different from those of the parts, and which cannot be predicted from knowledge of the parts.

Universal self-care requisites. (Orem) Those requisites, common to all human beings throughout life, associated with life processes and the integrity of human structure and function.

Well-being. (Paterson and Zderad) A steady state.

Wholly compensatory nursing system. (Orem) A situation in which the patient has no active role in the performance of self-care.

World view. (Leininger) The way in which people look at the world, or universe, and form a value stance about the world and their lives.

INDEX

■ ■ ■